Fertility, Conjuncture, Difference

Fertility, Reproduction and Sexuality

GENERAL EDITORS:

Soraya Tremayne, Founding Director, Fertility and Reproduction Studies Group and Research Associate, Institute of Social and Cultural Anthropology, University of Oxford.
Marcia C. Inhorn, William K. Lanman, Jr. Professor of Anthropology and International Affairs, Yale University.
Philip Kreager, Director, Fertility and Reproduction Studies Group, and Research Associate, Institute of Social and Cultural Anthropology and Institute of Human Sciences, University of Oxford.

Volume 1
Managing Reproductive Life: Cross-Cultural Themes in Fertility and Sexuality
Edited by Soraya Tremayne

Volume 2
Modern Babylon? Prostituting Children in Thailand
Heather Montgomery

Volume 3
Reproductive Agency, Medicine and the State: Cultural Transformations in Childbearing
Edited by Maya Unnithan-Kumar

Volume 4
A New Look at Thai AIDS: Perspectives from the Margin
Graham Fordham

Volume 5
Breast Feeding and Sexuality: Behaviour, Beliefs and Taboos among the Gogo Mothers in Tanzania
Mara Mabilia

Volume 6
Ageing without Children: European and Asian Perspectives on Elderly Access to Support Networks
Edited by Philip Kreager and Elisabeth Schröder-Butterfill

Volume 7
Nameless Relations: Anonymity, Melanesia and Reproductive Gift Exchange between British Ova Donors and Recipients
Monica Konrad

Volume 8
Population, Reproduction and Fertility in Melanesia
Edited by Stanley J. Ulijaszek

Volume 9
Conceiving Kinship: Assisted Conception, Procreation and Family in Southern Europe
Monica M.E. Bonaccorso

Volume 10
Where There Is No Midwife: Birth and Loss in Rural India
Sarah Pinto

Volume 11
Reproductive Disruptions: Gender, Technology, and Biopolitics in the New Millennium
Edited by Marcia C. Inhorn

Volume 12
Reconceiving the Second Sex: Men, Masculinity, and Reproduction
Edited by Marcia C. Inhorn, Tine Tjørnhøj-Thomsen, Helene Goldberg, and Maruska la Cour Mosegaard

Volume 13
Transgressive Sex: Subversion and Control in Erotic Encounters
Edited by Hastings Donnan and Fiona Macgowan

Volume 14
European Kinship in the Age of Biotechnology
Edited by Jeanette Edwards and Carles Salazar

Volume 15
Kinship and Beyond: The Genealogical Model Reconsidered
Edited by Sandra Bamford and James Leach

Volume 16
Islam and New Kinship: Reproductive Technology and the Shariah in Lebanon
Morgan Clarke

Volume 17
Childbirth, Midwifery and Concepts of Time
Edited by Christine McCourt

Volume 18
Assisting Reproduction, Testing Genes: Global Encounters with the New Biotechnologies
Edited by Daphna Birenbaum-Carmeli and Marcia C. Inhorn

Volume 19
Kin, Gene, Community: Reproductive Technologies among Jewish Israelis
Edited by Daphna Birenbaum-Carmeli and Yoram S. Carmeli

Volume 20
Abortion in Asia: Local Dilemmas, Global Politics
Edited by Andrea Whittaker

Volume 21
Unsafe Motherhood: Mayan Maternal Mortality and Subjectivity in Post-War Guatemala
Nicole S. Berry

Volume 22
Fatness and the Maternal Body: Women's Experiences of Corporeality and the Shaping of Social Policy
Edited by Maya Unnithan-Kumar and Soraya Tremayne

Volume 23
Islam and Assisted Reproductive Technologies: Sunni and Shia Perspectives
Edited by Marcia C. Inhorn and Soraya Tremayne

Volume 24
Militant Lactivism?: Infant Feeding and Maternal Accountability in the UK and France
Charlotte Faircloth

Volume 25
Pregnancy in Practice: Expectation and Experience in the Contemporary US
Sallie Han

Volume 26
Nighttime Breastfeeding: An American Cultural Dilemma
Cecília Tomori

Volume 27
Globalized Fatherhood
Edited by Marcia C. Inhorn, Wendy Chavkin, and José-Alberto Navarro

Volume 28
Cousin Marriages: Between Tradition, Genetic Risk and Cultural Change
Edited by Alison Shaw and Aviad Raz

Volume 29
Achieving Procreation: Childlessness and IVF in Turkey
Merve Demircioğlu Göknar

Volume 30
Thai in Vitro: Gender, Culture and Assisted Reproduction
Andrea Whittaker

Volume 31
Assisted Reproductive Technologies in the Third Phase: Global Encounters and Emerging Moral Worlds
Edited by Kate Hampshire and Bob Simpson

Volume 32
Parenthood between Generations: Transforming Reproductive Cultures
Edited by Siân Pooley and Kaveri Qureshi

Volume 33
Patient-Centred IVF: Bioethics and Care in a Dutch Clinic
Trudie Gerrits

Volume 34
Conceptions: Infertilities and Procreative Technologies in India
Aditya Bharadwaj

Volume 35
The Online World of Surrogacy
Zsuzsa Berend

Volume 36
Fertility, Conjuncture, Difference: Anthropological Approaches to the Heterogeneity of Modern Fertility Declines
Edited by Philip Kreager and Astrid Bochow

FERTILITY, CONJUNCTURE, DIFFERENCE

Anthropological Approaches to the Heterogeneity of Modern Fertility Declines

Edited by Philip Kreager and Astrid Bochow

berghahn
NEW YORK • OXFORD
www.berghahnbooks.com

First published in 2017 by
Berghahn Books
www.BerghahnBooks.com

Library of Congress Cataloging-in-Publication Data

Names: Kreager, Philip, editor. | Bochow, Astrid, editor.
Title: Fertility, conjuncture, difference : anthropological approaches to the heterogeneity of modern fertility declines / edited by Philip Kreager and Astrid Bochow.
Description: New York : Berghahn Books, [2017] | Series: Fertility, reproduction and sexuality : Social and cultural perspectives ; volume 36 | Includes bibliographical references and index.
Identifiers: LCCN 2017014885 (print) | LCCN 2017033857 (ebook) | ISBN 9781785336058 (e-book) | ISBN 9781785336041 (hardback : alk. paper)
Subjects: LCSH: Fertility, Human--Cross-cultural studies. | Human reproduction--Cross-cultural studies. | Demographic anthropology—Case studies.
Classification: LCC GN241 (ebook) | LCC GN241 .F47 2017 (print) | DDC 304.6/32--dc23
LC record available at https://lccn.loc.gov/2017014885

British Library Cataloguing in Publication Data

A catalogue record for this book is available from the British Library.

ISBN 978-1-78533-604-1 (hardback)
ISBN 978-1-78533-605-8 (ebook)

Contents

Illustrations, Figures and Tables

Illustrations

Figures

Tables

PREFACE

The impetus to comparative analysis in anthropology originated more than a century ago from observing the social, cultural and economic systems that societies build on the core facts of life – reproduction, death, age, sex, marriage, family and kin relationships. Over the last four decades, these systems have been buffeted in their demographic dimensions by unprecedented changes, of which population growth, the spread of contraceptive and abortion technology, HIV/AIDS, population ageing, IVF and related new reproductive technologies are well known. As this storm continues to play out, fertility in most of the world has entered a phase of declining trends that follow an immense diversity of patterns in their timing, pace and extent. Historical research has confirmed that this heterogeneity also characterized European fertility declines over more than two centuries. While it is true that, with declines, the range of fertility levels now experienced in different countries has narrowed, there is no sign of the kind of homogeneity at the level of 2.1 births per woman that population theorists once expected. The causes and implications of the unending renewal of population heterogeneity, and particularly the role of the diversity of fertility declines in this process, have thus become a central problematic in the study of population.

Seeking to shape these changes, national and international agencies have acted as policy drivers and funding conduits, to which anthropology, like other social and biological sciences, has duly responded. Without understating the importance of research as a basis for programmes that address suffering and try to improve life, it is obvious that for research to make fundamental contributions to human problems requires continued conceptual and empirical development. Anthropology's comparative approaches have required rethinking. Disciplines like anthropology and demography, which in the early postwar era were thought to have little in common, have been forcibly brought together. Indeed, as explanations of fertility decline fostered by postwar modernization and economic development theory have led to endless debate rather than adequate and agreed scientific explanations, the need to develop the common ground of these disciplines has grown. Therefore, it is very important to ask whether research is giving rise to new frameworks and evidence that can explain what mechanisms underlie the renewal of heterogeneity, and how they operate.

The chapters collected in this volume bring together ethnography and analysis that draw on two major advances in the conceptualization of population change. Anthropologists and historians have for some time broken from the usual population and development discourse which privileges stereotyped macro- and micro-levels of analysis. First, as national data are a composite of differing behaviour in the several subpopulations that compose states, we need to identify and explore the contours of these subpopulations separately and build a comparative approach – a compositional demography – which brings out their differences. The chapters demonstrate repeatedly the impact of inequalities that define different groups in society and their differing reproductive options. Longer-term processes that have led to the formation and continuance of groups, their relationships to each other and to the state have a direct bearing on reproduction and are shaped, in turn, by the ways in which people evaluate the set of reproductive options they, and those around them, have.

A second advance is addressed to this level of localized individuals and events. Taking account of subpopulation differences requires much more empirical content than standard micro-analyses of reproductive behaviour, in which all actors can be modelled as if they face stereotyped and discrete (usually economic and contraceptive) alternatives. Individuals situated differently in local hierarchies, having differing ties within subpopulation memberships and acting at different life course stages confront not single choices, but conjunctures of influences and multiple lines of possible action that carry ramifications across their own life courses and those of others. Vital conjunctures are the moments that shape the dynamics of subpopulations and hence the heterogeneity of reproductive trends and patterns that come to characterize them. Observation and analysis of conjuncture and difference together constitute building blocks of the compositional demography needed to disentangle and understand the continuing diversity of human fertility.

We are grateful to the Max Planck Institute for Social Anthropology (Halle) and the Institute of Social and Cultural Anthropology

(Oxford) for their support, with warm thanks in particular to Günther Schlee for his encouragement, and to the Fritz-Thyssen Foundation for additional support facilitating Astrid Bochow's visiting fellowship at the Fertility and Reproduction Studies Group (FRSG) in the Institute of Anthropology at Oxford. Simon Szreter kindly provided us with an insightful commentary on several of the chapters. We are grateful to Sasha Puchalski and Caroline Kuhtz at Berghahn for their superb work in expediting and editing the manuscript for publication.

We are particularly fortunate to be able to add the last two chapters in the volume, written by demographers with extensive field experience (Yves Charbit and Véronique Petit) and by an anthropological demographer (Jennifer A. Johnson-Hanks) whose work has provided a direct stimulus and inspiration to several of the chapters. These two chapters reflect on the collection as a whole. The first addresses the continuing role of measurement at the local level in achieving ethnographic acuity and conceptual clarity. The second gives a synthesis of the composition and conjuncture framework, which is of particular interest as it shows the integral relationship of the two main components and how they enable the wider field of population research to address emerging challenges.

Philip Kreager and Astrid Bochow
March 2017

INTRODUCTION

Philip Kreager and Astrid Bochow

> That faith in modern culture was a gloomy one . . . a kind of elastic prison which stretches on without ever setting us free.
> —José Ortega y Gasset

In the last forty years, anthropologists have made major contributions to understanding the heterogeneity of reproductive trends and the processes underlying them. Main approaches run sharply counter to conventional modernization and economic development models that continue to hold sway over demographic data systems and their analysis. In this, anthropological demography can simply be said to have taken demographers at their word. As is well known, a host of widely cited studies beginning in the early 1970s have revealed a great diversity of declining reproductive patterns, together with the inability of conventional modernization and socioeconomic measures and models to explain them adequately.[1] Fertility declines, rather than a story of the rise and triumphant spread of Western birth control rationality, in which modern contraceptive technology facilitates the spread of nuclear family values and 'stopping behaviour' everywhere, reveal instead a diversity of reproductive means, ends and institutional arrangements continuing before, during and after relatively lower reproductive levels are reached. As demographic transition theory has proven to give too simplified an account to serve as an adequate framework for explaining this diversity, the way is open to explore alternative comparative frameworks grounded in the evidence of contrasting case studies of populations at local and wider levels of society.

Recent developments have begun to crystallize around two complementary approaches. At a local level, reproductive 'choice' is experienced by persons and couples over their life course in what Johnson-Hanks (2006, 2015) has called 'vital conjunctures'. Events such as pregnancy and birth, alternatives such as abstinence, contraception and abortion, and ever-present concerns and constraints like infecundity, maternal health and age are the object of norms and expectations that reflect a complex intersection of family, kin, community, economic, religious, educational and other pressures. In the junctures that bring some or all of these forces together, women and men negotiate possible futures for themselves and their offspring, and do so in the awareness that these negotiations carry compound implications across their life courses. Observation and analysis of vital conjunctures thus enables consideration both of agency and social structure, and examination of their interrelations in the context of specific events – without supposing that people prioritize the demographic ideal type of parity-specific birth control, or that reproduction in all societies consists of a more or less linear trajectory to replacement level fertility. Similar reproductive trends and levels may be achieved in different ways and with differing motives. Evidently, to understand the realities of personal and collective fertility histories, we need to construct models that do not come down to a single stereotype – a supposed rational 'fertility decision-making' that is, as in the Gunter Grass parody (1982), a binary choice: 'baby/no baby'.

A second development helps us to place actors and conjunctures in relation to wider fertility change. Fertility declines across national and regional populations are commonly pre-empted by certain subgroups, with other subpopulations then following, but in a far from unitary fashion. These differences reflect the varying composition, structure and social position of subpopulations, which open up differing access to social, economic and political hierarchies, and the differing advantages and disadvantages that go with them. We may therefore expect that differences between subpopulations and the relationships that articulate these differences are of crucial importance in understanding the contrasting reproductive patterns observable in such groups. Social and economic inequalities between subpopulations and the relationships that some but not all group members have with those in other groups are, as we shall see, important examples.

Anthropological approaches here join a wider interest in compositional demography that has also become important to social history and theory, network sociology and historical demography (e.g. Garrett et al. 2001; Johnson-Hanks et al. 2011; Kreager 2011; Kohler et al. 2015). While disciplinary vocabularies vary, family dynamics and fertility change in these several approaches are helpfully understood in terms of 'communication communities' (Szreter 2015), i.e. subpopulations in which gender, class and other local hierarchies, network relationships and collective identities shape the flow of information and practices. Fertility trends may vary within and between communication communities according to how members are placed and relations between such groups.[2] Individuals' and families' negotiations of vital conjunctures are the micro-processes that effect reproductive and other adjustments within such groups and may incorporate other groups' influence on them.

With time, the accumulative impacts of conjunctural adjustments often come to be seen as important and even typical characteristics distinguishing some constituent groups in a society or state. The practice of highlighting reproductive differences has, of course, a notorious history, from the eugenic claims of colonial states and national socialist parties about dire implications of racial and lower-class fertility to the problems of Puerto Ricans as portrayed in *West Side Story*. Anthropological demography here adjoins a large body of writings on the nature and development of collective identities (e.g. Barth 1969; Anderson 1993). Looking at population change from the bottom up – i.e. beginning from individual and local conjunctures, and their agency in the context of group differences – carries implications on several levels. For example, at the level of relations between subpopulations, it provides some reality against which the often exaggerated discourses that try to stigmatize reproductive behaviour in certain class, ethnic, religious and other groups may be assessed critically (e.g. Cohn 1987; Kertzer and Arel 2002; Szreter et al. 2004; Pauli, this volume; Roche and Hohmann, this volume). As Basu (1997) remarks, there remains a need for some check on the tendency of party and governmental interests to employ fertility trends and theories to the political and economic advantage of some groups over others. And, at higher levels of analysis, taking a bottom-up approach to national population trends enables us to recognize them as the composite outcome of the agency of a number of different constituent groups with different reproductive values and associated behaviour.

In short, subpopulations and their differences are the collective building blocks that together compose demographic change at the national level and may be the locus of political and cultural identities that feed back differentially on the reproduction, mortality and migration of each subpopulation. Fertility trends, rather than standing as a monolithic outcome of externally stimulated 'modernization', reflect a more fundamental internal dynamism of conjunctures and social differentiation that varies across the several subpopulations or communication communities that make up a society or state and that respond differently to external factors.

History Confounds Modernity

As a research strategy addressed to reproduction, the study of conjuncture and difference draws on intellectual movements that began to take shape in the 1970s and 1980s. With the benefit of hindsight, we can say that three related movements in anthropology and related social sciences created the conceptual space in which this strategy, and anthropological demography more generally, became possible: (i) a rethinking of theories of social structure; (ii) a re-alignment with historical scholarship; and (iii) a reassessment of how qualitative and quantitative models and methods may be combined.

First, within the wider field of anthropology, there was considerable dissatisfaction with the rather static portrayal of cultural logics and social structures, whether in classic colonial ethnography or subsequent structuralist analysis. Rather, cultures are in a continual state of creation in which enduring institutions and forms of expression may be renegotiated repeatedly by groups and the actors that compose them (e.g. Bourdieu 1977; Hammel 1990). As the discipline developed from the 1970s, changing reproductive trends and behaviour provided anthropologists with one helpful focus for this critique, for example, by enabling anthropologists to consider how family and community institutions distribute people, power, information and practices, then observing the differing agency this process gives to specific groups, with consequently differing fertility levels and trends (e.g. Bourdieu 1972; Kertzer and Hogan 1989; Das Gupta 1997; Bledsoe and Banja 1999; Tremayne 2001). Over the latter decades of the twentieth century, reproduction further proved to be an important domain in emerging specialisms in anthropology and other disciplines that are also concerned with distributional issues and inequalities. Gender (Greenhalgh 1995), medical practices (Inhorn and Tremayne 2012), the political economy of development (Schneider and Schneider 1996) and the environment (Hill and Hurtado 1996) are well-known instances. It became common for anthropologists to note that, even when fertility change reflects the use of ostensibly 'the same' technologies in different cultures (whether those techniques are directed at reproduction, production or the market), their adoption means very different things to different social groups. 'Fertility transition', 'modernization' and 'development' are not unitary processes.

Second, historical demographers also noted the diversity of fertility declines, together with the inability of generalized modernization and economic development hypotheses to account for it (e.g. Wrigley 1972), making clear the power of historical examples to subvert prevailing assumptions. Of course, international and national institutions founded in the postwar era were predicated on modernization and development models, which in important respects accounts for these models' continuing prevalence despite their inability to explain heterogeneity (Demeny 1988; Szreter 1993; Greenhalgh 1996). The scientific and scholarly puzzle of why and how fertility variation is sustained nonetheless remains.[3] Historical demography, in opening up archival sources that enabled historians to move beyond histories confined to elite groups, facilitated collaboration with comparative studies of the family, local economy and politics, and created rich new avenues for collaborative research that revealed a diversity of mechanisms underlying European demography (e.g. Bonfield et al. 1986; Engelen and Wolf 2005). Anthropological demography made major contributions here too (e.g. Kertzer 1984; Segalen 1991).

The inadequacy of prevailing notions of modernization and economic development to explain heterogeneity (even in the restricted sense of broad levels or thresholds of development necessary to account consistently for fertility patterns, or 'explanation' as reliable, general statistical correlations between demographic and economic trends (e.g. Knodel and van de Walle 1979; Szreter 1993)), naturally led to a second strand of historical rethinking. It was realized that prevailing population concepts and hypotheses in the postwar era relied on an intellectual basis that privileged a narrow strand of nineteenth- and twentieth-century European social and economic theory. On the one hand, major traditions of population thought were ignored, notably developments before 1800, as well as later immensely fruitful ones in evolutionary biology (Kreager 2015).

These traditions rely on direct observation of local relationships between subpopulations as the source of population changes, establishing heterogeneity as a significant and inevitable force that needs to be accounted for. Observing the renewal of heterogeneity as it arises from subpopulation dynamics thus becomes a central object of inquiry and an essential element of scientific and historical explanation. Although these traditions of thought were marginalized in the nineteenth- and twentieth-century rise of statistics, major conceptual advances have continued to be made in them (Kreager et al. 2015a). On the other hand, the notion of modernity itself (or the conventional trope that opposes 'modern' to 'traditional' society) has been recognized as problematic – notably for erasing local institutions and their history, thus depriving them of agency. The 'modern theme', as Señor Ortega observed nearly a century ago ([1930] 1957), is a peculiarly tenacious habit of European thought.

An apt example of how ethnography combines fruitfully with awareness of longer-term conceptual developments is Tim Jenkins' (2010: 129–58) reconsideration of Pierre Bourdieu's analysis of family, marriage and reproduction in Béarn, southwest France. Bourdieu was, of course, a major player in the critique of postwar anthropology and sociology, and his seminal work on mechanisms of low fertility (1962) and marriage strategies (1972) exemplifies the role that demographic variables came to play in it. Bourdieu is an important advocate of bottom-up analysis of the dynamics of social and population change, arguing that key theoretical formulations – such as the conceptualization of habitus, practice and symbolic violence, for which his work is best known – should arise from sustained reflection on conjunctures revealed by ethnography and not simply from preconceived social and economic models. However, whether Bourdieu actually follows this method and whether his analysis is shaped more powerfully by the modern theme are important matters that Jenkins' own Béarn ethnography raises. His sympathetic but critical assessment of Bourdieu's approach is worth careful attention, as it clarifies not only the empirical and theoretical fallacy of modernism, but also how the tenacity that Ortega noted is perpetuated.

Bourdieu's early important work on Béarn, 'Célibat et condition paysanne' (1962), was a synthesis of ethnographic and census data: the former describes the strict system of marriage, property and gender norms characteristic of traditional Béarnais rural society; trends from the latter then reveal this system in crisis. Tradition focused on the central value of the transmission of family property to a single heir as the means of sustaining family position in local hierarchies. Demographic correlates of this system guaranteed its proper functioning: heirs married late; younger sons commonly did not marry; control over daughters' marriages, and especially the size of dowries, ensured that families did not get too much in debt; and fertility was kept low. However, census data revealed a mechanism that, in Bourdieu's view, spelled the terminal decline of this system: a steady rise in proportions of men, and hence of heirs, not married in rural areas. As the whole system is predicated on the controlled marriage of heirs, how could this happen?

A major consideration in Bourdieu's account is the changing balance of power and influence between market towns and the hamlets in which traditional farms are located. While heads of household and their heirs continued traditional marriage and reproductive controls, the opportunities for marriage expanded in the towns, such that celibacy there was seven times less for men and half of rural levels for women. Modern attractions and employment in towns contrasted with continued hard and long labour required on farms, and familiar tropes of modernization like the role of education, individualism and loss of parental authority are all noted – Bourdieu suggests that these attractions had particular appeal to mothers and daughters. The political power of towns likewise grew with the rise of commerce and a professional class of outsiders, French replaced patois in discussion of policy and the peasant proprietor came to feel himself an alien in social contexts outside rural farms.

Bourdieu's 1972 paper 'Les stratégies matrimoniales dans le système de reproduction' returns to his earlier ethnography, now presenting its conclusions as a systematic, general model of marriage; again, in a later analysis, he emphasizes this step as 'a break with the structuralist paradigm' (2002: 12), also remarking the essential role of low fertility in the maintenance of the system. Models, he argues, should thus be grounded in observed indigenous practices, not sociologists' externally hypothesized decision-making rules of behaviour. His term 'habitus' was coined to describe this ground, defined as 'the system of dispositions inculcated by the material conditions of existence and by familial education' (2002: 171). Jenkins notes the importance of this conceptual shift in terms that anticipate the anthropological demography of conjuncture noted above: habitus enables the choices made by actors in pursuit of their ends to result in the reproduction of wider group social structures (2010: 147). The model reveals both the strengths of the traditional system and how the limits imposed by its demography cannot compete with the opportunities that modernity offers.

For those familiar with the wider literature on modernization and fertility regulation, Bourdieu can be seen to have presented a sophisticated, locally grounded version of a wider orthodoxy in which modernity always trumps tradition. There are, however, problems. Jenkins carried out his own fieldwork in Béarn over an extended period from the 1970s to the 1990s and witnessed the demise of farms where no heir was available or willing to succeed to the entail. Yet, as his ethnography shows, the system continues to function. As he notes, its imminent demise was first forecast in the early nineteenth century, and a series of eminent sociologists including Le Play and Weber have continued for two centuries to believe they are witnessing its near-death throes, up to and including Bourdieu. Jenkins' combined historical and ethnographic account shows how marriage and property arrangements have varied between recognized subgroups, enabling more adaptive capacity than Bourdieu allows; as Jenkins demonstrates, the system continually projects an image of vulnerability, while in practice sustaining its existence. The workings of this and related processes are best left to the reader to investigate for himself or herself in Jenkins' book. However, his account of the chimera by which modernity displaces tradition and how it comes to infest Bourdieu's argument is of direct importance here and repays close attention.

Two main points in Jenkins' analysis may be summarized as follows. First, census categories do not reflect accurately the local groups or subpopulations in which conjunctures or adjustments in habitus are occurring, nor distinctions between them that are crucial to their demography. The census records large, medium and small properties according to area farmed, using arbitrary cut-off points between each; it is not possible from the records to identify the differing paths to marriage and non-marriage followed by siblings (2010: 138). As Jenkins shows, the categories that guide choices in the traditional system differ markedly from this classification. Local hierarchy is defined by 'great' and 'small' 'houses', 'house' being the term for ancestral property and family reputation that it is the objective of the system to preserve. The primary importance of ensuring the marriage of the heir (and marrying him or her well) that Bourdieu and Jenkins describe articulates the traditional system from the point of view of 'great' houses. This has always been the challenge that they face; 'small' houses, in contrast, are usually not in this position, are often reduced to tenancy or dissolution and thus frequently face a corresponding dispersal of members and capital. Thus, in the terms of local categories and agency, two main groups or subpopulations are understood to exist, the conjunctures they face are different, and their options and reputations vary accordingly. Dissolved 'small' properties create opportunities for 'great' ones to expand. Some 'great' houses decline, while the adroit marriage of a female heir and management of smallholdings can lead some members of the 'small' category to rise. The system has, in all history for which we have record, relied on an elasticity amongst units that is not apparent in Bourdieu's account and that clearly contains more options for preserving 'great' houses than he considers. Meanwhile, the continuing problems faced by 'small' houses are not a threat to the system, but are part of its normal adaptive variation.

Second, similar issues arise in the census distinction between towns and hamlets, and Jenkins remarks that Bourdieu's reliance on these categories is accompanied by a curious change in his account of local agency. Under the traditional system, peasants are wily managers of a complex demographic and property calculus. Yet, confronted with the modernity of the towns, they suddenly become automatons fixated only on marriage and heirship. However, as the dialectic of great and small houses indicates, the 'old' calculus was predicated on adaptation to circumstance. Jenkins notes a series of major changes in local economy and society that the two subpopulations of proprietors have had to adjust to. The area has accommodated the familiar transformation of agricultural techniques that comes with tractors, fertilizers, new crops and irrigation. Changing transportation means that work in local industries is accessible for younger sons, whether they reside in the towns or the hamlets, and important new industries have emerged. New sources of farm finance are readily available. And so forth. Farm families, in short, are mixed economies with several possible revenue streams that can be varied if necessary. It is difficult to believe that the contrasting measures of non-marriage between the market town and hamlets on which Bourdieu's argument depends exists independently of all of these adaptive elements in the system, but the census of course provides insufficient detail to enable tracking individual patterns of employment in relation to marriage, or to relate them in turn to the fate of houses or particular siblings' marriage patterns.[4]

The apparently inevitable triumph of modernity in Bourdieu's account thus depends not on the historical evolution of the system or on the experience of those participating in it, but rather on an elementary shift in the classifications on which description and analysis rely. Distinctive subpopulations like the great and small houses – which exist simultaneously and occupy differing places in the social structure – are replaced by an argument in which the analyst displaces these subpopulations and networks with standard census and other survey categories. A shift from one classificatory scheme of description to another is read onto society as a historical succession from one homogeneous ('traditional') form of existence to another ('modern') one. Where standard census and other survey categories displace the subpopulations and networks that actually shape people's experience and the options they are pursuing, not surprisingly, their agency disappears. With Jenkins we might ask: where do all of these bright, new modern people emerge from? The answer is that they are not produced merely by modern influences coming from outside local society (although people are, as noted above, able in some cases to adapt these influences their own purposes). Nor are they simply an artefact of analysis; they are one aspect of differences generated internally in a society by the differing positions of long-established subpopulations and their members, and their experience in handling the options available to them. Failure to recognize this, together with failure to give local categories and experience their due, dooms analysis, as Ortega observed, to the endless pursuit of a homogeneous modernity that never arrives.

Combined Methodologies

The example of Bourdieu's sociology is important not only because it shows how the agency and history of peoples can be erased by the classifications and measures of conventional quantitative databases. It also shows that, despite the efforts of anthropologists – indeed, the very ones who have taken a major role in trying to develop ethnographically grounded anthropological theory – this same erasure comes to prevail in their models. In the process, it is not only peasants' agency that disappears – it is anthropology's.

Under the circumstances, it can come as little surprise that the third intellectual movement underpinning anthropological demography has been recognition of the urgent need to reassess how qualitative and quantitative methods and models may best be combined. It is important, at the beginning, to note that what is at issue is not the competition or incompatibility of two methodological traditions. Just as the encounter of the peasant world and modernity is not the collision of two isolates, there is a long history or interface shared by qualitative and quantitative approaches.[5] The root of this relationship, as the doyen of modern demographic modelling, Alfred Lotka (1925: 35), insisted, is the same elementary fact that Jenkins emphasizes: the reliability of any quantitative compilation or model rests on the classification it employs; hence, classification powerfully shapes the lines along which formalization subsequently develops. The convention that opposes the quantitative and the qualitative is, in any case, recent. It obscures the priority that earlier thinkers gave to compositional factors – i.e. how the several differing groups that compose a society are formed, sustained and relate to each other – in the very emergence and development of the concept of population in European science and society, and its formalization as an object of scientific study.[6]

As ethnographers and historians from the 1970s onwards turned their attention increasingly to processes of fertility variation and decline, the question of the empirical validity of standard classification systems immediately became problematic. Census and survey demography offered potentially promising means of assessing the generality or particularity of local findings, with the possibility of giving them greater relevance and influence. However, when these sources were analysed in order to compare local data to the wider communities to which groups belonged and to national populations, analysts often found themselves blocked. Many subpopulations (variously ethnic communities, regional cultures, regionally defined labour sectors, religious groups, etc.) are not distinguished in survey and census compilations; even where such groups are recognized, considerable problems often confound the accuracy of their enumeration. A great many substantive and methodological shortcomings in consequence emerged, of which six may be briefly listed.

First, standard sources use conventional administrative and geographical units that cut across and subdivide a group's distribution. Second, provinces, household units, occupational and other categories in these sources generally reflect metropolitan or European models, or perhaps the dominant national culture. Such classifications tend to assimilate distinctive subpopulation patterns to external norms. Third, they also often become fixed over long periods, thus failing to pick up the emergence of significant new cultural and informal sector economic groups. Fourth, household classification schemes generally do not address population mobility and changing family composition across the lifecycle. For example, different types of marriage, which commonly have very different implications for fertility, are rarely noted, and factors that can strongly influence reproduction, like patterns of migration that differ between subpopulations, can be inferred only very approximately. A fifth problem, in consequence of these several shortcomings, is that demographic data systems do not capture key relationships (such as how networks link households and how different ethnic and occupational groups are linked in social and economic hierarchies). Finally, randomized samples used in national surveys may capture too few members of constituent subpopulations to enable a representative account of them to be given. Limitations such as these began to be noted as soon as combined historical anthropological and demographic perspectives became a major avenue of population research (e.g. Goody 1972; Berkner 1975), and they continue to attract important clarifications (e.g. Randall et al. 2011). As these problems affect demographers' interpretation and analysis in contemporary societies, a common ground of methodological concern has gradually emerged, with fruitful dialogues between disciplines (e.g. Caldwell et al 1988; Gillis et al. 1992; Jones et al. 1997; Szreter et al., 2004; Johnson-Hanks et al. 2011; Petit 2013).

As Walters (this volume) remarks, registration and other standardized population data systems have a powerful censoring capacity. That important subpopulations and social categories are left out, either permanently or over long periods, was a repeatedly debated concern of the nineteenth-century vital statisticians who erected national data systems in Europe; that no solution was found at the time has had the consequence that key economic and cultural variables are absent from the record – variables that the Princeton European Fertility Project (Coale 1969) and other research subsequently came to regard as essential to explaining European fertility declines (Kreager 1997). National statistics in the developing world are now based largely on European models and several chapters in this volume (Bochow; Roche and Hohmann; Hukin; Randall, Mondain and Diagne) note how censoring continues. Such systems need not be set in the concrete of past European norms; Kroeker (this volume), for example, notes how in Lesotho, classifications have been added to accommodate local reproductive and marital arrangements.

Arguably, the foremost problem facing the study of reproduction as a dimension of population heterogeneity is lack of agreement on which populations and subpopulations provide the best units for comparative purposes and how to characterize the several levels at which they function. From the bottom-up perspective of conjuncture and difference, key initial questions are: what local processes sustain, alter and give rise to groups, and how are childbearing and childrearing shaped by these processes? What feedbacks exist between reproduction and these processes? From the characteristically top-down perspective of statistical institutions and of historians and social scientists dependent on them, the corresponding questions are: how, given the welter of subpopulations contributing to national and provincial trends, can we arrive at accurate, regular and comparable units and classifications that together compose national levels and trends of reproduction? How can an understanding of local processes be integrated into surveys and census systems to provide accurate identification of subpopulations and their composition? Both bottom-up and top-down perspectives are clearly needed.[7] Given the diversity of subpopulations, it is inevitable that the way in which groups are specified in survey and census tabulations will in some cases oversimplify their distinctiveness, such that anthropologists are bound to remain critical of them. That said, there can be little doubt that if anthropologists addressed themselves concertedly to this issue, survey and census organizations would have to hand much more useful information and an incentive to clarify heterogeneity. Working together would then assist the design of classifications and data collection. Collaborative research is essential. No less important is critical historical work of the kind Jenkins provides in the Béarnais case, which is needed in most countries to help unpack oversimplifications that already exist and to understand what their impact has been on the perception of demographic and related change, and how such perceptions have influenced policy.

New Evidence

Historical demography, together with social and intellectual history, thus provide natural allies of anthropological demography. Historians have provided much of the energy and argument that the heterogeneity of declines forms the central problematic in understanding contemporary as well as long-term demographic change, and that this requires serious questioning of conventional population units and the development of new ones that can reflect local realities. The demographic history pursued in Cambridge has long been a fount of innovation in this respect and can serve as a brief case in point here, especially as the English case was supposed by Notestein (1945) to be the very model of fertility transition. In his view, transition was the more or less monolithic consequence of industrialization and modernization, leading to new reproductive institutions (small families) and rational contraceptive behaviour (parity-specific birth control). Parish reconstitution, however, soon began to build a more diverse picture of national population history from the bottom up. It demonstrated the contrary of what Notestein had supposed: small family forms were widespread more than two centuries before the spread of factory industry, together with reproductive patterns that varied considerably between groups before and during its spread; longstanding checks on reproduction relating to marriage, abstinence and contraception preceded industry and remained important during the marked fertility declines that began from 1870 (Wrigley 1961; Hajnal 1965; Flandrin 1976). As historians' attention turned to reanalysing nineteenth- and twentieth-century census data on declines, pioneering research showed that patterns varied significantly between subpopulations depending on gender, class and occupational sectors (Szreter 1996), with major declines in some subpopulations before 1870 (Szreter and Garrett 2000), together with distinctive regional patterns (Garrett et al. 2001). The need to explore local variations on several levels has thus become imperative and the important contributing evidence of oral history data is now recognized (Fisher 2008; Szreter and Fisher 2010). Recent availability of integrated census micro-data now enables analysis at the registration subdistrict level, opening up the reconstruction of local and regional fertility profiles that can be analysed in conjunction with other social data. 'A more finely grained geographical analysis, identifying the occupational or social mix of the smaller spatial units, is thus essential in the identification of the forces behind the fertility decline' (Reid and Garrett, in press).

In this approach, the population and subpopulation units in which demographic changes occur cannot be taken simply as those supplied by standard census reports or in conventional macro-/micro-level analyses. Identifying and tracking the boundaries and composition of groups in society that experience changes, whether similarly or differently, is a primary object of research. The study of conjunction and difference, as outlined in the preceding pages, parallels and complements this approach, since it is addressed to understanding processes that give rise to diversity in contemporary fertility declines. At present, the methodological issue of units and levels best suited for comparative purposes remains, as in historical demography, provisional. In anthropology, the identity, composition and structure of subpopulations making up a society are the product of ethnography and analysis, often also entailing specially designed local censuses and surveys.[8] As in evolutionary theory, units cannot be decided in advance.

To begin with, different subpopulations or constituent groups in society tend to be defined by anthropologists on the basis of local features that stand out in the ethnography. These commonly include socioeconomic hierarchies, communal, ethnic and religious groups, generations, gender, and an array of family and kin structures. The field enjoys one advantage over history (that reproductive processes can be observed and discussed with participants), but there can also be a relative disadvantage (lack of historical depth). In consequence, anthropological demographers – as several chapters in this volume show – commonly take considerable care to conduct research into historical contexts and use them to formulate their analyses. Contextual data are likewise critical to assessing national demographic survey series that may be relevant. Coming from the historical demographic side, Sarah Walter's chapter shows that longer-term demographic records that enable a bottom-up approach may actually be available in places like tropical Africa, where it has generally been assumed that they do not exist; as she notes, the experience of several generations of administrators, missionaries and anthropologists turns out to be very helpful in constructing and interpreting this long-term picture.

Ethnography brings together observation of local behaviour and of the way people express values and attitudes. Censuses and surveys can only record what people are prepared to say, subject to the inevitably artificial conditions of interviews based on structured questionnaires; such data record the outcomes of events and processes, not their direct observation. Because standardized sources commonly rely on household and official geographical units, they only explore some – and not necessarily the most relevant – subpopulations. People participate in multiple groups and networks, the boundaries or memberships of which can frequently change. Subpopulation or network memberships are by nature open and shifting, for example, across the life course or in the context of wider structural changes in society. Observing these processes is essential to understanding what factors are or are not included in standard data sources. Some but not all subpopulation memberships will be important to understanding reproductive patterns. Membership in some groups not directly concerned with reproduction – say, units of production or political hierarchies – may nonetheless be crucial to social statuses that have a real bearing on the conjunctures in which reproductive options are weighed. It is thus crucial not to confine research only to networks of communication about, say, reproduction, contraception or AIDS, but to study historical and contemporary relationships that bring people together into subpopulations for other purposes and that provide contexts in which people evaluate such communication (e.g. Bochow, this volume; Kroeker, this volume; Pauli, this volume; Roche and Hohmann, this volume; Gregson et al. 2011). While ethnography provides the means to identify memberships and observe how groups are formed and change their composition, at some point an analyst has to test whether such subpopulations have a reality beyond the case studies and communities he or she has observed. Local censuses and representative surveys designed to capture language categories and practices of local subpopulations provide means for checking group compositions and relationships. Where the validity of these units is confirmed, they can be compared or contrasted to findings that rely on standard units used in mainline survey programmes.

Combined approaches that begin in ethnography and historically documented contexts have proven undoubtedly rich in their capacity to generate new and surprising results, which lead, in turn, to a healthy questioning of widespread assumptions about fertility declines as a monolithic process of 'transition'. This capacity is evident in the chapters collected here. In the remainder of the introduction we will note some of the ways in which the chapters continue to develop the three principal movements from which recognition of the central importance of the heterogeneity of declines and the role of anthropological demography have grown.

Relations between Subpopulations as Mechanisms of Reproductive Change

Modernity arrives in different forms and has been arriving in a great many parts of the world for a long time – as Ortega's remarks, written nearly a century ago, remind us. Wrigley, in his seminal assessment (1972) of the concept of modernization, addressed the classic test case – the era of England's Industrial Revolution. Carefully and extensively reviewing its main components,[9] he noted two central problems that leave it unable to account sufficiently for England's pre-eminent modern development. One is that key technical innovations necessary for rapid economic growth did not derive solely from the general rationality that modernization is supposed always to entail, but were a consequence of specific, local circumstances. The second is that, amongst these circumstances, changes in the structure of social groups and of relationships between them (notably in the division of labour and in social conventions regarding acceptable living standards) were fundamental. The values and practices that came to be associated with modernity and thence with economic improvement spread unevenly; local valuation of what is 'modern' became part of what differentiated groups in society from a much earlier date than the emergence of key technical innovations. As Wrigley says, there was 'a long gathering process of change' that helped to prepare the way for economic growth; his observation that 'a society might become modernized without also becoming industrialized' (1972: 236–37) has with time become mainstream to the revision of standard development models and to understanding how and why fertility patterns have varied so widely.[10]

Earlier in this chapter, we noted that the social and life course issues arbitrated in vital conjunctures become basic characteristics that distinguish groups in society. Changes in the timing and arrangement of marriage, alternatives to marriage, the incidence of childbearing, schooling, the division of labour, the acceptability of different occupations and other family norms are bound up in wider social statuses and opportunities. Take-up of values and practices perceived as modern need not require general economic development and, indeed, began in many places under colonialism in which the incomes and material conditions of the great mass of people usually changed modestly (and not necessarily for the better). Beginning in the 1950s and 1960s, the international and governmental agencies that sought to promote family planning in the developing world, together with modern values associated with Western family, marriage, education and employment patterns, likewise belonged to the 'gathering process of change' that Wrigley noted. As this history is part of people's experience, it continues to be influential, and because their experience was far from uniform, the roots of modernity are often not what models used by population and development planners suppose.

We see, for example, in Julia Pauli's Namibian data how in early stages of modern development, a single society can give rise to a number of coexisting subpopulations in which the means and purposes of modern contraception, and consequent fertility levels, vary. The subpopulations are characterized by generational and emerging class differences, each with different forms of marriage and reproductive patterns. The relationships that came to define these groups in the late colonial period have continued to shape the conjunctures people faced in the ensuing decades. The historical context of this modernization is of particular note: modern methods of fertility control arrived in Namibia with the imposition of apartheid. The main methods available from the 1970s – sterilization and injections – were employed by the South African government to counter the 'black threat' posed by high fertility in local populations. The control policy was accompanied by administrative, educational and commercial development that created a small, wealthy African elite of 'big men' who cooperated with the government's strategy of rule by artificially created ethnic 'homelands'.

National demographic data on these generations show the onset of fertility declines, but also that declines were modest. Namibians maintained African patterns of early marriage and high fertility in differing ways. The situation on the ground, as indicated in Pauli's study of one 'homeland', clarifies this variation: distinctive life course and reproductive patterns emerged and came to characterize different subpopulations as people faced the conjunctures to which the context of the new regime gave rise. On the one hand, marriage became so expensive that it was largely an elite prerogative. Wives of big men became model housewives following a perceived Western pattern, although their fertility remained above four children per woman. Contraception was used in this group on the Western model of 'stopping', i.e. adopted once a sufficient number of children had been reached. However, their embrace of contraception and marital fidelity was not matched by their husbands, who maintained multiple relationships outside of marriage. Continuity of this widespread African pattern was possible because the 'homeland' structure created vulnerable lower strata subpopulations that provided services to the local elites. In these groups there was great economic insecurity and little prospect of upward mobility. Similar to the 'outside wife' pattern observed elsewhere in Africa (Bledsoe 1990), some of these women had continuing relationships with married big men, bearing them children and gaining some support from them, while others had children in multiple and usually brief affairs. The conjunctures of lower-strata women thus form two vulnerable subgroups and it is in these that most uptake of contraception has occurred – for spacing rather than stopping purposes. Their fertility is notably lower than among the elite. Meanwhile, there are signs of generational change in the latter group. Young daughters of elite women are now being discouraged by their mothers from accepting the unhappy inside/outside wife regime and encouraged instead to delay marriage and childbearing. The situation is aptly symbolized by a ceremonial key awarded to girls on reaching age 21 without children and that they see as a crucial step in shaping their life courses.

In sum, to understand the dynamics of fertility declines in Namibia, we need to identify a number of subpopulations and how reproduction has shaped the composition of these groups as part of the ongoing formation of classes in a particular political context. Lower strata, not higher, have led the decline; for these groups, modernization as a mechanism of fertility change works by increasing insecurity (economic and marital), not by the uniform and happy adoption of Western family size desires and values. Subsequent chapters by van der Sijpt, Kroeker and Hukin all show that this is a recurring theme: a wider historical conjuncture of nascent class formation and its inequalities impacts on the vulnerability of young women in lower strata, leading them to specific vital conjunctures in their lives in which they adopt abortion and modern contraceptive techniques in an attempt to limit the effects of vulnerability in their lives (cf. Johnson-Hanks 2006).

The second chapter, by Sarah Walters, is a groundbreaking synthesis of ethnography and long-term parish register demography in East Africa, which enables her to track attempts to introduce values and practices deriving from modern, Western culture for nearly a century. The agency of these changes is, again, not one that usually figures in the demographic literature: the colonial state and, more particularly, the Catholic Church. Since the end of the nineteenth century, missionaries brought to East Africa modern medicine and childcare, education, famine relief, agricultural improvements and systematic vital recordkeeping, together with Christian values of conjugality and individual choice in respect of matters of family and faith that are intimately bound up with modern, European values. As Walters says, the whole approach constituted a 'moral demography' in which Church teaching and other activities potentially opened wider access to opportunities in the colonial state and the later, independent nation-states.

Of course, not all of this package was immediately acceptable. The insistence on monogamy and that reproduction must follow rather than precede marriage proved to be a sticking point in polygynous societies. Pastoral activities naturally focus on principal life course events – birth, marriage, death – and adherence to Church teachings brought parishioners and priests into conflict with local secret society organizations also focused on the control of these conjunctures. The registers in consequence give us a detailed account only of one subpopulation – members of the faith – there being other groups who remained outside the church, or who joined other churches, with resulting tensions in the wider community. However, as Walters shows, the records do enable us to track events both at the individual and population levels, showing how vital conjunctures play out and how this constructs membership of the Church population. Because registers and ethnography together give us a detailed picture of the conjunctures of parishioners who struggled with key modern elements in the Church's teaching, they enable us to study an influential subpopulation in the process of its formation, how its composition grew not only by births but also by conversion (or was decreased by local conflicts, migration and excommunication), and how its age structure and other demographic features evolved.

Moreover, it shows how priests' long experience of working amongst several local subpopulations gradually produced a significant change in their understanding of their role. By the 1960s and 1970s, when social demographers began to write about the need for rapid population change and the imminent spread of modern nuclear family values across Africa (e.g. Goode 1963; Caldwell 1976), clergy were coming to accept that attempts to bring about rapid change in marriage, ritual and related practices could be counterproductive and that the normalization of modern Christian values would take a number of different forms in African cultures, as part of a long-term process. Priests' familiarity with indigenous moral codes and realities of marriage now gives them an important role to play as preservers of African culture.

Sophie Roche and Sophie Hohmann's Tajik study provides a third face of modernity: Soviet colonial policy and its impact from the 1920s. This chapter provides a major case study that reveals important processes and variations characterizing a wider system (cf. Hirsch 2005). In creating the 'republics' of Central Asia, the Soviet system separated historical centres of Tajik culture (Samarkand, Bukhara) from the area that became Tajikistan. Modern medical care, bureaucracy, education and central economic planning were introduced to replicate the model of Soviet identity elsewhere. Culture was part of this top-down project: each 'republic' was supposed to have its own folkloristic tradition, and therefore Tajik was declared a distinctive language and ethnicity shared by groups in the area. The methods employed to restructure local society on this model were, as elsewhere in the Stalinist period, brutal: better-off agriculturalists and their families were removed in the purge of 'kulaks'; whole villages were forcibly relocated to uncultivated regions to bring them into an expanded production model; the collectivization and mechanization of farming were intended to break down existing family structures by removing private property and replacing traditional family and community authority; instead, collective farms ('Kolkhoz') were organized as workers' 'brigades' in which local leaders were rewarded by links to the political elite in the new capital of Dushanbe. Women's equality as producers was not matched by equality in domestic and political spheres: they continued to bear the main family care and childbearing responsibilities, while their full-time employment was enforced by doctors who had exclusive right to attest women's age, pregnancy status and access to contraception – ensuring, for example, that they worked until childbirth and, from the 1960s, the promotion of sterilization.

However, the draconian enforcement of the Soviet ideal of modern identity could not erase local differences. As whole communities were often forcibly relocated, they could retain much of their internal structure; while a Kolkhoz might be formed from several such groups, all shared the experience of relocation and desire to retain their values. Roche and Hohmann's research combines ethnography and a carefully conducted local census to examine evolving relations between two subpopulations in one of the relocation sites. Data on marriage within and between these groups, their respective fertility levels and distinctive sibling-based family strategies show how relationships preserving subpopulation differences have continued. Tajik ethnicity as a uniform and primary locus of identity remained a construct of central authority; rather, reproductive and other norms followed the interests and relationships of the subpopulations. A striking feature of this research is that the addition of local census to ethnographic data enables Roche and Hohmann to disentangle precisely the kind of differing sibling life-course, marriage and procreation trajectories that Bourdieu's use of standard census data failed to track in the case of Béarn: older, middle and younger siblings exhibit distinctive patterns, a variation that is fundamental to the preservation of family and subpopulation identities and that reveal the composite nature of fertility adjustments.

Patrick Heady's study of Ovasta, a community in Carnia, north-east Italy, provides an example of the southern European family and community systems that Jenkins and Bourdieu describe. However, Heady's case study differs in two important respects. One is that

Ovasta appears to conform much more to a scenario in which modern developments in the regional economy appear to overwhelm traditional relationships. Fertility has fallen to a level well below that needed to sustain the community. At the same time, older patterns of seasonal migration have given way to permanent moves to urban areas, taking more than one in five young people from the community. Unlike Béarn, there was no core of big houses; the pastoral economy was more marginal and the community in consequence relied on labour pooled between households, for which bonds built up amongst men were instrumental. As sufficient solidarity and numbers no longer exist, principal economic activities, like cheese making, have become impossible. While Heady's analysis, like that of Walters, focuses on only a single subpopulation (in this case, those who stay in Ovasta, not those who leave), he adds a second focus by employing comparative data on nineteen communities in eight European countries (see Grandits 2010). This perspective opens up examination of a key component of reproductive change that cuts across the communities and that current approaches to European fertility declines have struggled to explain. Reduced fertility in itself is not surprising, given that reproductive controls, as Bourdieu and Jenkins describe, have long been a basic mechanism of these family systems. What demographers did not anticipate, however, and that remains unexplained by the several competing hypotheses Heady reviews, is why fertility has fallen so low – to levels of one child per woman.

A Malthusian take on emigration from Ovasta, for example, would expect the opposite outcome: as emigration opens up niches in the local economy, there should be no incentive to limit reproduction – on the contrary, Malthus would expect fertility levels to continue or even for a time increase, filling the empty productive places. However, as Heady describes, this kind of maximizing of reproductive numbers for economic purposes is a mentality that has no place in local economy and society. Social convention historically welcomed fertility somewhat above replacement as evidence of success and status, but levels were tempered by a collective recognition of environmental constraints on the pastoral economy. A compromise between reproductive success and environmental constraints was achieved, as Heady describes, by a balance of two mechanisms that appears to have worked in Ovasta and a wider set of Mediterranean communities. One was strong marriage endogamy: kin and family ties were focused on securing good local marriages and parenting that favoured investment in children and continuity of family honour. This habitus, as Bourdieu observed, was important long before the supposedly modern innovation of limiting reproduction to enhance child 'quality'. Local families in effect competed for good marriages, and secure childbearing and rearing, while recognizing that they could not maximize fertility if that undermined a second key factor – the solidarity with other community members necessary to achieve pooled labour in the context of limited production opportunities. There was thus awareness that moderate childbearing was an advantage amongst families in competition for limited resources, and this norm has not changed. Why, then, have fertility levels moved downwards to the point where the very continuity of families is in question?

Heady's thesis is that longstanding norms to moderate fertility remain strong, yet emigration has removed the second support to childbearing: the role of community solidarity. Family and kin certainly continue to focus on good marriages and parenting, but in current conditions this no longer extends to fertility somewhat above replacement as a correlate of status. Rather, with much greater tendency to emigrate, a key social and economic support for the security to reproduce (whether babies or family status) has been removed. It may thus be, as modernization theorists suggest, that the appeal of opportunities in the wider economy and of enhanced individualism work generally to lower fertility – but this is not all that is at issue, nor is it sufficient to account for specific reproductive levels, such as below-replacement fertility in rural communities. To explain why one level of reproduction occurs rather than another, we also need to consider which 'traditional' practices remain, together with the structural implications of the retreat of certain others. Heady provides a preliminary test of this model, which yields striking regional differences in kin networking between the European communities in his sample. As he notes, models then need to be tested by observation at the local level in order to examine and measure whether hypothesized mechanisms actually have the influence attributed to them.

Amongst the fundamental inequalities that modernity is supposed to alter are relations between genders. In general, modernization is believed to enhance female equality directly via the spread of education, wage labour and contraception, while patriarchal family structures are likewise supposed to be diminished. The issue is, of course, complicated by the many subpopulations and networks to which the two broad groups, men and women, also belong. Gendered inequalities also arise, as we have seen in the chapters by

Pauli, Walters, and Roche and Hohmann, where modernity was fostered by colonial, medical and professional models that carried their own structures of male dominance. Other examples in which 'traditional' and 'modern' male preferences combine are readily available in the literature (e.g. Das Gupta 2009). Tropical Africa has become an obvious focus for research on these issues, since it combines powerful indigenous male precedents (established in lineage and marriage systems that continue to shape family life), postcolonial states and limited national fertility declines. The seemingly obvious implication is that male-dominated structures remain an obstacle to African reproductive modernization. In their chapter, Sara Randall, Nathalie Mondain and Alioune Diagne show that the conjunctures in which men and women confront and try to resolve these issues in contemporary Senegal reveal a subtle balance in which normative male prerogatives are preserved while being extensively circumvented.

Randall, Mondain and Diagne completed two rounds (1999 and 2007) of in-depth interviewing of randomly selected men and women in a Senegalese town that has experienced extensive labour migration to Europe, education and integration into the national market economy. Women as well as men have been involved in the latter two developments, which have led to a general acceptance of modern material values and significant improvements in domestic standards, albeit with problems of recurring absence and unemployment that often make family life insecure. The town is also the locus of strict Muslim brotherhoods that uphold the conjunction of longstanding ethnic and Islamic gender values, both in the community and in migration sites. Married men are supposed to have unquestioned authority over their wives and economic responsibility for them; women's maternal role is idealized and sacred, and submission to their husbands is the foundation of their social reputation and spiritual wellbeing. As the authors note, this configuration leads men to answer questions posed in national survey programmes in strict conformity to Islamic norms, regardless of practice. The idea of controlling the number of births was in particular considered an act against God's will. In-depth interviewing in many cases showed a similar 'correct' line, but also revealed a wider range of secular attitudes, including acceptance of birth control, particularly for preserving wives' health. The 'correct' line, in other words, can often be something of a rhetorical stance. On the one hand, anything less than strict orthodoxy in public conveys disrespect for Islam and for others in positions of authority;

it is likely to be disastrous for the couple's reputation and runs counter to deeply held beliefs. On the other hand, there are many conjunctures in which the 'correct' line is unrealistic and private alternatives are quietly found – for example, periods of economic vulnerability in which women's continued productive role is critical, women's health and the role of spacing of children in preserving it, and sexual relations outside of marriage. These conjunctures are, in the author's view, slowly but steadily shifting reproductive norms, even while leaving wider cultural and religious norms in place. They also show that female agency is not produced simply by an external modernizing stimulus, but by the incorporation, for example, of new technologies and material improvements, into local ends.

Altering Life Courses

As all of these chapters demonstrate, diverse compositional demographies arise out of historical and personal conjunctures that need to be understood on several levels. At the level of the state and of constituent populations that compose it, conjunctures are defined by historical circumstances that bring together external agencies, local social structures and cultural modes of problem-solving. Local and external agents may each have their own view of what is modern and about what aspects of behaviour are appropriate for modern values and practices. Access to major benefits that can come with education, healthcare, improved economic infrastructure and social welfare is in most places very unequal. Such differences, as we have seen, often reflect the differing positions that groups and their members hold in local hierarchies. Adopting standard and national-level classifications of population units and indices to the exclusion of these differences frequently erases them. Population statistics, instead of an essential avenue to identifying mechanisms of population change, becomes a powerful censor.

At the local level, in which individuals, couples, families and kin are situated in the historical setting of the communities, regional identities, economic sectors or other subpopulations in which they live, there is the opportunity to observe actual processes of population change, the moments or, as Johnson-Hanks says, *vital conjunctures* in which people construe and arbitrate amongst the possible courses of action that wider and changing historical conjunctures pose. People do this through the medium of immediate issues in their lives, of which reproduction and its control are a prime instance. This process may sustain the subpopulations of which they are members, alter them or lead to the emergence of new groups and kinds of groups.

Reproduction is, of course, only one mechanism of subpopulation formation and change. As the chapters show, vital conjunctures that arbitrate different reproductive patterns are commonly bound up with other compositional processes like migration, the division of labour, alternative routes to forming marriages or partnerships and the formation of religious and community memberships. Reproductive choices are commonly guided by these processes, the opportunities and constraints they entail, and the group ties and identities they compose. At one extreme, as in Patrick Heady's Italian example, vital conjunctures combining migration with low fertility may imperil a longstanding local demographic system. More commonly, as in the studies by Pauli, Jenkins, and Roche and Hohmann, we see how marriage alternatives linked to differences in status, migration histories and the division of labour lead subpopulations to achieve a range of different reproductive outcomes that define the differing social positions of group members. Walters' chapter provides an example in which religious conversion and associated marriage and reproduction lead to the formation and development of new religious subpopulations, while Randall, Mondain and Diagne show how established religious groups maintain their values while adopting reproductive controls that many, if not most, members regard as forbidden.

Research that tracks population heterogeneity by showing how individual women's and men's reproductive trajectories evolve differently in particular subpopulations thus establishes an important baseline for understanding the dynamics of population change. First, it restores the agency of individuals and the groups to which they belong, rather than supposing that they are, in effect, mere unwitting followers of a uniform economic or other rationality. Second, within this compositional demography, it becomes possible to connect demographic differentials that are key to declining fertility (such as the timing of reproduction across individual and family life courses) to the actual problems of childbearing that people are trying to resolve. Declining fertility, like other trends, emerges as a composite outcome of many conjunctures that determine birth intervals and the priority amongst proximate determinants of fertility (Bongaarts et al. 1984) across the life course. Problematic conjunctures, how people cope with them and how their actions combine to change reproductive patterns are the subject of detailed case studies in the final four ethnographic chapters of this book, which address childlessness, delayed childbearing, abortion, partnership issues and why the prevalence of one or another contraceptive technique remains a matter of local moral demography.[11]

The anthropology of the colonial and postcolonial era laid down a comparative approach that anchored reproduction as a central object of control in societies across Sub-Saharan Africa (e.g. Evans-Pritchard 1951; Turner 1957; Douglas 1966; Godelier 2009). The status of lineages and their members was supported by higher numbers of children, the exchange of daughters and bridewealth in marriage, the advantages of multiple wives and their children in productive activities, and elaborate ritual and supernatural controls (e.g. witchcraft) over life course events like sex, pregnancy, childbirth, initiation into adulthood, inheritance and marriage. The relative success of men and their kin groups in managing this system defined local hierarchies; male dominance and female obedience, as described by Randall and her colleagues, defined gender relations. Underpinning this system were demographic controls expressly favourable to childbearing and rearing (early marriage and breastfeeding practices coupled with women's extended postpartum abstinence), as well as mechanisms for ensuring the prompt remarriage of widows and the incorporation of children conceived outside marriage. However, the anthropologists to whom we owe this important work were only secondarily concerned with tracking variations within and between subpopulations, or with the quantitative documentation of them.

The several chapters on Sub-Saharan Africa by Bochow, Kroeker and van der Sijpt (as well as by Pauli, Walters, and Randall, Mondain and Diagne, discussed above) show the considerable extent to which understanding of population and subpopulation variation has moved to the fore. In Erica van der Sijpt's Cameroonian ethnography, we find a fascinating, detailed account of how conjunctures pose a complex and often conflicting set of alternative life-course paths and how people navigate them. Plural marriage patterns, which were traditionally polygynous, have not been replaced by the Western norms of monogamy, education and nuclear family values. Rather, forms of plural partnership have proliferated, along the lines of 'inside and outside wives' described by Bledsoe (1990), with markedly different implications for women's career aspirations and reproductive trajectories. As van der Sijpt shows, the conjunctures in which young women find themselves pregnant in advance of formal marriage arrangements (a well-established African pattern) arbitrate the full range of potential life courses, from an urban life of educated formal sector employment, to a lifetime of shifting, provisional 'outside' statuses, to being a polygynous co-wife in an outlying village.

While some of these alternatives may appear new and radical, all of the life course paths that women follow and their fertility outcomes remain structured by parameters that have long shaped African compositional demography. Van der Sijpt lists five: whether women look to their patriline or matriline for support; sibling order and numbers of siblings (which determine whether marriage involves bridewealth as a key component); the position of a woman's kin group in political networks (relatively powerful ties providing greater or lesser social capital); a woman's position in the marriage market (e.g. whether she has multiple partners and therefore more options); and marriage order (e.g. being a second or third wife in a plural union, rather than the first, may provide more freedom in relation to childbearing). As van der Sijpt remarks, a woman's fertility is decided not in one, but in a series of vital conjunctures across her life course in which the relative importance of these five variables changes, for example, as she grows older and in consequence of previous conjunctures and their outcomes. Thus, a young woman who becomes pregnant outside of marriage has already passed through a conjuncture in which the possibility of having a child, whether to practise contraception, what implications pregnancy may have for her continuing education and job prospects, and whether one or another partner is likely to take parental and marital responsibility have been weighed. The five variables continue to arbitrate the conjuncture she now faces, e.g. of whether a man agrees to be her husband, which man, what kind of marital and material relationships that would entail, whether her education can continue, whether she could remain single and have the child raised by her mother or other kin, whether she should have an abortion and so forth. Successive conjunctures determine which proximate determinants regulate the spacing of children and her total fertility, as well as having a major impact on her social status, reputation and network memberships. Adopting a modern, Western model of monogamous conjugality remains a realistic option for very few women in this system, although many modernization variables like contraceptive technology, education, movement to urban areas and so forth are in play. However, these factors are not independent determinants, since their influence depends on which combination of the five parameters prevail in the subpopulation to which she belongs and which life stage she has reached.

Astrid Bochow's chapter describes the vital conjunctures of elite women in Botswana, a context that counters sharply the often-stated view that Sub-Saharan Africa remains a high fertility region strongly resistant to reproductive control. National surveys show that the country has experienced a dramatic fall in fertility, from 6.6 births per woman in 1985 to 2.9 in 2006. Her case study is of particular importance as the rise of an educated, relatively wealthy urban elite that identifies strongly with professionalism and modern nation-building and that sees fertility control as fundamental to a nationwide ethnic identity, is surely a context in which we would expect to see conventional modernization theories confirmed.[12] The reality, as Bochow shows, is a much more interesting demographic system than the usual modernization variables would lead us to believe.

Vital conjunctures currently faced by men and women are shaped, as we have seen in preceding chapters, by changes during the colonial era. Bochow draws on ethnography of the 1930s and 1970s, which included surveys, to outline the following historical sequence. Pregnancy before marriage and other arrangements to ensure ample reproduction remain common, without specific numerical family size norms being normative. However, the ways in which people go about this began to change with new economic developments under colonialism that removed young men, both married and unmarried, to work in South African mines. This complicated bridewealth arrangements, reducing traditional lineage power and opening up new living arrangements for women (cohabitation, matrifocality), which gave them greater choice and freedom of movement, whether for economic or reproductive purposes. Contraception, as well as longstanding abstinence and breastfeeding norms, was a regular part of this picture from the 1930s onwards. While women continued to have premarital children at a young age, they aimed at long intervals between children partly for traditional health reasons and partly reflecting opportunities of their new situation. A subpopulation emerged of higher-status women and men who adopted Christian models of childbearing after marriage and were able to take advantage of newly introduced schooling. In this group, childbearing might be postponed into a woman's mid twenties. This subpopulation was well-placed when government bureaucracy expanded upon national independence and with the discovery of rich mineral resources (diamonds) in Botswana, both of which led to economic expansion and demand for educated personnel. A widely recognized pattern of childbearing then emerged, in which a woman might have a premarital child or one early in a partnership, but would then postpone later childbearing until late in her fertile period. Partnerships often changed across the life course, as is characteristic of cohabiting and matrifocal family arrangements. This pattern was considered a characteristic national, Tswana ethnic pattern and, as it was widespread, census and survey data categories were modified to include a normative 'living together' pattern.

In sum, lower fertility came to be associated with an early and late childbearing pattern not typical of modernization scenarios. This was coupled with a fluid partnership pattern in which women and men might have a sequence of cohabitations over time. Meanwhile, other African norms not usually associated with modernization also prevail, for example, in which men may have multiple relationships, childbearing success is essential to status, and kin continue to exert strong pressures on couples to have children. Yet the elite have also entered into what is familiar in Western low-fertility scenarios, in which careers compete with childbearing, childrearing has become a major expense and conspicuous consumption is expected even though consequent debt is problematic. However, such stereotypical modern concerns depend for their influence on the three successive conjunctures that Bochow notes as defining the reproductive life course in this subpopulation: early, often unintended births before marriage; spacing and delaying during middle years, owing to uncertain partnerships and AIDS; and late attempts at childbearing, often to affirm an established partnership. Reduced fertility with modernization is thus bound up with multiple sources of insecurity, greatly augmented in recent decades by the AIDS epidemic, which the continuation of plural sexual relationships has undoubtedly helped to foster. For those women who did not succeed in having a child early in their reproductive years, the threat of childlessness is very real and may be a major factor in destabilizing partnerships. This situation is even worse for women not in the elite, who do not have adequate resources for medical assistance. Ironically, as Bochow notes, these several sources of insecurity enable elite couples to play different causes of low fertility off against each other: pressured by kin to have a child, they can plead career and financial causes for the 'delay', thus disguising the impact of AIDS on their reproduction.

Lena L. Kroeker's ethnography of urban and rural workers in a second southern African state, Lesotho, provides a striking contrast to Bochow's study of the Botswanan elite. Many of the circumstances over the last four decades are similar, including the theme of disguised fertility realities and motivations. Fertility decline, from

5.4 to 3.3 births per woman, is again impressive and has taken place against a long history of male labour migration to neighbouring South Africa, a rise of female-headed households and movement to urban areas, greater access to education (of which women have taken advantage) and the deadly impact of AIDS. As in all of the African chapters, available contraception, awareness of modern Western family ideals, desire for economic advancement into the waged economy and the implications of these values for longstanding premarital pregnancy patterns are all part of the picture. These changes coexist with the continuing influence of wider kin groups over marriage, reproduction as an indigenous criterion of full personhood (usually entailing several children) and gender relationships that continue to disadvantage women. The 'long gathering process of change' of which Wrigley wrote is thus much in evidence, yet the reality of fertility declines is bound up not in a wholesale shift to modern, Western family norms, but in a complex set of vulnerabilities that very slow and incomplete integration into the global economy have created.

The first shock was the serious decline from the 1980s in the demand for male labour, which returned many men to local unemployment. Unlike Botswana, major new male opportunities have not emerged to fill the gap. Women, meanwhile, have become increasingly accustomed to managing their own households, and major employment opportunities emerged in urban areas of Lesotho for women's economic independence based on textile production. Men have continued to head households in rural areas and to exercise power over marriage arrangements and sexuality, but have lost respect owing to their inability to provide for their families; growing domestic violence arising from this situation has provided further incentives for women to move to the towns. It is there that women, whether married or not, confront the vital conjunctures that, as Kroeker describes, create opportunities for 'secret family planning'. The theme of covert contraception use here echoes what Randall and her colleagues found in Senegal, but is part of a different compositional demography. Women may hide their marital status from lovers; single women may cease contraception and get pregnant in an attempt to 'entrap' men in marriage; contraception and abortion arise in the attempt to balance economic uncertainties, partnership issues and the desire for independence, as well as health issues. The Christian ideal of stable, marital monogamy may be an object of desire for some, but neither the economy nor gender relations make it a reality for more than a very small minority. Conjunctures vary, as women in rural and urban subpopulations face different vulnerabilities and possibilities. The second shock, evidently, is the rapid and extensive spread of AIDS, which has complicated successful childbearing, childrearing, continued partnership and economic security.

Eleanor Hukin takes the issues raised in the several African chapters a step further, looking more specifically at how different contraceptive methods become part of the vital conjunctures that women and men face. The context of her research – Cambodian towns and countryside – is obviously very different from Africa, belonging to an Asian region noted for rapid economic growth and fertility declines. While Cambodia has not been a regional leader,[13] the last four decades have witnessed a fall from 6.7 to 3.0 births per woman. Hukin begins by applying accepted statistical estimates of risk to national survey data and, at first glance, the picture appears to conform unambiguously to the standard modernization story: women in higher educational and income groups, living in urban areas, have lower fertility, and there has been a significant increase in modern contraceptive use. However, other findings indicate that a closer look is needed, pointing to some interesting parallels to preceding chapters. Thus, the take-up of modern contraceptive technology (in Cambodia, usually injections or the IUD) is more characteristic of women in lower than higher economic strata; women with more education and belonging to higher income and social strata continue to employ a range of traditional methods for controlling fertility; birth regulation is not new and reflects a range of priorities other than aiming at a particular, small family size, of which women's personal and child health is a primary concern. Interestingly, there has been a greater increase in the use of traditional than of modern methods of birth control during the fertility decline, which has evidently not kept women from having fewer children.

Hukin's ethnography reveals the rich, varied and subtle awareness of ways of avoiding pregnancy in Khmer culture that lies beneath broad national trends, and uses this knowledge to unpack the reasons for the seeming puzzle of an educated, urban elite that prefers traditional methods, while the lower strata readily accept new Western technologies. Often multiple methods of reproductive control are involved, but Hukin's central finding is that Khmer culture turns the Western idea of contraceptive modernity upside-down. Central to reproductive controls is the calendar method, which requires periodic abstinence and may be backed up by withdrawal and (sometimes, Hukin suggests) an apparently long-standing recourse to abortion. All groups agreed that the calendar approach was a 'modern' method, often called 'the doctor's way': it requires knowledge (e.g. of the Gregorian calendar, as opposed to the lunar cycle known to women with little or no schooling), and reinforces Buddhist models of moral and physical balance and of female discipline and restraint. The management of reproduction is women's responsibility, and educated and better-off men may expect, by the same moral codes, to play a supportive role. These women are likely to employ other birth-limiting practices as is consonant with good health and wellbeing, but not for the purpose of trying to control numbers of children; thus, breastfeeding is recognized to inhibit ovulation, and terminal abstinence (for older women) and complete abstinence (for the unmarried) are enjoined.[14] More educated, upper-strata women are also more likely to have access to a hospital abortion, although this is concealed as it is a sin under Buddhism. Poorer, less educated women are considered, and consider themselves, less able to practise the 'modern' calendar approach and therefore use methods like the IUD and injections that do not require them or their husbands to exercise so much restraint. They may be concerned, like upper-strata women, about the negative health effects of Western contraceptive technology, which is seen as unnatural and interventionist, but they lack the modern knowledge that calendar methods require. Abortion pills are easily available in the marketplace, and traditional massage practices and medicines are also used; the vulnerability of women in the poorer strata is once again an important theme.

In sum, an important theme in these four chapters, as in all contributions to the book, is to show that modern values and technologies are normally integrated into societies under the continuing influence of extant moral and gender norms, and how this process varies because of fundamental inequalities and the ways by which people search for flexible means to adjust to economic constraints and other social and personal uncertainties. Indeed, in all of the chapters, the social and economic insecurities that people face in the course of modernization loom much larger in determining the course of their reproductive behaviour than the advantages generally presumed in the demographic literature to follow directly from the embrace of modern values and economic development. Definition of the conjunctures people face and the alternative courses of action they pursue tell us a lot about how different groups in society cope, why the demography of subpopulations differs and why the supposed homogenization of fertility behaviour does not emerge.

The more general importance of this approach is clear. One gain is to rebalance empirically our understanding of fertility change, so that the idealized vision of modernization is checked against the inequalities and vulnerabilities that people actually face. Second, from the standpoint of population theory, an approach to understanding fertility change grounded in subpopulation differences and in the several vital conjunctures that compose them helps us to understand why the modernization and demographic transition framework proved indeterminate. Moreover, the several examples provided in this book show how it is possible to rethink trajectories of demographic change once historical differences have been recognized. Of longer-term interest is the possibility of revitalizing the analysis of past census and survey series along the lines currently being developed by Cambridge historical demographers. Combining the basically bottom-up methodologies of anthropology with top-down demographic and other social science methods opens up research strategies of considerable empirical potential. What is likely to be entailed is a shift for anthropologists from the continuing preference for single community studies by individual researchers to multi-site research involving teams of anthropologists, local researchers, historians and demographers. The purposes include not only identification of significant subpopulation differences and the processes that produce them, but assisting census and survey design in order to better identify them. Applicability to pressing environmental, epidemiological, genetic and evolutionary questions is also likely to be greatly enhanced.

Philip Kreager is Senior Research Fellow in Human Sciences, Somerville College; Director, Fertility and Reproductive Studies Group, Institute of Social and Cultural Anthropology; and Research Associate, Department of Sociology, University of Oxford. His recent publications include *Population in the Human Sciences: Concepts, Models, Evidence* (Oxford University Press, 2015) and *Ageing without Children* (Berghahn Books, 2005).

Astrid Bochow is Lecturer in Social Anthropology, Georg August Universität Göttingen, an Associate of the Fertility and Reproductive Studies Group, Institute of Social and Cultural Anthropology, Oxford University, and a Member of the Steering Committee of the Research Network: Religion, HIV/AIDS and

Social Transformation. She has conducted extensive field research in Botswana and Ghana.

Notes

1. Fertility declines as the *idée fixe* of postwar demography begins, of course, with Notestein's formulation of 'demographic transition' (1945). A shortlist of papers documenting the heterogeneity of declines and the incapacity of Notestein's framework to explain them, would begin with Coale (1969) and proceed through Knodel and van de Walle (1979), Chesnais ([1987] 1992), Cleland and Wilson (1987), Gillis et al. (1992) and Kohler et al. (2002).
2. Much more might be said here about the potential role of network analysis to assist in the identification and exploration of subpopulations and of how differences between them (of which fertility declines are but one aspect) are altered or sustained. This is a substantial topic in its own right, with many conceptual and methodological issues yet to be answered (see e.g. McLean 2007) that go beyond what can be encompassed in this volume.
3. However, substantial progress has been made on this puzzle in evolutionary biology, since the latter systematically employs population concepts largely ignored in population statistics (Kreager 2009; Kreager et al. 2015b).
4. This abbreviated account leaves out Jenkins' more detailed observations on Bourdieu's ethnography, and particularly the absence of important constituent groups in his primary interview data. As he also remarks, Bourdieu's account, together with those of LePlay and other sociologists, need to be seen as part of a French political discourse on *soi-disant* economic and social development in which there have long been party interests. The theme of sibling variation recurs in this volume, in the chapters by Roche and Hohmann, and van der Sijpt.
5. Hence, it is not only the supposedly imminent disappearance of the traditional peasant world of southwest France that has a two hundred-year history. That history coincides with the period of the emergence and long rise and spread of statistics in European government and research. The two are no doubt related, as, for example, LePlay's account of the supposed disappearance of important peasant family forms was based on his early quantitative approach. The story that Jenkins tells is without doubt general and not peculiarly French.
6. The aggregate nature of human societies and their constituent groups was the subject of sophisticated reasoning from the Greeks to the late eighteenth century, in which the principal concern was not enumeration, but balanced and imbalanced proportional relationships between

groups' composition and size as instrumental to the formation, sustenance and decline of states. It was this reasoning that gave rise to population arithmetic as a potential science and instrument of policy from the mid seventeenth century, and has remained fundamental to evolutionary biology, in which the origin and evolution of species is defined by the way in which subpopulations are formed, sustained or decline (Kreager 2009, 2015). The science of statistics that emerged from population arithmetic beginning in the early nineteenth century took over the measures and models of population arithmetic, but assigned them an entirely different basis. Statistical methods, grounded in ostensibly complete and precise census and other databases were considered to provide a universal and completely objective basis for a science of society. In this, statistical reform was seen as an intrinsically modernizing force (Porter 1986).

7. For further discussion and examples, see Kreager et al. (2015b).
8. In addition to the chapters by Roche and Hohmann, and Pauli (this volume), see Schröder-Butterfill (2004) for examples.
9. As Wrigley details, modernization as a mechanism of economic growth focuses primarily on a conception of the inherent rationality of development, comprising a linked set of changes that come as a package, including: economic maximization of returns; development of markets, monetization and division of labour; replacing customary arrangements with legal systems; development of governmental bureaucracy; individual self-interest taking priority over the demands of kin and community memberships; and so forth.
10. As Szreter (1993) remarks, some demographers, notably Notestein, found it necessary to very quickly revise the priority of different aspects of modernization, putting the possibility of the diffusion of contraceptives ahead of industrialization. Put bluntly, if countries like Burkina Faso have to industrialize in order to go through fertility transition, the wait will be rather long. As Szreter also notes, once the idea of modernization became plastic in this way, it was conceptually indeterminate (1993: 685–86).
11. A third major gain from recognizing the renewal of population heterogeneity as a baseline for explaining population change lies beyond the scope of this book, although it is clearly implied by the first four of the topics just listed. Differing patterns of fertility decline carry implications for population ageing, as differently placed subpopulations are likely to experience correspondingly different resources in children and access to other members of younger generations (Kreager and Schröder-Butterfill 2010); the causes of this heterogeneity may be tracked in intergenerational relations and the many different shifts in support flows across the life course (Kreager and Schröder-Butterfill 2008).
12. Ethnicity as a population unit here has a different construction compared to Roche and Hohmanns' Tajik example, a reminder that the

significance of an ethnic label can be very different depending on its source and political uses.

13. The Khmer Rouge government of 1975–79 embarked on its own definition of modern socialist state formation, entailing the genocide of some two million Cambodians, including most of the existing professional classes.
14. Cambodian recourse to multiple methods of birth control, including periodic abstinence, suggests interesting parallels to European history (see e.g. Szreter 1996: 392–94; Szreter and Fisher 2010: Chapter 6).

References

Anderson, B. 1993. *Imagined Communities*. London: Verso.

Barth, F. 1969. *Ethnic Groups and Boundaries*. Boston: Little, Brown.

Basu, A.M. 1997. 'The "Politicization" of Fertility to Achieve Non-demographic Objectives', *Population Studies* 51(10): 5–18.

Berkner, L. 1975. 'The Use and Misuse of Census Data for the Historical Analysis of Family Structure', *Journal of Interdisciplinary History* 5(4): 721–38.

Bledsoe, C. 1990. 'Transformations in Sub-Saharan African Marriage and Fertility', *Annals AAPSS* 510: 115–25.

Bledsoe, C.H., and F. Banja. 1999. *Contingent Lives*. Chicago: Chicago University Press.

Bonfield, L., R.M. Smith and K. Wrightson (eds). 1986. *The World We Have Gained*. Oxford: Basil Blackwell.

Bongaarts, J., Frank, O. and Lesthealghe, R. 1984. 'The Proximate Determinants of Fertility in Sub-Saharan Africa', *Population and Development Review* 10(3): 511–37.

Bourdieu, P. 1962. 'Célibat et condition paysanne', *Etudes rurales* 5/6: 32–135.

———. 1972. 'Les stratégies matrimoniales dans le système de reproduction', *Annales E.S.C.* 27: 1105–25 [1976 translation: 'Marriage Strategies as Strategies of Social Reproduction', in R. Forster and O Raunum (eds), *Family and Society*. Baltimore: Johns Hopkins University Press].

———. 1977. *Outline of a Theory of Practice*. Cambridge: Cambridge University Press.

———. 2002. *Le bal des célibataires: Crise de la société paysanne en Béarn*. Paris: Éditions du Seuil.

Caldwell, J.C. 1976. 'Toward a Restatement of Demographic Transition Theory', *Population and Development Review* 2(3–4): 321–66.

Caldwell, J.C., A.G. Hill and V.J. Hull (eds). 1988. *Micro-approaches to Demographic Research*. London: Kegan Paul International.

Chesnais, J.-C. [1987] 1992. *The Demographic Transition*, Oxford: Clarendon Press.

Cleland J., and C. Wilson. 1987. 'Demand Theories of Fertility Transition', *Population Studies* 41(1): 5–30.

Coale, A.J. 1969. 'The Decline of Fertility in Europe from the French Revolution to World War II', in S.J. Behrman, L. Corsa and R. Freedman (eds), *Fertility and Family Planning*. Ann Arbor: University of Michigan Press, pp. 3–24.

Cohn, B. 1987. 'The Census, Social Structure and Objectification in South Asia', in B. Cohn, *An Anthropologist amongst the Historians and Other Essays*. Delhi: Oxford University Press, pp. 224–54.

Das Gupta, M. 1997. 'Kinship Systems and Demographic Regimes', in D.I. Kertzer and T. Fricke (eds), *Anthropological Demography: Toward a New Synthesis*. Chicago: University of Chicago Press, pp. 36–52.

———. 2009. *Family Systems, Political Systems, and Asia's 'Missing Girls': The Construction of Son Preference and its Unravelling*. Policy Research Working Paper 5148. Washington DC: World Bank.

Demeny, P. 1988. 'Social Science and Population Policy', *Population and Development Review* 14(3): 451–79.

Douglas, M. 1966. *Purity and Danger*. London: Routledge & Kegan Paul.

Engelen, T., and A. Wolf (eds). 2005. *Marriage and the Family in Eurasia*. Amsterdam: Aksant.

Evans-Pritchard, E.E. 1951. *Kinship and Marriage among the Nuer*. Oxford: Clarendon Press.

Fisher, K. 2008. *Birth Control, Sex and Marriage in Britain 1918–60*. Oxford: Oxford University Press.

Flandrin, J.-L. 1976. *Families in Former Times*. Cambridge: Cambridge University Press.

Garrett, E., A. Reid, K. Schürer and S. Szreter. 2001. *Changing Family Size in England and Wales, 1891–1911*. Cambridge: Cambridge University Press.

Gillis, J.R., L.A. Tilly and D. Levine (eds). 1992. *The European Experience of Declining Fertility, 1850–1970*. Oxford: Blackwell.

Godelier, M. 2009. 'It Always Takes More than a Man and a Woman to Make a Child', in M. Godelier (ed.), *In and Out of the West: Reconstructing Anthropology*. Charlottesville, VA: University of Virginia Press, pp. 80–100.

Goode, W.J. 1963. *World Revolution and Family Patterns*. New York: Free Press.

Goody, J. 1972. 'The Evolution of the Family', in P. Laslett and R. Wall (eds), *Household and Family in Past Time*. Cambridge: Cambridge University Press, pp. 103–124.

Grandits, H. (ed.). 2010. *Family, Kinship and State in Contemporary Europe*, vol. I. Frankfurt: Campus Verlag.

Grass, G. 1982. *Headbirths, or, The Germans are Dying Out*. London: Secker & Warburg.

Greenhalgh, S. 1990. 'Toward a Political Economy of Fertility: Anthropological Contributions', *Population and Development Review* 16(1): 85–106.

———. (ed.). 1995. 'Anthropology Theorizes Reproduction: Integrating Practice, Political Economic, and Feminist Perspectives', in S. Greenhalgh (ed.), *Situating Fertility*. Cambridge: Cambridge University Press, 3–28.

———. 1996. 'The Social Construction of Population Science: An Intellectual, Institutional and Political History of 20th-Century Demography', *Comparative Studies in Society and History* 38(1): 26–66.

Gregson, S., P. Mushati, H. Grusin, M. Nhamo, C. Schumacher, M. Skovdal, C.A. Nyamukapa and C. Campbell. 2011. 'Social Capital and Reduced Female Vulnerability to HIV Infection in Rural Zimbabwe', *Population and Development Review* 37(2): 333–59.

Hajnal, J. 1965, 'European Marriage Patterns in Perspective', in D.V. Glass and D.E.C. Eversley (eds), *Population in History.* London: E. Arnold, pp. 101–43.

Hammel, E.A. 1990. 'A Theory of Culture for Demography', *Population and Development Review* 16(1): 455–86.

Hill, K., and A.M. Hurtado. 1996. *Ache Life History: The Ecology and Demography of a Foraging People.* New York: Aldine de Gruyter.

Hirsch, F. 2005. *Empire of Nations: Ethnographic Knowledge and the Making of the Soviet Union.* Ithaca: Cornell University Press.

Inhorn, M.C., and S. Tremayne. 2012. *Islam and Assisted Reproductive Technologies: Sunni and Shia Perspectives.* Oxford: Berghahn Books.

Jenkins, T. 2010. *The Life of Property. House, Family and Inheritance in Béarn, South-West France.* Oxford: Berghahn Books.

Johnson-Hanks, J. 2006. *Uncertain Honour: Modern Motherhood in an African Crisis.* Chicago: University of Chicago Press.

———. 2015. 'Populations are Composed One Event at a Time', in P. Kreager, B. Winney, S. Ulijaszek and C. Capelli (eds), *Population in the Human Sciences: Concepts, Models, Evidence*. Oxford: Oxford University Press, pp. 238–56.

Johnson-Hanks, J.A., C.A. Bachrach, S.P. Morgan and H-P. Kohler. 2011. *Understanding Family Change and Variation: Toward a Theory of Conjunctural Action*. Dordrecht: Springer.

Jones, G.W., R.M. Douglas, J.C. Caldwell and R.M. D'Souza (eds). 1997. *The Continuing Demographic Transition.* Oxford: Clarendon Press.

Kertzer, D.I. 1984. *Family Life in Central Italy, 1880–1910.* Brunswick, NJ: Rutgers University Press.

Kertzer, D.I., and D. Arel. 2002. *Census and Identity: The Politics of Race, Ethnicity, and Language in National Censuses.* Cambridge: Cambridge University Press.

Kertzer, D.I., and D.P. Hogan, 1989. *Family, Political Economy, and Demographic Change.* Madison: University of Wisconsin Press.

Knodel, J., and E. van de Walle. 1979. 'Lessons from the Past: Policy Implications of Historical Fertility Studies', *Population and Development Review* 5(2): 217–45.

Kohler, H-P., F.C. Billari and J.A. Ortega. 2002. 'The Emergence of Lowest-Low Fertility in Europe during the 1990s', *Population and Development Review* 28(4): 641–80.

Kohler, H-P., S. Helleringer, J.R. Behrman and S.C. Watkins. 2015. 'The Social and the Sexual: Networks in Contemporary Demographic Research', in P. Kreager, B. Winney, S. Ulijaszek and C. Capelli (eds), *Population in the Human Sciences: Concepts, Models, Evidence.* Oxford: Oxford University Press, pp. 196–237.

Kreager, P. 1997. 'Population and Identity', in D.I. Kertzer and T. Fricke (eds), *Anthropological Demography.* Chicago: University of Chicago Press. pp. 139–74.

———. 2009. 'Darwin and Lotka: Two Concepts of Population', *Demographic Research* 21(16): 469–502.

———. 2011. 'The Challenge of Compositional Demography', *Asian Population Studies* 7(2): 85–88.

———. 2015. 'Population and the Making of the Human Sciences: A Historical Outline', in P. Kreager, B. Winney, S. Ulijaszek and C. Capelli (eds), *Population in the Human Sciences: Concepts, Models, Evidence.* Oxford: Oxford University Press, pp. 55–85.

Kreager, P., and E. Schröder-Butterfill. 2008. 'Indonesia against the Trend? Ageing and Inter-generational Wealth Flows in Two Indonesian Communities', *Demographic Research* (Special Issue on Strong Family Ties), 19(52): 1781–810.

———. 2010. 'Age-Structural Transition in Indonesia: A Comparison of Macro- and Micro-level Evidence', *Asian Population Studies* 6(1): 25–45.

Kreager, P., B. Winney, S. Ulijaszek and C. Capelli. 2015a. 'Introduction', in P. Kreager, B. Winney, S. Ulijaszek and C. Capelli (eds), *Population in the Human Sciences: Concepts, Models, Evidence.* Oxford: Oxford University Press, pp. 3–51.

———. (eds). 2015b. *Population in the Human Sciences: Concepts, Models, Evidence.* Oxford: Oxford University Press.

Lotka, A.J. 1925. *Elements of Physical Biology.* Baltimore: Williams & Wilkins.

McLean, P.D. 2007. 'The Principles of Networking as a Social Process', in *The Art of Network.* Durham, NC: Duke University Press, pp. 1–34.

Notestein, F. 1945. 'Population – The Long View', in T.W. Schultz (ed.), *Food for the World.* Chicago: Chicago University Press, pp. 36–57.

Ortega y Gasset, J. [1930] 1957. *The Revolt of the Masses.* New York: W.W. Norton & Co.

Petit, V. 2013. *Counting Populations, Understanding Societies: Towards an Interpretative Demography.* Dordrecht: Springer.

Porter, T.M. 1986. *The Rise of Statistical Thinking 1820–1900.* Princeton: Princeton University Press.

Randall, S., E. Coast, E. and T. Leone. 2011 'Cultural Constructions of the Concept of Household in Sample Surveys', *Population Studies* 65(2): 217–29.

Reid, A., and E. Garrett (in press). 'The British Fertility Decline: A View from the British Censuses, 1851–1911', paper presented at the 50th Anniversary Conference of the Cambridge Group for the Study of Population and Social Structure, Cambridge, 16–18 September, 2014, to appear in R.M. Smith (ed.), *Population Histories in Context*. Cambridge: Cambridge University Press.

Schneider, J.C., and P.T. Schneider. 1996. *Festival of the Poor: Fertility Decline and the Ideology of Class in Sicily, 1860–1980*. Tucson: University of Arizona Press.

Schröder-Butterfill, E. 2004. 'Intergenerational Family Support Provided by Older People in Indonesia', *Ageing and Society* 24: 497–530.

Segalen, M. 1991. *Fifteen Generations of Bretons: Kinship and Society in Lower Brittany, 1720–1980*. Cambridge: Cambridge University Press.

Szreter, S. 1993. 'The Idea of Demographic Transition and the Study of Fertility Change: A Critical Intellectual History', *Population and Development Review* 19(4): 659–702.

———. 1996. *Fertility, Class and Gender in Britain, 1860–1940*. Cambridge: Cambridge University Press.

———. 2015. 'Populations for Studying the Causes of Britain's Fertility Decline: Communication Communities', in P. Kreager, B. Winney, S. Ulijaszek and C. Capelli (eds), *Population in the Human Sciences: Concepts, Models, Evidence*. Oxford: Oxford University Press, pp. 172–95.

Szreter, S., and E. Garrett 2000. 'Reproduction, Compositional Demography and Economic Growth: Family Planning in England Long before the Fertility Decline', *Population and Development Review* 26(1): 45–80.

Szreter, S., and K. Fisher. 2010. *Sex before the Sexual Revolution: Intimate Life in England 1918–1963*. Cambridge: Cambridge University Press.

Szreter, S., H. Sholkamy and A. Dharmalingam (eds). 2004. *Categories and Contexts: Anthropological and Historical Studies in Critical Demography*. Oxford: Oxford University Press.

Tremayne, S. 2001. *Managing Reproductive Life: Cross-cultural Themes in Sexuality and Fertility*. Oxford: Berghahn Books.

Turner, V. 1957. *The Forest of Symbols: Aspects of Ndembu Ritual*. Ithaca: Cornell University Press.

Wrigley, E.A. 1961.'Family Limitation in Pre-Industrial England' *Economic History Review* 19(1): 82–109.

———. 1972. 'The Process of Modernization and the Industrial Revolution in England', *Journal of Interdisciplinary History* 3: 225–59.

Chapter 1

The Key to Fertility

Generation, Reproduction and Class Formation in a Namibian Community

Julia Pauli

Introduction

In Namibia, middle and upper-class families often celebrate the twenty-first birthday of a daughter or a son with an especially splendid birthday party. During these occasions, one or more keys are given to the birthday child. The key(s) symbolize the opening up of his or her future. This ritual practice reflects the legal fact that in Namibia, the age of majority is twenty-one. Only a person who has reached the age of twenty-one can independently bring or defend a court case or enter into a civil marriage without parental consent, among other rights (see Coomer and Hubbard 2009).

When I heard about the 'twenty-first birthday key' for the first time in Fransfontein, a rural community located in northwest Namibia, another symbolic dimension appeared. In Fransfontein, 'the key' represents not only future possibilities but also past accomplishments, especially in moral and reproductive terms. It was May 2004 and I was visiting our neighbours. We talked about pregnancy and giving birth. In Fransfontein, as elsewhere in Namibia, an early age at first birth (around 19 years) is very common. I asked what the women considered a good age for a first pregnancy. Without any hesitation, all women present said: 'twenty-one'. I was surprised and looked at the youngest woman, Isabel. She smiled and

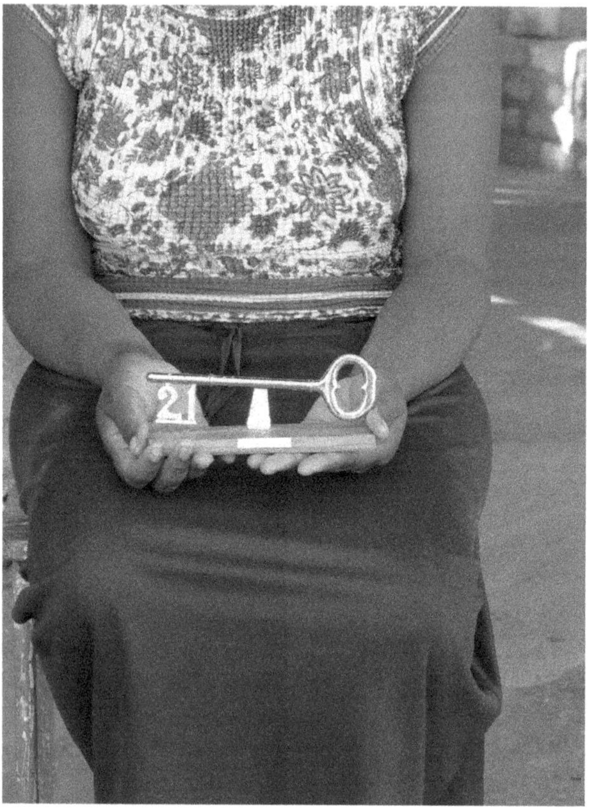

ILLUSTRATION 1.1 The Key

said: 'Yes, twenty-one, because then you get the key.' Isabel went inside the house and came back with her key: 'You see, Julia, I got the key at twenty-one and my daughter was born at twenty-two.' She stressed that if she had become pregnant earlier, she would not have received 'the key' at her twenty-first birthday. Her key is made out of plastic and is painted silver. Her name is engraved on the little plate on which the key is mounted (see Illustration 1.1).

Isabel received the key from her small mother, her *maros* (mother's younger sister). Isabel's mother remarked to me that the key can be given by anyone in the family; it does not have to be the *maros*. Isabel's *maros* also organized a celebration for her. At that time, Isabel was living with the *maros* in Windhoek. I asked the women what the key means. Isabel's mother explained to me that the key means that a woman is now open, that she can have children. However, she continued, most Fransfontein women do not receive a key and celebrate a twenty-first birthday party. The majority of people have no money to celebrate. Further, at the age of twenty-one, most Fransfontein women are already mothers (Fieldnotes, 5 May 2004).

Interestingly, the key connects the first birth to age and not to marriage. What is being rewarded is not Christian 'purity' defined as conception only within marriage, but a later age at pregnancy and birth. Actually, in my interviews on 'the key', marriage was never mentioned in respect to 'the key'. Although an average age at first birth around nineteen years has been the norm for most of the twentieth century in Fransfontein, this pattern is subtly being questioned through 'the key'. While the social becoming of most Fransfontein women is marked by their first pregnancy and their first birth (see also Upton 2001), younger women from wealthy Fransfontein families now define their entrance into adulthood not through pregnancy, but through nonpregnancy, symbolized by 'the key'. At the age of twenty-one, only the daughters of the elite are still studying, delaying their first pregnancies.

Isabel's mother did not receive a key. When I asked her why not, she laughed, as if this was a very absurd question. She reflected that when she gave birth to her children in the 1970s and 1980s, there were no keys around. The first keys only appeared in the village during the 1990s. The women stressed that now the keys are important because they indicate which women behave themselves and which do not.

In my chapter I want to scrutinize how this moral categorization of female reproductive behaviour slowly and subtly emerged during the last decades in Fransfontein. According to Philip Kreager (1986), the construction of differences between groups, between 'us' and 'them', is often connected to the moralization of central vital events, especially giving birth. Along similar lines, Jane and Peter Schneider (1996) have analysed in great detail the reproductive stigmatization of certain groups and classes by other groups and classes throughout more than a century in Sicily, Italy. Specific groups, in the Sicilian case the peasantry, are turned into the demographic 'other'. These demographic others are being classified as promiscuous and uncontrolled, exhibiting a dangerous sexuality resulting in too high numbers of children. The Fransfontein 'key' to fertility likewise classifies the reproductive behaviour of Fransfontein women and is an expression of comparable dynamics. But why and when did this reproductive stigma emerge? As the above narrative indicates, women who gave birth to their children before the 1990s were not yet confronted with the giving of 'keys' as a reward for nonfertility and the associated moral evaluations of reproductive behaviour. Nevertheless, it was during the years in which Isabel's mother had her children that fertility started to decline in both Namibia and in Fransfontein. How then can this decline be understood? And how do the reproductive experiences of Isabel's mother and other women of her generation relate to the creation of reproductive stigma expressed through 'the key'?

Even without 'keys', substantial reconfigurations of family structures and gender roles were framing the reproduction of women who gave birth during the 1970s and 1980s. During the 1970s and 1980s, new social categories emerged in the village. The establishment of apartheid and the creation of 'homelands' resulted in a strong increase in power and possibilities for a few influential men (Pauli 2009, 2010, 2011). Many of the wives of these men, locally called big men (*kai aogu* in the region's main language Khoekhoegowab), increasingly stayed home, following a new gender ideal, the housewife. Virtually all of the big men had one or more outside wives (Pauli 2010, 2012). The spread of infrastructure and new bureaucratic structures accompanying the establishment of the homeland not only resulted in white-collar jobs like teachers, administrators or politicians; unskilled work, especially in the cleaning sector, also became available. During the 1970s and 1980s, a significant number of outside wives received permanent employment as domestic workers in one of the new government institutions through their influential lovers. Most of these women remained unmarried. Locally, they are labelled as 'the hostel workers'. These women describe themselves as 'in the middle'. They are neither on top of the social strata, like the married elite women, mostly housewives, nor are they as vulnerable as other unmarried women with no permanent employment. This third group of unmarried and economically vulnerable women is not as clearly defined as the other two groups. Further, the boundaries of all three groups are permeable, e.g. some hostel workers married influential big men and became married housewives.

Jennifer Johnson-Hanks (2015) has recently highlighted how the categories and groups constructed for the explanation of demographic patterns and outcomes may influence explanations. She concludes that for an understanding of demographic dynamics, the processes through which groups and categories are formed are pivotal. To grasp these processes analytically, Johnson-Hanks has introduced the concept of vital conjunctures (2006, 2007, 2015).

Building on the works of Giddens, Bourdieu and especially Sewell, she defines vital conjunctures as 'structures of possibilities that emerge around specific periods of potential transformation in the lives of one or more participant' (2006: 3). As the brief discussion above indicates, a central moment of transformation in the lives of the people discussed here was the establishment of apartheid in the 1970s and 1980s. Using generations as an analytic frame, I will distinguish three generations of women. The first generation of elder women born between 1915 and 1944 bore most of their children up to the end of the 1960s and before the establishment of apartheid politics and the homeland. Almost all of these women are married. As the three subgroups of women introduced above show, the lives of the second generation of women born around the middle of the twentieth century, i.e. between 1945 and 1964, are much more heterogeneous. These women started their childbearing years with the establishment of the South African homeland politics. The majority of their children were born during the 1970s and 1980s. Finally, I distinguish a third generation consisting of young women born at the end of the 1960s and later. These women have started their reproductive lives in the new era of Namibian Independence and are still in their childbearing years. Like Isabel, they are the daughters of the second generation of women. This approach combines the use of generations as groups of cohorts experiencing significant events together and the use of generations as genealogical groups, e.g. comparing mothers and daughters (cf. Alber and Häberlein 2010; Pauli 2009: Chapter 2)

The aim of my chapter is twofold. First, I want to ask how the three female subgroups, i.e. housewives, hostel workers and economically vulnerable women, that emerged during the 1970s and 1980s are entangled with changing reproductive behaviour and fertility decline. Following Johnson-Hanks, I want to analyse how far vital conjunctures may vary for the different subgroups and throughout their life courses. The use of these three subgroups as analytical categories can be justified on the grounds that they are indeed of great importance for the women themselves and for local social ordering. As in most research in anthropological demography and demography, I am focusing on the fertility of subgroups of women. Men, of course, are considered in different roles throughout this chapter. However, their fertility (and possible related subgroups) will not be analysed in detail. Using 'the key' as an analytic starting point, my second aim will then be to scrutinize why the fertility of the third generation, the daughters, is being evaluated in specific moral categories. The key to an understanding of fertility is thus the understanding of complex and dynamic webs of social, economic and normative conjunctures that shape the reproductive behaviour of the different generations and subgroups of women.

Namibian Demographic Transitions: Changing Marital and Fertility Regimes

Demographic research locates the beginning of the Namibian and South African fertility decline around the 1970s (Moultrie and Timaeus 2003; Garenne and Zwang 2005). Kirk and Pillet have classified Namibia into the group of African countries with a steady fertility decline (Kirk and Pillet 1998; Shemeikka et al. 2005). The total fertility rate (TFR) of the 1991 and 2001 national census has declined from 6.1 children per woman in 1991 to 4.1 children per woman in 2001 (Republic of Namibia 2003: 63). Analysing both the first national census of 1991 and the first Demographic and Health Survey (DHS) in 1992, Raitis (1994) finds several variations in fertility levels. Of special importance here, she finds that more education leads to lower levels of fertility and that marriage affects fertility. Although the never-married women have a high total fertility rate of 4.4, this rate is nevertheless one child less than the TFR of all women (Raitis 1994: 113).

In 2003, the Namibian Ministry of Health and Social Services published a report on the main findings of the 2000 Namibian DHS (MOHSS 2003). The Ministry of Health and Social Services (MOHSS) reports that marriage rates have been declining and that only forty-six per cent of all women in 2000 can be classified as married (MOHSS 2003: 80). On the macro-level, both fertility and marriage are declining in Namibia. To better understand these declines and their possible interconnections, I will now discuss those factors that centrally frame fertility, i.e. age at first birth (the onset of a woman's reproductive life), birth intervals (the time between a woman's births) and age at last birth (the end of a woman's reproductive life) (Bongaarts 1978).

The report of the 2000 DHS by the MOHSS states that the median age at first birth has not changed from 1992 to 2000 (MOHSS 2003: 53). Further, the report finds that the median age at first birth is twenty-one years. The MOHSS report (2003: 51) also finds an increase in the length of birth intervals from a median birth interval of thirty-four months in 1992 to a median birth interval of forty months in 2000. Unfortunately, for the age at last birth I have no information at the national level. The DHS only interviews women of childbearing age. However, I will include a discussion of the age at last birth in my analysis of the Fransfontein data below.

Demographers agree that the spread of Western-type contraceptives was the most important factor for the decline in fertility (Raitis 1994; Garenne and Zwang 2005). However, the spread and use of these types of contraceptives in Namibia since the 1970s was often not voluntary; rather, family planning was part of a racist population policy of the colonial South African state (Lindsay 1989). Lindsay has stressed that the euphemistic term 'family planning programme' is actually not very well suited to understanding the scope of the South African programme. 'Population control policies' is more fitting, underscoring the central goal of controlling the African population by the 'white' community and state.

The establishment of South Africa's population control programme in Namibia during the 1970s was triggered by multiple factors. During the 1960s and 1970s, the international perception of a 'Third World population explosion' or 'population bomb', threatening the wealth and livelihoods of the so-called developed world, led to the establishment of numerous population programmes throughout the so-called developing world (Szreter 1996: 21–44). As Lindsay (1989: 3) shows, South African population policies varied this general theme insofar as the arguments for ('black' African) population control were highly racist, focusing on the ban of a *swart gevaar* (a black threat) that might result in the loss of white minority power.

The population programme of the 1970s was mainly based in hospitals and clinics. Until today, contraception is provided at no cost by the state. Since the establishment of the state-run 'family planning programme', Depo-Provera, a hormonal injection with often strong side-effects and exclusively manufactured by the multinational Upjohn Corporation, is by far the most common contraceptive available for 'black' women (Lindsay 1989: 26–43).[1] Hormonal pills are sometimes available. Sterilizations have also been practised since the 1970s. The IUD, or 'loop', is very uncommon. In general, during apartheid, 'black' Namibian women had very little effective choice (1989: 26). With the dramatic spread of HIV/AIDS, condoms, until the 1980s primarily used by 'whites', have become common throughout Namibia. Thus, in the 2000 DHS, the most commonly used method is injectables (thirty-nine per cent), then the male condom (twenty-eight per cent) and the pill (twenty-four per cent)

(MOHSS 2003: 59). According to the 2000 Namibian DHS (MOHSS 2003: 59–63), sixty-one per cent of all Namibian women age fifteen to forty-nine have used a 'modern' contraceptive method at some time in their lives. This percentage only increases slightly (to sixty-three per cent) when one includes other, traditional' methods (MOHSS 2003: 59).

Before relating these macro-demographic findings to changes in marriage and reproduction in Fransfontein, I will now provide some information on the fieldwork and on the community's main political economic transformations.

From Farm Worker to Hostel Worker: Fransfontein's Ongoing Class Formation

The findings presented here are based on eighteen months of collaborative field research (sixteen months during 2003–2004, and two shorter stays in 2005 and 2006) with Michael Schnegg in the rural region of Fransfontein, Kunene South, northwest Namibia. The community of Fransfontein is located approximately five hundred kilometres away from the country's capital, Windhoek.[2] Information on marriage and reproduction is based on participation observation during a dozen engagement and wedding celebrations, several focus group discussions with married and unmarried women, twenty life histories with married and unmarried women and men, and several 'expert' interviews with medical personnel and political authorities from the Fransfontein region. In addition to these qualitative data, in 2004 we conducted an ethnographic census and detailed fertility histories in 329 households of the Fransfontein region (Fransfontein community and its rural hinterland), including 750 individuals, 388 women and 362 men. A total of 137 of these households are located in Fransfontein village itself. If not otherwise indicated, I will focus on these households and not the rural hinterland. The Fransfontein region is multiethnic and multilingual. With the help of local interviewers, we were able to conduct our census interviews in Khoekhoegowab, English, Afrikaans and Otjiherero.

The demographic changes of the 1970s have to be understood against the background of the political economic history of the region.[3] The beginnings of Fransfontein as a community in the 1890s, and Namibia as a German colony in the second half of the nineteenth century, were characterized by a certain level of fluidity and flexibility in terms of land use rights, boundaries, mobility and ethnic categorization. However, divisions, restrictions and constraints on the indigenous population become increasingly pronounced as white settlers extended their territorial and labour demands in the first half of the twentieth century. As a result of racist politics and land grabbing by the white settler community, most elder Fransfonteiners had to stop their pastoral way of life and were forced to work on 'white' commercial farms. Further, until the 1960s 'blacks in Namibia were totally excluded from all positions of influence or authority within the Namibian polity' (Abrahams 1982: 21). The extent of the changes of the 1970s and 1980s has to be perceived against this historical background. Since the 1960s, Namibia was administered as a fifth province by South Africa. The South African annexation also implied the establishment of apartheid and the creation of 'homelands' based on ethnic criteria (Rohde 1997: 258; Wallace 2011: 261–71). One of these homelands was 'Damaraland', including the Fransfontein reserve. While for many the situation became even worse with apartheid, for a happy few the establishment of infrastructure and bureaucracy meant new and longlasting possibilities to enhance their living conditions (Tötemeyer 1978; Rohde 1997; Fumanti 2007).

A 'modern' elite of 'style-setters' (Plotnicov 1970: 293), i.e. administrators, businessmen, politicians and teachers, emerged in Fransfontein and the other homelands (Tötemeyer 1978). As I have described in detail elsewhere (Pauli 2009, 2011), their desire for conspicuous consumption and modernity became especially visible in the new ways in which weddings were being celebrated. From the mid 1970s onwards, weddings became incredibly expensive and complex, and marriage rates dropped sharply (Pauli 2009, 2011). In addition to splendid and expensive weddings, elite couples increasingly preferred a new form of division of labour, with the wife staying at home and becoming a housewife. Further, divorce and separation are extremely rare (only three per cent of all marriages). If a couple marries, they will stay together. Consequently, only the wealthy are married today in Fransfontein. Almost seventy per cent of the population is unmarried. As I have outlined in my summary of the macro-demographic trends in Namibia above, marriage rates have also declined at the national level. Additionally, several anthropological case studies describe similar declines for other parts of Namibia (Gordon 1972; Iken 1999; Tersbøl 2002) and other Southern African countries (Kuper 2002; Mokomane 2005; Hunter 2010; van Dijk 2010). While for the elder Fransfontein couples now in their sixties, seventies and eighties, marriage was still a very common rite of passage, marriage today is the most important indicator of upper-class belonging.

However, it was not only marriage that changed substantially from the 1970s onwards. New family structures and gender roles emerged as well. Beginning in the 1960s, job opportunities increased significantly in Fransfontein. This applied not only to white-collar work. Less-qualified and lower-paying jobs, especially as domestic servants, also became available. New buildings, like health stations, administrative buildings and schools, were built in Damaraland. In Fransfontein, a primary school, a new state-financed hostel, a large community hall and a health station were all built between the mid 1960s and the beginning of the 1980s. The distribution of new jobs fostered by these changes was a central element in an emerging patronage system. From the 1960s onwards, the new bureaucratic homeland elites had a certain autonomy regarding public funds. Through these local power structures, i.e. so-called big men (*kai aogu*), employment was distributed (cf. Pauli 2010). On the one hand, patrons used these resources in exchange for political support and loyalty. On the other hand, there was also a gender dimension within the patronage system. In all of the newly built institutions, unskilled women were employed as cleaners, cooks or hostel matrons. Many of them were lovers of influential *kai aogu*. Out of 194 Fransfontein women aged fifteen or older in 2004, twenty-five women (thirteen per cent) found employment as hostel workers during the 1970s and 1980s. Twenty-two (eighty-eight per cent) of these women were born between 1945 and 1964, and were thus in their twenties and thirties in the 1970s and 1980s. Most of them had children with men who were influential at that time and who worked in the homeland's administration. Very few of them ever married. Instead, they preferred to live on their own, together with their children. Only two women born after 1964 have been hired as hostel workers. Younger women never had a chance to work in this sector. Thus, the phenomenon of this female local 'middle class', the 'hostel workers', is bound to a historically situated, very specific economic and political conjuncture.

Finally, many women who were temporarily lovers of big men (and other men) became neither wives nor hostel workers. Many of these women are living in matrifocal household structures and survive on a mixture of economic strategies, combining monthly pension payments for the eldest women in the household, small stock husbandry, remittances and petty economic activities like collecting firewood, washing clothes and selling locally brewed beer

(Pauli 2007; Schnegg 2009). Their economic situation is extremely difficult. About half of all 137 Fransfontein households are headed by a woman. However, not all female-headed households can be classified as poor. The hostel workers described above are also household heads.

These two groups of unmarried women (i.e. hostel workers and 'poor' women) are connected through sometimes dense food-sharing networks, locally called *Augu* (Schnegg and Bolten 2007; Schnegg 2009). Many of these unmarried women are also living in close proximity to each other in a neighbourhood called *ǂoabatere*, i.e. 'go out!'. This local term reflects the circumstance that most of the women living in *ǂoabatere* have children with different men, but that hardly any of them are living together with a man (Pauli 2007). Because of quarrels relating to alcohol abuse, cheating and domestic violence, women from *ǂoabatere* separate from their male partners quite often.

To conclude, in terms of livelihoods and family patterns, unmarried women are rather different from married women. Fransfontein married elite women enjoy economic security, stay with their husbands and live in nuclear families. Contrary to this, unmarried women often face economic insecurity, have changing partners and live in matrifocal households. In all of these respects, the differences between hostel workers and women with no permanent income are not significant; they are only the legacy of relationships of thirty or forty years ago. In the next step of my analysis, I will therefore first describe general trends in fertility for all women and will then focus on differences and similarities between married and unmarried women. Only then will I scrutinize similarities and differences between all three subgroups of women.

The Fransfontein Fertility Decline

During in-depth interviews with elder women and their daughters and granddaughters, the decline in fertility was often commented upon. The women clearly perceived the decline and in general linked it to the availability of contraceptives. Younger women expressed relief at not having to go through the burden of as many births as their grandmothers. In total, we have interviewed 364 women about their fertility histories. Table 1.1 gives an overview of the development of achieved parity for eight birth cohorts recorded in our local census data.

TABLE 1.1 Total Fertility Rates of 364 Fransfontein Women

Birth cohorts	N	Per cent	TFR
1915–24	11	3.0	3.5
1925–34	26	7.1	7.0
1935–44	41	11.3	6.6
1945–54	47	12.9	5.7
1955–64	59	16.2	4.8
1965–74	65	17.9	4.6
1975–84	89	24.5	2.7
1985–94	26	7.1	0.6
All women	364	100	5.2

The first cohort (1915–24) is much smaller than the others. The low total fertility rate for this cohort is thus likely to need some critical adjustment, as it is likely to be subject to other influences (e.g. patterns of survivorship not available in the data). The last cohort is also problematic. We only interviewed women aged fifteen and older in 2004. Consequently, the last cohort actually ends with the year 1990 and only covers five rather than ten years. If one excludes the first cohort, a clear trend becomes visible in Table 1.1. The population is experiencing a fertility decline, at least amongst those women who have finished their reproductive phase, for whom total fertility rates have dropped from a high 7.0 to a moderate level of 4.8.[4]

Like the national results described above, there is a remarkable stability in the average age at first birth across time in Fransfontein. First births for Fransfontein women of all generations occur between nineteen and twenty years of age (average 19.5).[5] Longer birth intervals can be observed for Fransfontein women and at the national level. While elder women on average gave birth every two years, the time between births for younger women is on average three years. The average age at last birth has dropped from thirty-eight years for women born between 1925 and 1934 to thirty-six years for women born between 1955 and 1964. The changes in the length of birth intervals and the average age at last birth are gradual, every cohort adding a little more to the lengthening of birth intervals while progressively reducing the age at which reproduction ceases.

After having described the general development of fertility during the last few decades for both the macro-context and the micro-context, I will now compare fertility rates for married and never-married women. The reasons for this are twofold. First, I follow Jennifer Johnson-Hanks' suggestion not to take marriage as one among other independent variables explaining fertility differences, but rather to understand the different social contexts that marriage creates and does not create for reproduction: 'When we calculate birth rates separately for the married and the unmarried, rather than including a marital status variable in a regression model, we are explicitly claiming that marriage constitutes a key factor of the social context relevant for childbearing' (Johnson-Hanks 2007: 13). Second, as I have described in previous paragraphs, marriage has changed substantially in Fransfontein. While marriage was the common frame for women's reproduction until the 1970s, with the emergence of new elites and the parallel decline in marriage rates, most reproduction is now taking place outside marriage. To be married has turned into a marker of class distinction, and it is mostly people from local elite families who marry today. How far, then, and since when did the fertility of the unmarried majority start to differ from the fertility of the married elite minority?

Of the 364 women for whom I have information on marital status, thirty-two per cent (115 women) are or have been married, and sixty-eight per cent have never married (249 women).[6] In a similar fashion to findings at the national level discussed above, unmarried women in the Fransfontein area have approximately one child less than ever-married women. The total fertility rate for ever-married women is 5.9 compared to 4.7 for never-married women. Major differences in age-specific fertility rates between married and never-married Fransfontein women can be found between the ages of twenty-five and forty (see Figure 1.1 below).

Figure 1.1 shows that marital status affects fertility only *after* the beginning of childbearing. Unsurprisingly, then, there is no difference in the average age at first birth between ever-married and never-married women. After the onset of reproduction, fertility is higher for married than for never-married women. A more detailed analysis of birth intervals reveals that, from the 1970s onwards, unmarried mothers have spread their births across the reproductive span more than their married counterparts (see Pauli 2009: Chapter 6). These longer birth intervals also lead to a lower overall fertility level of unmarried women. Further, unmarried women increasingly had children with three or more reproductive partners, a pattern Jane Guyer (1994) has described as 'polyandrous motherhood'. This reproductive practice further increased the average time between births for unmarried women because it took the women

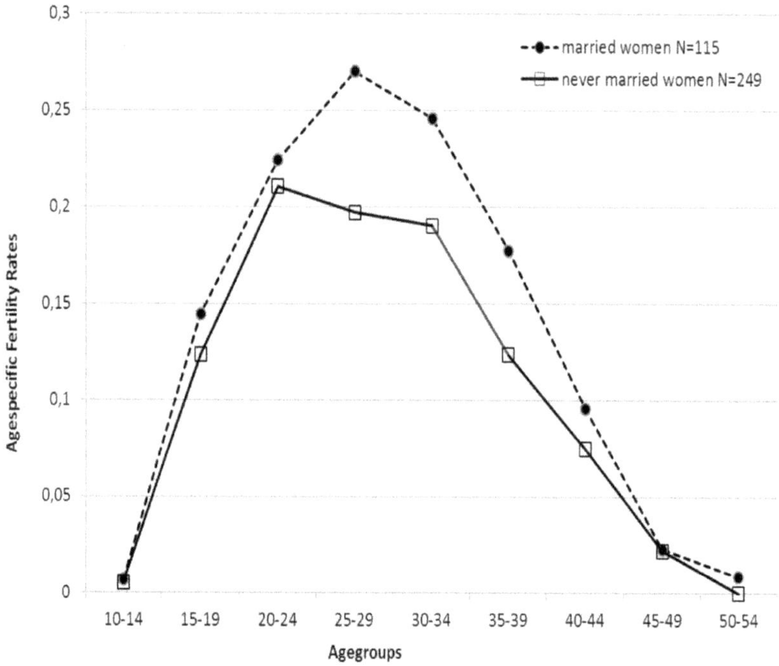

FIGURE 1.1 Age-Specific Fertility Rates for Never-Married and Ever-Married Women (N=364)

time to meet a new partner. The average age at last birth also started to differ for married and unmarried women from the 1970s onwards. Married women born between 1945 and 1964 on average gave birth for the last time between the ages of thirty-seven and thirty-eight, while their unmarried counterparts did so at age thirty-five. The fertility decline of the 1970s and 1980s described above has thus mainly resulted from changes in the reproductive practices of unmarried women.

Comparable to the national level, the availability and use of Western contraceptives since the mid 1970s strongly influenced the average length of all birth intervals and the age at last birth of married and unmarried women. The percentage of women who have used a 'modern' contraceptive method in Fransfontein (sixty-four per cent) is almost equivalent to the national results (sixty-one per cent – 2000 Namibian Demographic and Health Survey). In the 1970s and 1980s, married women used Western contraceptives mainly to stop their childbearing altogether, while unmarried women used Western contraceptives for child spacing and stopping. The most common contraceptive method per cohort and marital status underscores this finding. While the most common contraceptive method for married women of the cohort 1945–54 is sterilization, most unmarried women of this cohort used hormonal injections. Several married women also commented that in the 1970s, medical personnel recommended sterilization to married women with several children.

To sum up, generations of women differ in their reproductive behaviours. Women of the oldest generation, born up to the mid 1940s, were almost all married, had short birth intervals and high fertility. When these women bore their children, Western contraceptive methods were non-existent. In the 1970s, things started to change. Western contraceptives became an option. Further, the 1970s mark the beginning of significant changes in the economic, social and political fields. The emerging elite gradually transformed marriage. Although they are trendsetters in other social domains (like weddings), elite women who married in the 1970s and 1980s are rather conservative, their fertility behaviour resembling the reproductive pattern of their mothers. Like them, the married women had many children and short birth intervals. Western contraceptives were only used at the end of the reproductive lives, often in the form of sterilizations. Unlike these married women, the growing number of unmarried women started using Western contraceptives mainly for spacing and had several reproductive partners. Despite these emerging reproductive differences, age at first birth differs neither by generation nor by marital status, and is very similar for all women. The question thus emerges why married women since the 1970s followed the reproductive models of those generations preceding them, while their unmarried counterparts were more likely to adopt and enact new technologies and behaviour.

Different Futures, Different Subgroups: Life Course Trajectories and Reproduction

According to Jennifer Johnson-Hanks, in order to understand reproductive decision-making, we have to understand the structures of possibilities, the specific conjunctures and also the 'kind of futures [that] are imagined, hoped for, or feared' (2006: 25). The three subgroups of women born from the mid 1940s and until the 1960s, i.e. elite married women, unmarried hostel workers and unmarried poor women, faced different structures of possibilities and imagined varying futures when they bore their children. Importantly, however, there were hardly any differences between them at the beginning of their reproductive lives. They did not systematically differ in terms of their family backgrounds or their educational achievements. The differences between the groups of women only emerged in the course of their lives, the constraints they were facing and the decisions they made. To illuminate the entanglements between different life course trajectories and reproduction for each of the three subgroups, I will discuss some specific cases in more detail.

Lina's life is in many respects a typical example of the Fransfontein elite housewife.[7] Lina was born in 1959. She finished primary school, but did not complete high school. In the mid 1970s, she met her future husband in Khorixas, the administrative centre of the homeland, approximately twenty kilometres away from Fransfontein. He was an influential politician. Lina received a job as a hostel worker in Khorixas. At the age of nineteen, she became pregnant for the first time. Her next child was born three years later, in 1981. Then, in 1982, she married the five-years-older wealthy politician. It was one of the biggest wedding celebrations at that time. Lina stopped working in the hostel and became a housewife. In 1985, 1990, 1991 and 1993, four more children were born. On average, Lina's birth intervals are 2.5 years long. The time from her first to her last birth spans fifteen years of Lina's life. In the 1990s, the family built a beautiful and (compared to local standards) luxurious house and moved to Fransfontein. Almost throughout the whole marriage, her husband cheated on Lina. He fathered several out-of-wedlock children. When I met her in 2003, she had somehow accepted the situation. However, she told me that several years ago and out of a feeling of hopelessness, she had tried to commit suicide. She never used any contraceptives between births. For her, she said, every child was a gift from God. Nothing should prevent that. And with her decision to become a married woman, she also decided on having her husband's children. However, at the age of thirty-four and after the birth of her last child in 1993, a doctor suggested sterilization, and Lina agreed.

Except for her sterilization, Lina's fertility history in many respects resembles that of her mother's generation. Women like Lina's mother, born up to the mid 1940s, also married, had high fertility, short birth intervals and never used contraceptive methods. Although Lina's reproductive behaviour resembles an older fertility pattern, the underlying motives are nevertheless new, only emerging from the 1970s onwards: For a housewife, there is really no need to control fertility. This also hints at the moral dimension of the category. For the married housewives, fidelity is a central value. Linda, a fifty-year-old married housewife, stated that unlike all those unmarried women 'running after men', housewives are 'faithful to their partner' (for comparable moral dynamics in Northern Namibia, cf. Becker 2004). Lina, Linda and other married housewives construct a moral discourse distinguishing the faithful married women from the uncontrolled unmarried women. One central difference between the two groups is their fertility. While married women like Lina and Linda have many children with one man, the unmarried women have fewer children with several men, among these the unfaithful husbands of the married women. The vital conjunctures between these groups are consequently very different. The imagined futures are also different, as the narrative of Hertha, a hostel worker, indicates.

Hertha, born in 1956, was one of the very few women I interviewed who said that she never wanted to marry. She stressed that she had had enough of men. Almost completely on her own, she raised five children by five different men. At the age of seventeen, while still in school in Fransfontein, she became pregnant with her first child and quit school. A few years later, she met the father of her second child, an influential politician. In 1978, she gave birth to his child. With his help, she received permanent employment in the Fransfontein school hostel. Up to this point, her life story is similar to that of Lina narrated above. However, while Lina married the influential big man and later quit working in a hostel, the relationship between Hertha and her *kai aob* did not last much longer after the birth of their child. Nevertheless, the *kai aob*'s child is the only one of Hertha's children who ever received maintenance from the father. The four fathers of her other four children never paid any maintenance.

The relationships with the fathers of Hertha's three following children, born in 1979, 1982 and 1990, were all short-lived. Like Lina, Hertha's reproductive life spans fifteen years. But Hertha's average birth interval is longer than that of Lina. On average, Lina's birth intervals are 2.5 years long, while Hertha's birth intervals are on average 3.2 years long. Hertha stressed that, except for the *kai aob*, all of her other men were poor and tried to live off her money. There was a lot of fighting. With every new man and every pregnancy, Hertha said she hoped the relationship would last. Her narratives are characterized by uncertainty, hopes for a better future, disappointments and revisions. Yet, contrary to Lina, who told her story in a depressed way, and despite the fact that Hertha experienced so much uncertainty in her relations with men and her birth giving, Hertha did not regret the decisions she took. When things went badly, she did not wait for too long and kicked the men out of her house. Tellingly, she lived in the Fransfontein neighbourhood *ǂoabatere*, i.e. 'go out!', described above. Hertha's last son was born when she was thirty-four. Before his birth, she had used both hormonal injections and pills to space her children. I asked her if she took any Western contraceptives after the age of thirty-four. She replied 'no'. Until the time of our interview, i.e. 2005, she had no new partner. Hertha said that her greatest joy was her economic independence. Although not earning a lot, she owned a small, well-kept house. All other unmarried hostel workers I interviewed narrated variations of Hertha's story. All of them were fed up with men at a certain point in their lives and thanked their economic independence for not having to deal with them anymore. Sana, born in 1950, unmarried with four children from three men who worked in a health clinic, said when I asked her how she feels about men: 'Men? Hm, I don't even trust men anymore. The fathers of my last two children disappointed me very, very much. It's maybe from there on that I got a feeling of "no".'

Although the beginnings of Lina's and Hertha's reproductive lives are similar, their life course trajectories and reproductive decisions diverged with marriage. While Lina became a married housewife, Hertha turned into an economically independent, local middle-class woman. This divergence is also reflected in their reproductive differences, i.e. variations in the total number of children, length of birth intervals, number of reproductive partners and use of contraception. One of the main reasons Hertha gave me as an explanation for her age at last birth was her decision to, from now on, 'stay off men'. For many unmarried women without a permanent income, this decision is much more difficult, as Tanja's narrative indicates.

Tanja was born in 1965. She finished primary school and had her first child at the age of nineteen. Until the age of twenty, Tanja's life was not very different from the other two women described above. Tanja had five children by five different men. The children were born in 1984, 1986, 1993, 2001 and 2004. In between births, Tanja used hormonal injections and condoms. In contrast to Lina and Hertha, Tanja's reproductive span is twenty years. Similarly, Tanja's average birth interval of four years was also much longer and her age at last birth (thirty-nine) was several years later than the other two women.

Tanja was one of the poorest women in the village. During an interview in November 2003, she told me that in the preceding week, she was so hungry that she fainted while carrying her baby girl. Luckily, she said, nothing happened to the child. The house that Tanja, her then nineteen-year-old daughter and three of her other children were staying in consisted of two very small rooms, with a small fireplace in front of the house. Once a week, Tanja helped one of the married elite women with her laundry. From time to time, Tanja's daughter was hired as a barmaid in one of the local *shebeens* (bars). However, these salaries were not enough to survive. In order not to starve, Tanja was part of one of the local food-sharing networks (*augu*). Although none of the five fathers of Tanja's children paid maintenance, they occasionally sent food, candles, matches or clothes. When these goods arrived, Tanja shared them within her *augu* network (cf. Schnegg and Bolten 2007; Schnegg 2009). In return, her female *augu* partners helped her with food and other items. When I asked her if she would like to marry, Tanja said with very strong emphasis 'yes'! This was her big dream. She told me that sometimes she peeked into the window of one of the Fransfontein *shebeens* and watched soap operas on TV. She was happy when the TV couple finally married. She did not care if a man was ugly. If he just stays and takes care of the woman and the children, that would be sufficient. She lamented that she had hoped that the father of her last child, who was employed in a tourist shop, would eventually marry her. However, after many nice words, he left her for another woman when she was five months' pregnant. Despite all her hardships and the many disappointments she had endured, Tanja still hoped that she would eventually marry.

This endurance may be the most substantial difference between the three women and the subgroups they represent. While the married housewife, Lina, and the 'middle-class' hostel worker, Hertha, have both, albeit in varying ways, given up on men and lost all hopes that a relationship with a man might lead to anything good, Tanja continues to hope. Not only that, Tanja continues to have children. Lina and Hertha stopped childbearing at the age of thirty-four. Although above forty when I met Tanja for the last time in 2006, she nevertheless had a new boyfriend and was prepared to get pregnant again.

For the explanation of the fertility decline since the 1970s, all three women and their respective groups are important. Although the reproductive behaviour of married housewives was rather conservative and 'backward', their earlier stopping of childbearing through sterilization lowered the absolute number of births. Unmarried hostel workers likewise stopped their childbearing much earlier than the previous generation. Additionally, they also started spacing their children and consequently had longer birth intervals. Explanations for this spacing behaviour include the search for new partners (expressed in the high average number of reproductive partners per unmarried woman) and women's willingness to use 'modern' contraception. Finally, the subgroup of women without marriage and employment is similar to the hostel workers in that they space their children. However, many of these poorer women do not stop childbearing as radically as their married and employed counterparts.

Remarkably, there are no differences between the three groups of women regarding the beginning of their reproductive lives. I could not find any statistical differences between the three subgroups of women for this generation (born between 1945 and the 1960s). Thus, when these women came of age in the 1960s to 1980s, having their first sex, their first love and their first child, it was not possible to tell which one of them would eventually become a married housewife, an independent working woman or a starving woman. For the daughters of these women, life chances are much more bound to family background. It is this emerging and worrying class-based foreshadowing of life trajectories, and its entanglement with fertility and reproductive stigma, which I shall discuss in the last part of this chapter.

The Reproduction of Differences and the Key to Fertility

While married housewives promoted a moral discourse of chastity, monogamy and high fertility for themselves, they all had to live with husbands who were practising the opposite (cf. Delius and Glaser 2009: 30; Hirsch, Wardlow and Smith, 2009). This may explain why many married elite women did not promote their lifestyles as role models for their daughters. On the contrary, elite mothers outspokenly told their daughters that it is better to imagine a different future. During a conversation in August 2004 with four married elite women near the end of their forties, I asked them if they hoped that their children would marry. None of them answered enthusiastically and one of them was openly against marriage and the life of a housewife:

> Woman 1: 'Mhm. I don't know.'
> Julia: 'Yes?'
> Woman 2: 'It is not so nice.'
> Julia: 'You are not so sure?'
> Woman 3: 'I don't know. My daughter should learn and be independent. Better no boys. Married she would just stay in the house and be silenced – silence until your heart becomes sick. I don't want that for my child.'

Thus, many of the elite mothers preached to their daughters that if they want a good life, then education and a well-paid job are the key to it. Some of the daughters followed these suggestions, among them Lotta, who happily received 'the key' at her twenty-first birthday. Lotta, born in 1975, was the youngest daughter of one of the few local elite families that emerged in Fransfontein during the 1970s and 1980s. At her twenty-first birthday, she lived and studied in Windhoek:

> Lotta: 'Yeah, I was with my sisters and brothers in Windhoek. Then I became twenty-one and my brothers – I don't know, it was really a surprise, they never told me, they just called each other. You know they ordered the cake, they prepared the meat.'
> Julia: 'Did you get a key?'
> Lotta: 'Yeah. Two! One from my elder brother from my father's side and one from my four siblings, my two sisters and two brothers . . . I was very proud. And they told me that: "Now we are proud of you! You finished your school and you are not a mother yet and you have turned twenty-one!" So really it was a good thing; something special, exceptional.' (Life history interview, 28 August 2004)

Lotta clearly realized that her behaviour was exceptional and deviated from what was normal, i.e. an early age at first pregnancy and first birth. The accomplishments celebrated at her twenty-first birthday were twofold: having finished school and not having become pregnant. Both were taken as markers of (elite) social becoming and entrance into adulthood. In our talks she continuously compared herself to other women her own age. She held the firm belief that for her generation, family formation matters if a woman wants to get ahead. This belief is confirmed ethnographically by comparison to the reproductive decisions and life courses of the daughters of the two unmarried women discussed earlier, Tanja and Hertha. Like her mother, Tanja's eldest daughter, Susanne, only finished primary school and then started working as a barmaid in Fransfontein. She became pregnant at the age of nineteen. In 2003, hostel worker Hertha's eldest daughter had finished high school and was looking for a job in Khorixas. She was twenty at that time. She stressed that when one lacks connections, even with her education it was difficult to get a good job. She had a boyfriend and when I asked her if she would mind getting pregnant, she shrugged her shoulders. Although her twenty-first birthday was coming up, there were no plans to celebrate and to give keys. Earlier, Hertha had told me that she had no money for such celebrations.

As these three narratives of the youngest generation of women indicate, the influence of family background and education on reproduction is increasing. It seems that differences that emerged during the 1970s and 1980s are being reproduced and consolidated in the youngest generation of women. However, because many of the women in the daughters' generation are still too young, it is not possible to calculate average age at first birth for the different subgroups within this generation. Thus, my results may better be taken as indictors of emerging reproductive and cultural trends rather than as conclusive findings. Nevertheless, the trend to delay age at first birth and instead pursue a prolonged education is also reflected in Table 1.2.

TABLE 1.2 Average Age at First Birth for Four Cohorts of Fransfontein Women (N=238)

Birth cohort	Education	Average age at first birth	N	Std.
1945–54	No schooling	19.00	6	4.000
	1–6 years of schooling	19.07	29	2.802
	7–10 years of schooling	19.55	11	2.382
1955–64	No schooling	18.88	8	4.155
	1–6 years of schooling	18.47	19	2.480
	7–10 years of schooling	20.85	26	4.487
	11–18 years of schooling	23.00	3	4.583
1965–74	No schooling	21.50	2	0.707
	1–6 years of schooling	18.21	19	3.867
	7–10 years of schooling	19.87	38	3.458
	11–18 years of schooling	22.60	5	4.506
1975–84	1–6 years of schooling	18.46	13	3.733
	7–10 years of schooling	20.15	52	3.038
	11–18 years of schooling	23.29	7	4.030

Women born before 1945 do not differ in their age at first birth from women born between 1945 and 1954. I have thus excluded these elder women from the table. Table 1.2 shows that only the highest level of education, a school duration of between eleven and eighteen years, substantially delays the age at first birth. The number of women in this category gradually increases over time. The often-found correlation between education and a later age at first birth also applies to Fransfontein (Johnson-Hanks 2006). All of the women with the highest level of education and born during the 1970s and 1980s are daughters of the Fransfontein elite. Like Lotta, introduced above, they have studied to become nurses, teachers, secretaries or politicians. They earn their own money and enjoy being the one who decides how to spend it. At a certain point in their lives, they feel that it may be time to give birth to a child. This decision is vastly different from the first pregnancy of their mothers at the age of nineteen. Lotta, for example, waited another five years after receiving her twenty-first-birthday keys before she got pregnant for the first time. Before that, she had a number of boyfriends and had tried different types of contraceptives. Then, at the age of twenty-six and in her last year of education, she decided that she wanted a baby:

> Julia: 'Did you plan to get pregnant?'
> Lotta: 'Yeah. I wanted a baby, because, Julia, I was already twenty-seven; no, I was turning twenty-seven. And I decided: twenty-seven without a kid! And these days even a nineteen or a sixteen-year-old lady or girl is having a kid. So let me have a kid, because now at least I am finishing studying, this is my last year and then I will be able to support my baby.'
> Julia: 'And what did the father think? Did he also want a kid?'
> Lotta: 'His father wanted a kid. And although we were not together anymore he wanted me to give the baby his name and surname. I said no. My baby is mine and he will stay mine.'

The key to Lotta's fertility is thus her economic, social and also moral independence, an independence she achieved through a specific structure of possibilities and imaginings. Lotta's mother followed a very different life trajectory, having had very little education or economic independence, but many children and a life as a housewife of a successful administrator and businessman. Lotta, however, wanted something different. Today, mother and daughter continue to be very close. The mother supports Lotta with childcare. Both women clearly view themselves as part of the local elite. However, the effect of their elite status on their fertility varies strongly. While the mother became one of the first Fransfontein housewives, subsequently living a life of gender-based privilege and dependency, the social becoming of her daughter, her dreams and hopes, are centred on her own economic and social independence. The vital conjunctures of first birth have substantially changed for the daughters of married elite housewives more than for any other group of women.

Conclusion

Becoming a mother continues to be one of the most central ways in which adult identity is formed in many regions of Southern Africa. Rebecca Upton underscores this connection between fertility and identity: 'If we are to be successful in understanding the cultural significance of fertility in southern Africa, a central concern should be an understanding of how concepts such as fertility and childbearing, versus infertility and lack of children, relate to the negotiation of identity' (Upton 2001: 362). A delay or lack of this important marker and event of social becoming can cause substantial suffering and crisis, as Astrid Bochow's (2012) and Rebecca Upton's (2001) work on infertility in Botswana shows.

The continuity of widespread early age at first birth in Namibia confirms this marker, as this pathway to adulthood remains the most common route taken by Namibian women. However, as I have tried to show, this common reproductive practice is being subtly contested both ideologically and demographically. For the youngest generation of Fransfontein women, waiting before first pregnancy has emerged as a value. The giving of symbolic keys at the twenty-first birthday of these young elite women publicly rewards their break from previous forms of social becoming through reproduction. This is all the more remarkable as the beginnings of reproductive life and the ages at first birth of the previous generation of Fransfontein women, the mothers of the 1970s and 1980s, do not differ for the three subgroups of women, i.e. married elite housewives, economically independent unmarried hostel workers and economically deprived unmarried women. Only after the birth of a first child, and with or without marriage, do the life trajectories and vital conjunctures of these three groups of women diverge. For their daughters, the reproduction of differences starts earlier.

Through their delay of first pregnancy, which is rewarded by the receiving of a key at their twenty-first birthday parties, young elite women promote reproductive waiting as a value; at the same time, the fertility behaviour of their not-so-controlled and educationally dedicated peers is also being scrutinized. Their reproduction is becoming a public issue of concern and even an object of stigmatization (cf. Schneider and Schneider 1996). For example, growing awareness of 'teenage pregnancies' as a social problem is being debated both in public and academic forums. On 25 July 2012, the most important national newspaper, *The Namibian,* featured a cover story entitled 'Gov't Revamps Policy on Pregnant Schoolgirls'. Deputy Minister of Education David Namwandi stated: 'We should let these girls continue with their education. We cannot afford to terminate their future at an early stage.'[8] Similarly, demographers have been worrying for some time about Namibian teenage pregnancies (Chimere-Dan 1997; Gage 1998). I certainly do not want to play down the difficulties that teenage pregnancies can cause for young women. Moreover, educating teenagers about HIV/AIDS and other STDs is of great importance in Namibia. However, what is conceptualized as 'the new problem of teenage pregnancies' is not a new development. As stated above, an early age at first birth has been common in Namibia and beyond for a long time. Thus, it is not so much the reproductive behaviour of the majority of Namibian women that has changed, but its moral evaluation. Young women today, who like their mothers and grandmother have their first child before the age of twenty, are being turned into demographic 'others' (Kreager 1986), a category of concern for the new political, economic and intellectual elites. I have tried to show how these transformations are embedded in class formation processes and generational dynamics.

Simon Szreter has stressed the centrality of local cultures and social structures for an understanding of reproductive dynamics: 'Changing fertility should be related, as in this case, to the local politics and social divisions within specific communities' (Szreter 1996: 537). As reproductive dynamics in Fransfontein show, only when taking the political, economic and ideational transformations since the 1970s into account is it possible to understand variations in fertility between women of different socioeconomic subgroups and generations. It is not the socioeconomic status per se that frames and forms the vital conjunctures at different times and throughout the life courses. A parallel can be made here to Jennifer Johnson-Hanks' (2007) observation that marriage or class (or socioeconomic status) is not simply one among many independent variables that explain fertility differences. Rather, the fact of belonging to specific socioeconomic subgroups and generations has to be scrutinized for the different contexts and conjunctures that form and frame reproduction over time.

Julia Pauli is Professor of Social and Cultural Anthropology at Hamburg University. Her main research interests are gender and kinship studies, anthropological demography, transnational migration, consumption and class formation processes. She has carried out extensive fieldwork in Mexico (since 1995) and Namibia (since 2003).

Notes

I thank Astrid Bochow and especially Philip Kreager for their important and inspiring comments on an earlier version of the chapter. The research was funded by the DFG (German Research Foundation), for which I am thankful. As ever, Michael Schnegg provided many important insights. Susanne Lea Radt helped with editing. Many Fransfontein women and men allowed me to ask them about their lives. I am very thankful for their trust and their help.

1. Until 1990, the situation was very different for 'white' women. For these women, the principle forms of birth control were pills and condoms (Lindsay 1989:26). I have no information on the behaviour of 'white' women after 1990.
2. The project has focused on the demographic, social, political, and economic transformations the region went through during the 20th century from both an ethnographic and a historical perspective. The project has been part of the interdisciplinary research project ACACIA (SFB 389), based at the Universities of Cologne and Bonn, Germany, and funded by the German National Science Foundation (Deutsche Forschungsgemeinschaft) from 2003-2007.
3. For more information on the general history of the region see (Pauli 2009; Pauli 2010).
4. Defined as women forty years and older at the time of the census in 2004, i.e. up to the birth cohort 1955–1964. Very few births occur after the age of forty.
5. Elsewhere (Pauli 2009: chapter 6) I have described the changes in fertility in detail. Here, I only present a summary of the main findings.
6. For detailed information on types of wedding and marriage see Pauli (2009, 2011, 2012).
7. All names are pseudonyms.
8. *The Namibian*, http://www.namibian.com.na/index.php?id=28&tx_ttnews[tt_news]=99758&no_cache=1 (accessed 19 October 2012).

References

Abrahams, K. 1982. 'The "Waserauta" Phenomenon: Additional Notes on the Namibian Elite', *Namibian Review* 25: 21–31.

Alber, E., and T. Häberlein. 2010. 'Ethnologische Generationenforschung in Afrika', in E. Alber, B. Beer, J. Pauli and M. Schnegg (eds), *Verwandtschaft Heute*. Berlin: Reimer Verlag, pp. 281–304.

Becker, H. 2004. 'Efundula: Women's Initiation, Gender and Sexual Identities in Colonial and Post-colonial Northern Namibia', in S. Arnfred (ed.), *Re-thinking Sexualities in Africa*. Uppsala, Nordiska Afrikainstitutet, pp. 35–58.

Bochow, A. 2012. 'Quest for Conception in Times of HIV/AIDS – (In)fertility Care in Botswana. Facts, Views & Vision', in T. von Gerrits, W. Ombelet and F. van Balen (eds), *Biomedical Infertility Care in Poor Resource Countries: Barriers, Access and Ethics*. Wetteren: Universa, pp. 81–86.

Bongaarts, J. 1978. 'A Framework for Analyzing the Proximate Determinants of Fertility', *Population and Development Review* 4: 105–13.

Chimere-Dan, O. 1997. 'Non-marital Teenage Childbearing in Southern Africa: The Case of Namibia', *African Population Studies* 12(2): 1–20.

Coomer, R., and D. Hubbard. 2009. 'A Major Decision: Considering the Age of Majority in Namibia', in O.C. Ruppel (ed.), *Children's Rights in Namibia*. Windhoek: Macmillan Education Namibia, pp. 101–20.

Delius, P., and C. Glaser. 2009. 'Sex, Disease and Stigma in South Africa: Historical Perspectives', *African Journal of AIDS Research* 4(1): 29–36.

Fumanti, M. 2007. 'Burying E.S.: Educated Elites, Subjectivity and Distinction in Rundu, Namibia', *Journal of Southern African Studies* 33(3): 469–83.

Gage, A.J. 1998. 'Sexual Activity and Contraceptive Use: The Components of the Decisionmaking Process', *Studies in Family Planning* 29(2): 154–66.

Garenne, M., and J. Zwang. 2005. 'Premarital Fertility in Namibia: Trends, Factors and Consequences', *Journal of Biosocial Science* 38: 145–67.

Gordon, R.J. 1972. *Some Sociological Aspects of Verbal Communication in Okombahe, S.W.A.: A Community Study*. Stellenbosch: University of Stellenbosch.

Guyer, J.I. 1994. 'Lineal Identities and Lateral Networks: The Logic of Polyandrous Motherhood', in C. Bledsoe and G. Pison (eds), *Nuptiality in Sub-Saharan Africa*. Oxford: Clarendon Press, pp. 231–52.

Hirsch, J.S., H. Wardlow and D.J. Smith. 2009. *The Secret: Love, Marriage and HIV*. Nashville: Vanderbilt University Press.

Hunter, M. 2010. *Love in the Times of AIDS: Inequality, Gender, and Rights in South Africa*. Bloomington: Indiana University Press.

Iken, A. 1999. *Woman-Headed Households in Southern Namibia: Causes, Patterns and Consequences*. Frankfurt and Windhoek: IKO and Gamsberg Macmillan Publishers.

Johnson-Hanks, J. 2006. *Uncertain Honor: Modern Motherhood in an African Crisis*. Chicago: University of Chicago Press.
———. 2007. 'What Kind of Theory for Anthropological Demography?', *Demographic Research* 16: 1–26.
———. 2015. 'Populations are Composed One Event at a Time', in P. Kreager, B. Winney, S. Ulijaszek and C. Capelli (eds), *Population in the Human Sciences: Concepts, Models, Evidence*. Oxford: Oxford University Press: 238–253.
Kirk, D. and B. Pillet. 1998. 'Fertility Levels, Trends, and Differentials in Sub-Saharan Africa in the 1980s and 1990s', *Studies in Family Planning* 29(1): 1–22.
Kreager, P. 1986. 'Demographic Regimes as Cultural Systems', in D. Coleman and R. Schofield (eds), *The State of Population Theory: Forward from Malthus*. Oxford: Basil Blackwell, pp. 131–56.
Kuper, A. 2002. 'Comparison and Contextualization: Reflections on South Africa', in A. Gingrich and R.G. Fox (eds), *Anthropology, by Comparison*. London: Routledge, pp. 143–66.
Lindsay, J. 1989. *Population Control Policies in Namibia*. Leeds: University of Leeds.
MOHSS. 2003. *Namibia Demographic and Health Survey 2000*. Windhoek: MOHSS (Ministry of Health and Social Services).
Mokomane, Z. 2005. 'Cohabitation in Botswana: An Alternative or a Prelude to Marriage?', *African Population Studies* 20(1): 19–37.
Moultrie, T.A., and I.M. Timaeus. 2003. 'The South African Fertility Decline: Evidence from Two Censuses and Demographic and Health Surveys', *Population Studies* 57(3): 265–83.
Pauli, J. 2007. 'Gendered Space: Female Headed Households in Fransfontein, Northwest Namibia', in O. Bubenzer, A. Bolten and F. Darius (eds), *Atlas of Cultural and Environmental Change in Arid Africa*. Cologne: Heinrich-Barth-Institute, pp. 186–89.
———. 2009. 'Celebrating Distinctions: Marriage, Elites and Reproduction in Rural Namibia', Habilitation Manuscript. Cologne: University of Cologne.
———. 2010. 'The Female Side of Male Patronage: Gendered Perspectives on Elite Formation Processes in Northwest Namibia', *Journal of Namibian Studies* 8: 28–47.
———. 2011. 'Celebrating Distinctions: Common and Conspicuous Weddings in Rural Namibia', *Ethnology* 50: 153–67.
———. 2012. 'Creating Illegitimacy: Negotiating Relations and Reproduction within Christian Contexts in Northwest Namibia', *Journal of Religion in Africa* 4: 408–32.
Plotnicov, L. 1970. 'The Modern African Elite of Jos, Nigeria', in A. Tuden and L. Plotnicov (eds), *Social Stratification in Africa*. New York: Free Press, pp. 269–302.
Raitis, R. 1994. 'Fertility in the Northwest Region of Namibia', *Yearbook of Population Research in Finland* 32: 106–17.

Republic of Namibia. 2003. *2001 Population and Housing Census. National Report*. Windhoek: National Planning Commission, Central Statistics Office.

Rohde, R. 1997. 'Nature, Cattle Thieves and Various Other Midnight Robbers: Images of People, Place and Landscape in Damaraland, Namibia', unpublished Ph.D. thesis. Centre of African Studies: University of Edinburgh.

Schnegg, M. 2009. 'It's the Combination that Counts: Diversification of Pastoral Livelihoods in Northwest Namibia', in C. Greiner and W. Kokot (eds), *Networks, Resources and Economic Action*. Berlin: Reimer, pp. 229–49.

Schnegg, M., and A. Bolten. 2007. 'Sharing Space and Food', in O. Bubenzer, A. Bolten and F. Darius (eds), *Atlas of Cultural and Environmental Change in Arid Africa*. Cologne: Heinrich-Barth-Institute, pp. 194–97.

Schneider, J.C. and P.T. Schneider. 1996. *Festival of the Poor: Fertility Decline and the Ideology of Class in Sicily 1960–1980*. Tucson: University of Arizona Press.

Shemeikka, R., V. Notkola and H. Siiskonen. 2005. 'Fertility Decline in North-Central Namibia: An Assessment of Fertility in the Period 1960–2000 Based on Parish Registers', *Demographic Research* 13(4): 83–116.

Szreter, S. 1996. *Fertility, Class and Gender in Britain, 1860–1940*. Cambridge, Cambridge University Press.

Tersbøl, B.P. 2002. 'How to Make Sense of Lover Relationships: Kwanyama Culture and Reproductive Health', in V. Winterfeldt, T. Fox and P. Mufune (eds), *Namibia. Society. Sociology*. Windhoek: University of Namibia Press, pp. 347–59.

Tötemeyer, G. 1978. *Namibia Old and New: Traditional and Modern Leaders in Ovamboland*. New York: St Martin's Press.

Upton, R.L. 2001. '"Infertility Makes You Invisible": Gender, Health and the Negotiation of Fertility in Northern Botswana', *Journal of Southern African Studies* 27(2): 349–62.

Van Dijk, R. 2010. 'Marriage, Commodification and Romantic Ethics in Botswana', in M. Dekker and R. van Dijk (eds), *Markets of Well-Being*. Leiden: Brill, pp. 282–305.

Wallace, M. 2011. *A History of Namibia: From the Beginning to 1990*. London: Hurst & Company.

Chapter 2

Becoming and Belonging in African Historical Demography, 1900–2000

Sarah Walters

As young Beti women memorize the catechism, they learn to entreat God to make them honourable women, despite their school and modernity. But in other contexts, they hope that education and modernity themselves will have this power, making them honourable in a new way.
—Johnson-Hanks, *Uncertain Honor*

Beginnings

It was pouring with rain. It was more than pouring. It was pounding so hard that it was bouncing off the veranda and in through the open shutters and spattering my laptop. The laptop was useless anyway. It had died that morning and there was no power. I was in the Catholic parish of Itira, on the northern side of Ukerewe Island in Lake Victoria, Tanzania. I could smell the rain and I could smell the lake. Everything was damp, and I was being interrogated.

Why would the Archbishop have given me permission to access the parish archive if I wasn't even Catholic? Was I Anglican? No. Presbyterian? No. Lutheran? No. But I must be something! It was an examination I had been through before, but my standard response – that in my home country not everyone had a religion – was not working and the parish priest was getting frustrated. In following years, I faced the same question repeatedly in parishes across East and Central Africa. Clergy and parish staff found my lack of religion in turns an evangelical challenge, a curious novelty and simply a shame. At church services, I joined the singing and the prayers, partly because I liked them, but also to avoid confusing the children and the nuns who thought they could at least assume religious affinity with the stranger who had landed in their village to copy parish registers day after day – they could at least place me.

Explaining my own identity in religious communities in Africa made it clear that what had seemed a straightforward, contained, doctoral thesis topic was a tangle of meaning and personhood that would take years to unravel and to understand. I had posed what seemed a simple problem and solution: little is known about Africa's demographic past because of the lack of data (Kuczynski 1948; Brass 1968), so I wanted to reconstruct a series of micro-demographic histories using church records, as was achieved for historical Europe (Fleury and Henry 1956; Knodel 1979; Wrigley and Schofield 1989). It soon became clear that more profound questions had to be answered first about the nature of Catholic and religious identity in Africa, the meaning of Christian conversion in an expanding church, and the interrelationships between morality, power and evidence in colonial contexts and in demographic research.

In this chapter, I address these questions in relation to the Counting Souls Project[1] through two frameworks described by Kreager and Bochow in the introduction to this volume. The first speaks to the literature on compositional demography. I consider how the categories imposed by missionaries dictated the population in observation, and how that population changed over time as evangelization progressed and the church expanded (Szreter, Sholkamy and Dharmalingam 2004; Kreager 2011). The second framework borrows from Jennifer Johnson-Hanks' work on vital conjunctures – which she defines as 'the full set of conditions relevant to the ongoing flow of action at a given time . . . the historically specific situations in which structure is mobilized and social action takes place' – and construal – 'the actor's interpretation of, and engagement with, the conjuncture in the form of demographically relevant action' (Johnson-Hanks 2007: 13–14). I argue that in nineteenth- and twentieth-century Africa, it was often the very contingency of life that led people to associate with the church, and that association not only had the power – through economic empowerment, education and healthcare – to change fortunes and conjuncture, but also affected on a deeper level the construal through which people responded, decided and enacted reproductive choice. I propose a concept of moral demography that operates in the space between the individual and the social, at the interface where populations are made by a series of micro-events arising from individual-level decisions themselves shaped by and shaping the macro-hegemonic context. It is a framework that enables 'problematic' evidence to speak the stories it is best suited to tell. I aim to show that the value of church archives in colonial and missionary contexts may be their ability to illuminate the structuring and restructuring of moral codes governing reproduction, as much as their role in estimating demographic rates.

Moral Demography: Towards a Framework

If '"moral economy" is the study of how economic activities of all kinds are influenced and structured by moral dispositions and norms, and how in turn those norms may be compromised, overridden or reinforced by economic pressures' (Sayer 2000), moral demography is the study of how demographic decision-making is structured by a set of codes about honour and respectability ('moral dispositions'), which interact with people's contingent circumstances to produce demographic outcomes (Bledsoe and Banja 2002; Johnson-Hanks 2004, 2006). Let us simplify to the basic units of individuals and events, the confluence of which represents a 'vital conjuncture'. We can consider those conjunctures from two perspectives. The first is reality: what is the actual occurrence of conjunctures in the world and over time? The second is from the perspective of what we can measure (Figure 2.1). As demographers, we try to make the measurement and occurrence circles overlap, and if they do not, we try to describe the extent of the discrepancy (e.g. bias).

Describing the discrepancy (or planning a study to minimize the discrepancy) requires consideration of context. Context affects two things. First, context should influence the categories that we choose for our measurement instruments. In order for our tools to have sensitivity for capture, they must be designed appropriately to identify all relevant events and individuals in a specific place and time. Prospectively, we try to be aware of how our own expectations might affect our imagining of local categories. Retrospectively, we identify shortcomings in measurement categories as a reason for bias. Second, context affects the construal through which (a) demographic action occurs and (b) its measurement may be determined.

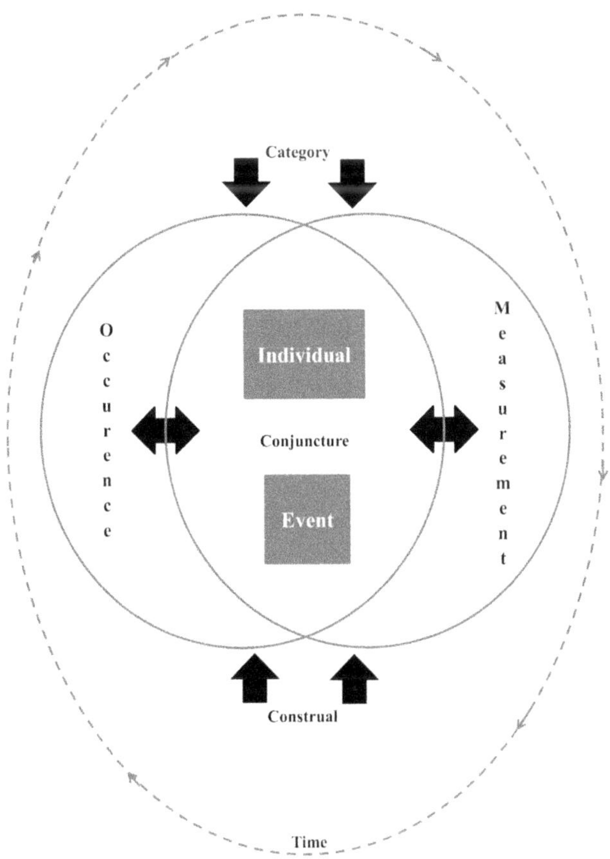

FIGURE 2.1 Moral Demography Framework

Construal is the sociomoral framework within which individual decisions about reproduction/family formation/health take place. It is also the lens through which demographic measurement tools are designed (i.e. it affects how we categorize). There is a feedback loop between occurrence, measurement and construal, in that as events/conjunctures become normative, they also become more measurable. In the moral demography framework, it is to be expected that the occurrence and measurement circles would increasingly overlap with time, all other things remaining equal.

In a longitudinal study, the outer circle, 'time', plays a complicating role. People may start acting or reporting more in line with the measurement categories, as those categories are increasingly seen as 'condoned', or in order to avoid lengthy additional questionnaires to document complex scenarios, or because they become aware of incentives. Equally, the construal may change over time, affecting both occurrence and measurement. For example, in Demographic Surveillance Sites in Sub-Saharan Africa, the provision of antiretroviral therapies affects people's willingness to present for HIV testing (by providing incentive and reducing stigma), as well as the transmission rate, thereby affecting both occurrence and measurement (Roura et al. 2009a, 2009b). Often the institution defining the measurement tool has considerable influence over the construal, with the power to 'normalize' and incentivize, even in an observational study. While the feedback loop between occurrence, construal and measurement draws the occurrence and measurement circles closer, it can also lead to increasing atypicality in relation to a wider population.

In using church registers to measure long-term demographic trends in Africa, these relationships become starker because the records were not designed specifically for demographic research, and the Roman Catholic Church played a deliberate and active role in (re)defining moral codes governing reproduction (Hunt 1999; Smythe 2006). The church created measurement categories and deliberately sought to change the construal context of reproductive decision-making (Hunt 1988, 1991). The categories it employed and the attitude it fostered were not constant over time, and understanding the outer loop of the framework (representing time) is crucial to comprehending censoring effects for different cohorts. In Figure 2.2, key aspects of the church's relationship with local people are overlaid on the original framework and they will be considered here from three interlinked perspectives: first, from the point of view of categorization; second, in relation to composition and censoring; and, third, from the perspective of conjuncture.

Categorization

I was in the passenger seat of the priest's pickup driving back to Mua Parish from Sunday mass at an outstation. In between dodging chickens and potholes, he was telling me about his decision to join the White Fathers and to devote his life to ministry in Malawi. He was reflecting on the enormous privilege of being a parish priest in rural Africa, of the opportunity it offered to be present at the most important junctures of a person's life: to baptize a newborn, to officiate at the marriage ceremony, to visit people in time of sickness and to be present at the time of death. He contrasted his

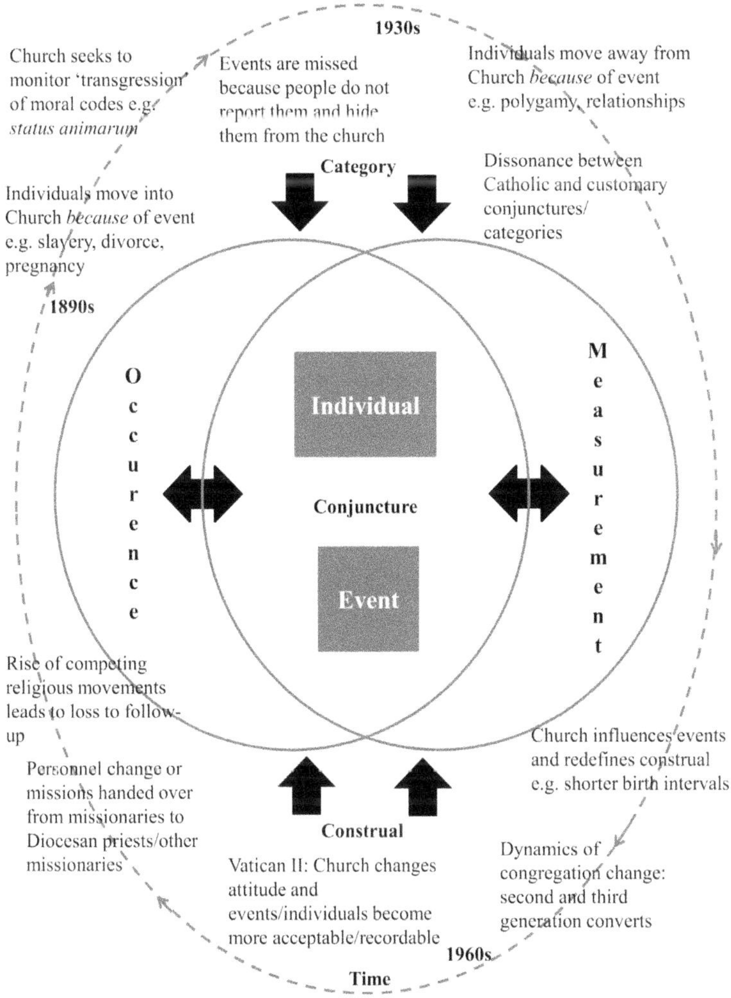

FIGURE 2.2 Moral Demography Framework, with Timeline

situation with that of other volunteers working all over Africa. All were 'outsiders', but he had the advantage of working through the well-constructed system of the Roman Catholic Church and the White Fathers' mission.[2] This allowed him instant access into those most intimate moments of a person's life, without question as to his authenticity or doubt as to his intentions.

Given my plan to reconstruct long-term trends in African demography using the records of baptism, marriage and burial kept by a missionary church, I was happy to hear of the missionary's presence and acceptance at these junctures. Yet, underlying his words was a theme that had been playing on my mind for some time. The theme was one of cultural encounter and, in particular, encounter around the contested and morally-charged moments of reproduction and family formation. The church and traditional authority all over Africa are deeply concerned with those moments. They mark them in various ways, they understand them in various ways and in turn they influence them in various ways. I wanted to know how those different conceptions of being and becoming could lead to restrictions in categorization and in turn to possible shortcomings in the parish record.

Even in Europe, the use of parish registers for demographic reconstruction has been critiqued for missing data on particular categories of people (Ruggles 1992). In order to convert parish counts of baptisms, marriages and deaths into demographic rates, a technique known as family reconstitution is applied, through which female marital fertility histories are re-created via record linkage (Wrigley 1966; Wrigley et al. 1997; Wrigley and Schofield 1973). Any woman not known to be resident throughout her married life (i.e. with no remarriage or burial date) is therefore discarded from analysis, as are illegitimate children. Certain demographic aspects of life were also underrecorded or not recorded, such as stillbirths and extramarital/premarital sexual relationships. Hence, in Europe, the ability to reconstruct 'realistic' demographic histories is constrained by (a) what the church considered 'legitimate' family formation and sexuality and (b) the logical confines of family reconstitution.

In Africa, the gap between reality and record is larger because of the greater dissonance between Christian and customary conceptions of the family and moral sexuality. Catholic dreams of stable, nuclear, patrilocal family structures were confronted with realities where extended families were the norm, where pater and genitor were often conflated, fostering was common, life was short, divorce was frequent, and extramarital and premarital sex were more accepted than in Europe (Goody 1976; Vaughan 1983). Polygamy was traditionally practised in many of the parishes studied, and was associated with long periods of postpartum abstinence and breastfeeding (Page and Lesthaeghe 1981; Schoenmaeckers 1981; van de Walle 1988). These traditional modes of reproduction were censured by Catholic priests. Polygamy was a barrier to baptism, and men were forced to 'put away' additional wives before they could receive the sacraments (Hastings 1974). Temptation into polygamous unions was seen as a considerable threat to the church, as described by a colonial official on his visit to one of the parishes in this study in the 1930s: 'The converts, according to the Father Superior, number 1800 but only one thousand are considered to be satisfactory members of the church. Plural wives, which are, as usual, the chief stumbling block are said to have increased in numbers among the Christians in late years – probably since the Chief set the example of polygamy' (Baker 1931: 19–20).

Given that the structure of the church registers was imported from Europe, there is a potential problem of only being able to measure 'satisfactory' Catholics in this context of fluidity between Catholic and customary modes of family organization. Given that the church was actively trying to instil Catholic family ideals and morals of reproduction in Africa, and intervened directly and indirectly to achieve those aims, we not only risk losing data on unsatisfactory Catholics, but we may also be blinkered to the influence of the church and the direction of change (Walters 2016). Examples of church intervention in reproduction include attempts to institutionalize maternity and childcare and campaigns to change feeding patterns and to reduce birth spacing and abstinence (which was considered to be linked to the 'problem' of polygamy), and the excommunication or censure of those who did not conform (Hunt 1988, Summers 1991). In the first half of the twentieth century, the church also tried to prevent male and female initiation and coming-of-age ceremonies, where much instruction about sexual and marital behaviour was traditionally transmitted (Varkevisser 1973). We are therefore trying to measure change using sources created by the very agents who were promoting and influencing that change (with some success, according to anthropological studies) (Wilson 1957: 257, Raum 1972: 43, see also Hunt 1988: 408). However, before dismissing the registers as biased or unreliable, it is worth exploring in more detail the records that were kept and the priestly motivations.

The nine parishes included in the Counting Souls Project are some of the oldest and most important parishes in Catholic East Africa (Figure 2.3). They were all founded by the White Fathers in the late nineteenth and early twentieth centuries, and Villa Maria, Mua, Bukumbi and Chilubula were the first Archdiocesan seats in their respective territories. The founding principles of the White Fathers emphasized good recordkeeping, language learning and deep knowledge of specific communities, with some missionaries spending most of their adult lives living and working in a single parish or linguistic area (Burridge 1966; Shorter 2006; Ceillier 2008; Nolan 2012).

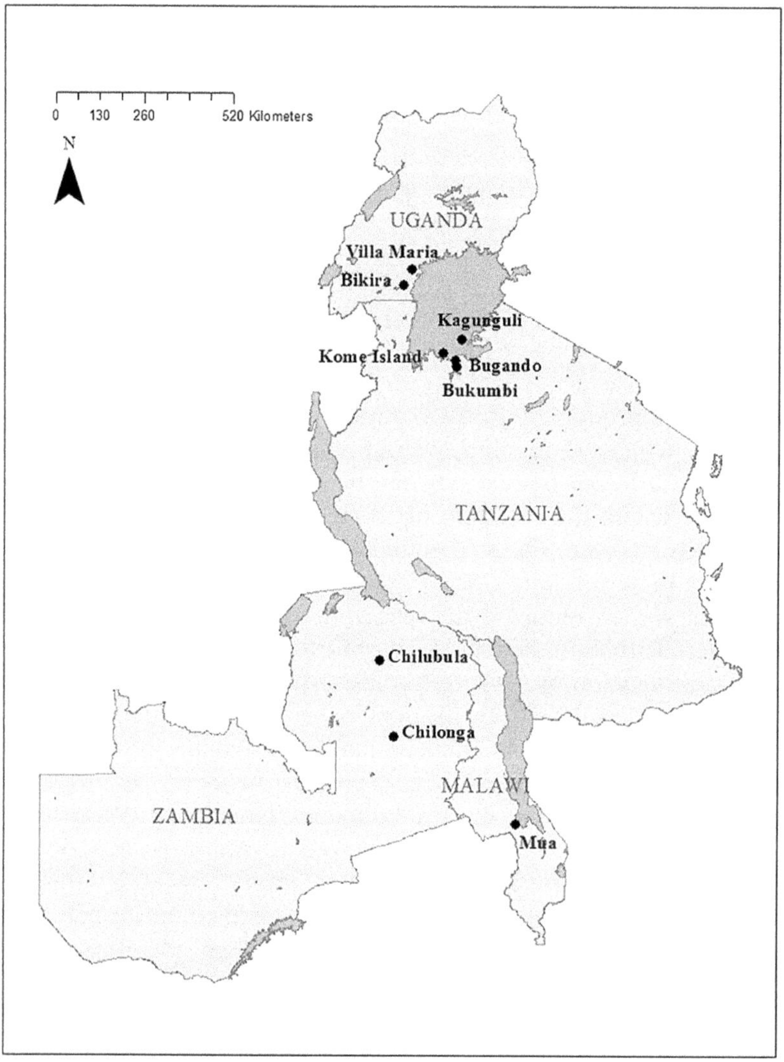

FIGURE 2.3 Map of the Nine Parishes Included in the Counting Souls Project (Including the Four Tanzanian Parishes in the Mwanza Historical Demographic Database)

Priests became skilled (often unsung) Africanist linguists, historians and anthropologists, and claimed greater understanding of those communities than the colonial authorities, often acting as mediators and translators between people and the state (Garvey 1994; Hinfelaar 2004). Their superior cognisance extended to demographic issues, and missionaries were aware of the demographic value of their parish register data: White Fathers in western Tanzania critiqued the 1948 census on the basis of their parish counts and in 1980s Zambia they were reading the latest publications in European historical demography (copies of papers by Peter Laslett and Tony Wrigley exist in their archive in Lusaka). The parish register data kept by the White Fathers are particularly suited to demographic reconstruction because they founded some of the earliest parishes in the interior of the continent (thereby reducing the problem of censoring); there is an extensive system of cross-referencing and family record cards; and the archives are well maintained (at least in parishes where the White Fathers have remained resident) (Feltz 1990; Shorter 2006). Lutheran missions in African kept family books similar to the Catholic *status animarum*, and these have been used previously for historical demography in East and South Africa (Colwell 2000; Notkola 2000; Notkola and Siiskonen 2000).

The archives of all parishes were fully digitized, resulting in an archive of more than 175,000 photographs and about half a million events (Walters 2016). Data were extracted manually into a database and family reconstitution was performed.[3]

In Uganda, records were found of baptism (including of people in danger of dying), confirmation and marriage. In all other parishes, additional records included death registers and the family cards known as *libri status animarum*. In Malawi and Zambia, in- and out-migration records were also located, although these were not kept as consistently as the other books. All parishes keep records of premarriage enquiries and interviews with potential spouses. Record linkage is facilitated by numerical cross-referencing between the books and by the *status animarum*. These *libri status animarum* ('states of souls' registers) were used to determine whether or not a person was eligible to receive communion (Laslett 1977; Del Panta, Rettaroli and Rosental 2006). They therefore contain extensive comment about people's actual circumstances, including living arrangements, relationships and moral character. For example, in Mua (the Malawi), *stati animarum* contain remarks such as 'Pedro is in South Africa, he left a girl here pregnant', or 'Michaeli is lazy and does not pray nor care for his wife', or 'Sofia is in Golomoti with Juventus. Juventus is Anglican', or 'Frances has gone mad and run away to Blantyre'. In the Zambian parishes, *stati animarum* were kept in book form, with approximately half a page for each family. Although fewer remarks were found in the Zambian books about moral character, there is detail of relationship histories, with foster/stepchildren listed, with parents' names (even if those parents were themselves not baptized). In Likoma (Malawi), Anglican records included a 'person book', wherein were recorded a person's attendance at church and any periods of absence or excommunication (suspension from church or from receiving the sacraments) (Walters, Helleringer and Masquelier 2013).[4] Considerable detail is given, including dates of excommunication and restoration, description of repentance and outcome, and the priests' assessment of peoples' shifting moral character (Walters 2016). Similarly, Tanzanian and Zambian Catholic records note attendance at specific services and the amount paid in tithes, opening the possibility of distinguishing between active, practising Christians and those who had simply been baptized.

Therefore, in demanding that people conform to Catholic structures, priests worked hard to document transgression of those structures. Missionary accounts and scholarly articles reflected on such topics as 'The Christian Who Does Not Practise' and the problems of polygamy, illegitimacy and divorce (Tanner 1969). Priests saw the lack of adherence to Catholic structures not as something to hide, but as something to record, understand and ultimately overcome, meaning that the 'problem' of categorization is not as severe as might be expected. Indeed, the documentation of transgression enabled missionaries to make estimates of illegitimacy, polygamy and divorce in their parishes (Linden and Linden 1974: 189).[5]

Although categorization might be a lesser problem than expected, the White Fathers' proclivity for probing into the intimate lives of their parishioners was not constant over time and place. Some priests were more inclined to interrogate and to document than others and, in general, the earlier registers are more detailed than later ones. This could be because congregations were smaller, and therefore it was easier to keep track of individuals, or because missionaries had a greater interest and incentive to follow the lives of the earlier (hard-won) generations of converts. Certainly, there was a wider decline in recording (diaries, letters, etc.) over time, and it became less common for follow-up data to be recorded in multiple places (e.g. for the marriage to appear on a person's baptism record as well as in the marriage register). As literacy improved, priests passed aspects of parish administration to local clerks, and there was a concomitant decline in the extent and consistency of recording, particularly of the informal detailing of people's actual living arrangements and transgression of Catholic structures. The decline was particularly noticeable when parishes were handed over to the diocese, a transmission that accords with the White Fathers' sustainability policy, but that had an effect on the continuity of recording. This gives rise to the paradox that the parishes where Catholicism spread most successfully were also those with the weakest recording and the least detail on the actual lives and relationships of parishioners (Walters 2016).

The varied intensity and quality of recording means that censoring does not always happen at specific time points, which gives rise to compositional effects. For example, while finite censoring – such as the start or end of a particular register or the founding/closing of a parish – can be accounted for in the analysis, more gradual change – such as increasing literacy and use of local clerks or the slow simplification of recording due to the expansion of the parish – is much harder to deal with statistically. If not accounted for, demographic rates appear to change when the driver is in fact the changing constitution of the population in observation (i.e. usually an increasing loss of information on less committed Catholics). There are ways to mitigate this, such as restricting observation to those baptized as infants or to those who have attended a church service in the past year. However, care needs to be taken to achieve consistency over time and place, and additional information beyond the basic parish books of baptism, marriage and burial is required, such as books of tithes or services where an individual's presence at church is recorded. The compositional effects of not accounting for censoring due to changing conceptual categories over time would compound actual compositional effects in the population.

Composition

There is no doubt that the composition of the Catholic population of East Africa changed over time, and that change has implications for the demographic analysis (Hastings 1979, 1996; Hinfelaar 1994; Isichei 1995; Peel and Falola 2005; Sundkler and Steed 2000). We can take both an individual and a population-based approach to composition. The former entails examining individual life histories and conversion narratives to understand why and when people converted, and what factors led them to disassociate. The latter entails understanding how the shape and structure of the Catholic population evolved. Both perspectives are revealing of the censoring effects and may also help us understand the degree of 'typicality' in relation to the wider population.

Taking the individual-level perspective, missionary diaries document the missionaries' relationship with the surrounding population and how it developed. Early diaries describe life histories of some of the first converts. They note reasons for conversion, including the missions' work freeing people from slavery (Austen 1968; Nolan 2008), its attraction to people trying to escape from their marriages or families (Larsson 1991; Grondin 1995; Hodgson 2005), and the use of medicine and material aid by the mission to draw people to the church (Smythe 1999), early converts therefore often had atypical demographic or economic profiles, and faced significant struggles with traditional authority and sometimes their own families about their decision to join the church (Waliggo 1976; Hunt 1999: 43). There were also many baptisms in danger of death in the late-nineteenth century, and these were sometimes recorded in the standard baptism register, further complicating the profile of the early Catholic population.[6]

Later missionary diaries depict how increasing competition from other denominations as well as increased mobility and (male) migration became a threat to Catholicism, both in terms of physical attrition to the congregation and through exposure to immoral living. An example from the Chilubula parish diary of 29 October 1907 is one among many describing the priests' worries about how their congregations would be affected by labour migration and the growing draw of Protestantism:

> In the course of the dry season, several young men from Chilubula and the surroundings left for the Mines District. They left more or less on the sly, without explaining to us the reasons why they were moving out. We are informed in a letter from ****** ******* that three of our Christians . . . are planning to go to the Protestant Mission of Kadowe to learn English. This desire to learn English is very common among the youth, and perfectly legitimate, and we shall have, sooner or later, to take steps to satisfy this demand . . . Others have signed in for service in the militia. We are not particularly pleased with their decision, for we are convinced there was no need for them to look for work outside their villages. There is plenty of work in the villages. In other words we are convinced that they are needlessly exposing themselves to lose their faith and their souls in the process. Far from the Mission and the spiritual care we lavishly bestow on them, they are exposed to constant and serious dangers to their souls and their salvation. We are greatly upset by their decision, for they are our spiritual children and we are their spiritual fathers. What is going to happen to the wives they leave behind unprotected? For they won't be back very soon. All those who signed in for work in faraway places are all married men.

Another reason that people left (or were pushed from) the church in parishes such as Mua (Malawi), Chilubula (Zambia) and Bukumbi (Tanzania) was growing antagonism between the mission and local secret societies and traditional authority (Linden and Linden 1974, Garvey 1994; Hintelaar 1994). These societies were seen as a direct threat to the mission's influence, and the excommunication of certain individuals known to be active members is detailed, as well as competition with secret societies for control over important moments in peoples' lives. Death was a particularly contested moment, a time when priests wanted to be present to hear confession and to perform the last rites, but people also wanted to ensure the safe passage of their ancestors into the spirit world. In Mua, the local population went so far as to hide people who were dying in the bush from the priests in order to ensure control over the passage of the soul and the funeral proceedings (Linden and Linden 1974).[7] When, as in this case, points of rupture between mission and people are also moments of demographic conjuncture, there is a real risk that demographic events are missed from the record; battles for control over transitional moments in the life course lead to informative censoring.

Further loss to follow-up occurs when people were forced from the church due to 'immoral' behaviour. The missionary diaries abound with such stories. For example, in Chilubula it was noted that:

> Some Christians have begun to shame their Church by their behaviour. One left his lawful wife to go and live with a woman in Kasama. Another who was married in church with a non-baptized woman chased her to marry another outside the church. There is another one that is on the point of doing the same. Two others, whose marriage in church was delayed until their former traditional union was declared nil [*sic*] and void by the court in Kasama, could not wait for their cases to be properly solved and came to cohabit together in the sight of the whole Christian community. The guilty couples were warned they were to mend their ways, or they would be excommunicated. (Chilubula diary, 8 September 1907)

Excommunications did indeed subsequently occur and because this happened at the point of relationship change (conjuncture), this once again points to informative censoring.

From the point of view of censoring, the strength (and length) of conversion to Christianity is also relevant, and this is documented in the diaries. Several priests noted that although the very earliest

Catholics may have been 'atypical' as far as the wider population was concerned because their motivation for conversion was some form of crisis – their deliverance from crisis through the mission may have inspired greater loyalty and commitment than among later generations. One missionary in Tanzania noted that by 1907, Christianity 'was becoming a pleasantly approved social custom, lacking all the ardour and conviction shown by the first converts' (quoted in Iliffe 1979: 231). Similarly, in Chilubula, a priest wondered: 'Is the euphoria that marked the beginning of Christianity at Chilubula, the fervour of the first Christians, coming to an end?' (Chilubula diary, 8 September 1907). The worry for demographers is that a decline in religious fervour may imply a decline in follow-up rates. Luckily, in African Catholic registers the problem of censoring is mitigated to some degree by the collection of cross-sectional information on attendance at services and in the periodic parish censuses that enable a means of censoring that is independent of outcome.

At the population level, the annual patterning of new baptisms shows significant jumps in certain years, often coincident with specific events (Figure 2.4). For example, the postwar peak in 1918–20 in the Tanzanian parishes occurred at a time of famine and epidemic, when the mission was extremely active in providing food and material aid to the parish. The earlier peak in the 1890s coincided with a missionary policy of baptizing people when they were in danger

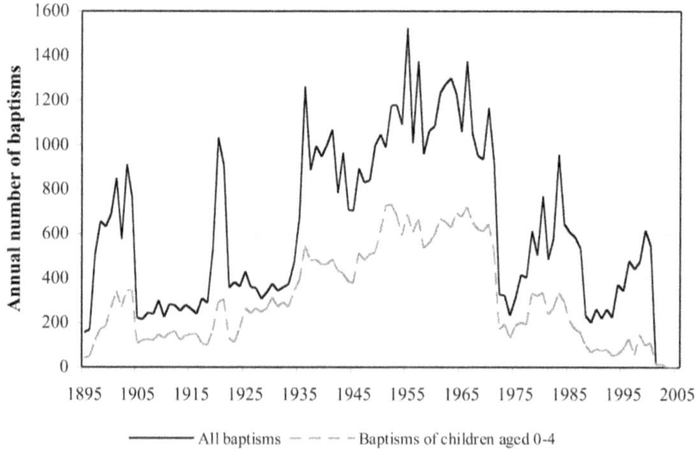

FIGURE 2.4 Annual Number of New Baptisms to Children and Adults in the Four Tanzanian Parishes (Source: Mwanza Historical Demographic Database (MHDD); see Walters 2008)

of dying, and many of those early converts did not survive. The trough during the Second World War occurred because of upheavals at that time due to the conflict in East Africa, and the internment or departure of German and Italian missionaries. In the 1970s, Julius Nyerere's Villagization policy caused considerable upheaval and population movement, which clearly impacted both on people's tendency to baptize their children (the number of new baptisms to children fell by two-thirds), as well as the ability of the church to attract new adult converts (Yeager 1989). Changing rates of baptism imply changing censoring effects for fertility analysis, and changing motivation (e.g. for food aid or for spiritual reasons) imply differing populations of converts. This graph looks rather different if plotted for each of the four Tanzanian parishes separately, and different again if plotted for the Zambian, Ugandan and Malawian parishes. Dealing systematically with this type of parish-specific compositional change is not straightforward and requires additional information on follow-up and church attendance.

The first decades of this missionary church were a time of expansion (Hastings 1996). The first converts aside from those baptized in danger of dying were adults, who were able to understand the missionaries' explanations and make rational decisions about whether or not to join the church. As those first-generation converts began to have their own families, the profile of the population changed and increasing numbers of infants and children (second-generation Christians) were baptized (Figure 2.5). There are limits to the analysis that can be conducted using the first-generation converts because of their potential 'atypicality' (i.e. many were freed slaves/runaways) and because their life histories are left-censored at the time they join the church. This censoring is mitigated in some parishes – for example, in Zambia, the wider history of each family is documented in the *status animarum*, and in most parishes the marriage enquiry books contain details of the relationship history of converts. The surest means of dealing with censoring is to restrict analysis to people baptized as children, but much of the earlier data must be discarded in this case.

Another compositional effect is the change in the balance of men and women seeking baptism over time. In the Tanzanian parishes, more men than women sought baptism as adults in the colonial period (with a dip in the adult sex ratio during the Second World War), but following independence in 1961, the sex ratio reversed, and women became the primary converts, with their majority increasing in every decade between the 1960s and 1990s (Figure 2.6). The

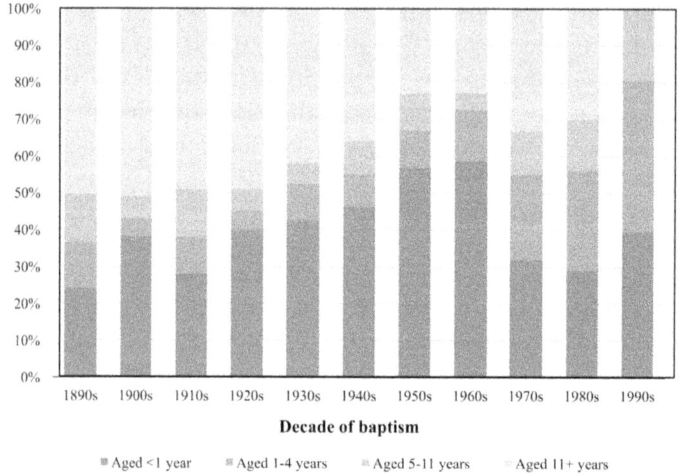

FIGURE 2.5 Age Profile of New Baptisms in the Tanzanian Parishes (*Source*: MHDD; see Walters 2008)

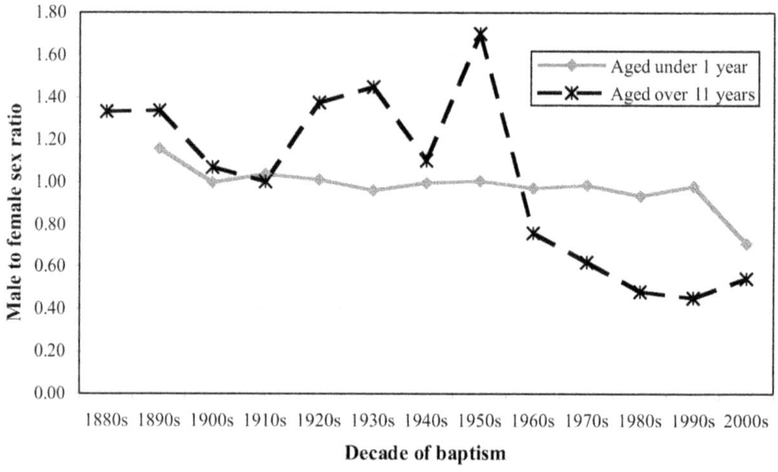

FIGURE 2.6 Adult and Infant Sex Ratios of New Baptisms in the Tanzanian Parishes (*Source*: MHDD; see Walters 2008)

proportion of male baptisms is at odds with observations that have been made elsewhere of a female bias in colonial African Christianity (Hodgson 2005). Hodgson describes 'a significant paradox of the missionary endeavour in many parts of Africa . . . as the preponderance of female adherents to Christianity despite concerted efforts by most mainstream missionary groups to convert men' (2005: 1).

One wonders if the export-oriented nature of the cotton market in Sukumaland could have led more men to seek affiliation with the church than in other areas, given their increased interaction with the colonial state (Austen 1968). This hypothesis would also explain the particular rise in male adherence in the 1950s, during the Sukumaland development scheme and the period of political activism in Mwanza prior to independence (Iliffe 1979).

The first century of a new church is clearly therefore one of significant instability in the composition of the congregation. Sixfold increases/decreases in the numbers of new converts can occur in the space of a decade, the proportion of new baptisms to adults can halve and the sex ratio of new adult baptisms can reverse (Figures 2.4–2.6). These effects are not random and can be explained by the wider historical context. Taken together with the individual-level descriptions of reasons for moving in and out of the church in conversion narratives, and the priests' diary accounts of the mission's relation with the wider population, a picture can be drawn of the likely censoring and compositional effects in each parish. Accounting for those censoring effects statistically should be achieved at the parish level, given that variability was so dependent on the local context.

The description thus far of categorization, censoring and composition has rested to a large degree on the use of missionary sources. It is clear that missionary attitudes and motivations need to be considered in reading those sources, and we also need to consider the mission's changing attitude over time. Just as local perceptions of the mission changed over the twentieth century and Christianity shifted from an exotic creed to the established norm, so the attitude of missionaries to local practice changed, from one of censure and intrigue to one of syncretism and respect. These changing attitudes affect what is recorded both in the parish registers and more widely in the historical documentation, and it is examined below.

Conjuncture, Construal and Change

I was sitting with about twenty medical students from the Malawi College of Medicine in a large round room in the Kungoni Centre for Arts and Culture at Mua Mission, central Malawi. They were from a mixture of backgrounds: some Chewa, some Yao, some Ngoni and some from neighbouring countries. We could hear the rustle of costumes as the dancers prepared themselves in the wings, and while we waited, we listened to the missionary priest, telling us about the meaning of the Chewa *gule wamkulu* and Ngoni dances we were about to see. This priest is a White Father who has lived in Malawi since the 1960s, working as a missionary, artist and anthropologist. At the Chamare Museum in the Kungoni Centre, he has assembled the world's largest collection of *gule wamkulu* masks and the museum is described to tourists as 'the finest ethnographic museum in Malawi' (Briggs and Bartlett 2010: 127). He was explaining to the students the Chewa *mwambo*, the traditional moral code and teachings about how to become and be a responsible and honourable Chewa.

Historically, the Mua Mission was not intent on preserving Chewa culture. Indeed, the battle between the Catholic missionaries at Mua and the secret *nyau* societies of the Chewa is well-documented (Linden and Linden 1974; Kachipila 2006). Frequent campaigns were launched by the missionaries to stop the dances and to outlaw the secret society; being *nyau* was seen as incompatible with being Catholic.[8] In turn, early twentieth-century *gule wamkulu* characters mocked the mission, and *nyau* pitted themselves against priests to gain control over Chewa souls in transitional moments such as birth and death (Linden and Linden 1974; Boucher et al. 2012). As I listened to the Malawian (including Chewa) medical students asking the priest questions about their own history and traditions, and to their professor thanking him for his work preserving their culture and artefacts, I reflected on the great shift the church has made from cultural colonialist to conservator of customs. It was a shift that occurred all over Catholic Africa, and similar institutions housing ethnographic and historical artefacts and documents have been established by White Fathers in Zambia (e.g. the Faith and Encounter Cultural Centre (FENZA)) and Tanzania (e.g. the Sukuma Museum at Bujora). The shift began in the 1950s and in particular following the Second Vatican Council of the 1960s, which laid the foundation for 'inculturation': the policy of relating Catholic teachings, symbolism and values to traditional teachings and culture, and promoting syncretism (Hastings 1990). David Clement (one of the founders of the Sukuma Museum) described the extent of this attitudinal (and policy) change:

> When all this started some twenty years ago, it was a revolution; and it required a lot of courage on the part of the pioneers to conduct that peaceful and religious revolution at a time when nobody imagined that the beating of a drum could be as pious as the sound of an organ,

> and what today everybody considers normal was at that time condemned by short-sighted persons as irreligious and even too profane for a Christian to even consider. This research team (Chama cha St. Cecilia) of the Sukuma Museum was created naturally from the desire to utilize African features in an African context; that is the Sukuma Christian should not feel strange in his own Christian church, he should not be obliged to renounce at any time his legitimate taste, habits, the beauty of his environment or the skills of his artisans . . . These [Sukuma dance] societies do not only deal with dance but also with the cult of the ancestors. Everything being so meshed it was a very delicate task for the researchers, who are devout Christians to investigate their origins, history, and development without being denounced by their fellow Christians of apostasy. (Clement 1977)

This changing church attitude to African culture has implications for censoring in the parish registers, but the direction of effect is unclear. It is to be expected that growing openness to and integration with customary practice would make the parish registers increasingly representative and sensitive over time. However, as described above, earlier missionaries were so intent on censuring customary practice that they actually kept quite detailed records on transgressions of Catholic codes in their *status animarum*. This is certainly true in relation to marriage. It is perhaps less true in relation to other demographic events, which were marked differently by Catholic and customary celebrations of being and becoming. Where conceptions of the life course differed, events of significance to the reproductive lives of parishioners (vital conjunctures) might be missed. For example, in many traditional African societies a newborn was not considered fully present in the world until a certain period of danger had passed. In Mua, people traditionally kept their infants enclosed in the hut for the first couple of months of life, until the child could smile or display other signs of growth and strength (van Breugel and Ott 2001). At that point, the infant would be brought out of the hut and a naming ceremony conducted to officially welcome the child into the world. If the child were to die before that time, he or she was not given a funeral or burial in the same way as would a 'full' human being. The treatment of newborns as on-loan spirit beings until that point conflicts with the practice of infant baptism in the church, and it is likely that the mortality of many of the newborns was missed if they died prior to their naming ceremony. Over time, naming ceremonies became less common and baptism more so, but determining exact dates of this shift to allow for censoring is difficult.

Other important moments of becoming and growth missed historically by the church are the male and female initiation ceremonies in which a person's passage to adulthood (and reproductive life) was marked. If we had a record of these ceremonies, it would be a more meaningful start date for the observation of fertility histories than the date of Catholic marriage. They are in that sense conjunctural moments, and ones that were not merely missed by the church, but actively censured (Varkevisser 1973). In Mua (Malawi), missionary diarists complained frequently about the initiation ceremonies because of what they considered improper and immoral teachings, and in Sukumaland (Tanzania), missionaries tried to close the huts where young people lived during initiation (Cory 1953: 39–40). Over time, the church changed its attitude, increasingly coming to understand that these ceremonies could be used as a conduit for moral teachings. Today initiation ceremonies are conducted with a Catholic blessing and some control. For example, at the White Fathers' Faith and Encounter Centre in Lusaka, Zambia, the church provides a hall and a priest for the ceremonies. There remains no record of these events in the standard parish books, but the growing harmonization between the Catholic and customary life course and the confluence between the Catholic and customary construal around reproduction and demographic conjuncture determines the extent of overlap of the occurrence and measurement circles in the moral demography framework.

The spread of Christianity in Africa was a process of negotiation and conversation between mission and people (Comaroff and Comaroff 1991). At the heart of that conversation was debate over moral codes of becoming: traditional religion and Christianity presented parallel and competing (sometimes conflicting) ideologies of honour and growth. Both described a moral life course and celebrated its proper passage while censuring deviance. Prior to Vatican II, these ideologies were presented as incompatible. People were asked to choose between the two, and markers of growth and being that had importance in one worldview were not necessarily celebrated in the other. In reality, people lived (and still live) between the two worlds, veering from mission to custom depending on the context.

Even today, most people who marry in church are already married according to customary law. I was staying at Mua Parish in June 2012 when marriage ceremonies were taking place. I spent one evening sitting at the long hardwood table in the dining room with the three parish priests filling in the forms for the eighty couples who were staying in the parish hall preparing for their wedding ceremonies the following day. I was in charge of the parish stamp and, as I stamped, I chatted to the priests about the couples in the hall. Nearly all had children with them and nearly all had been married in their village for the last couple of years. The priests spoke of the difficulty of translating the traditional Catholic marriage teachings into the local context, accounting for the fact that these couples already knew a great deal about the realities of married life. The Catholic marriage was not the true marker of that transition and clearly there are implications for demography: using this marriage date is likely to underestimate marital fertility, unless great care is taken to specify the population in observation and ensure the exclusion of people who were already married according to customary law. One option is to identify those subpopulations as far as possible and to create upper and lower bounds for demographic estimates. For example, in calculating marriage age, we might compare the age at Catholic wedding for couples baptized as children to the age at first birth for all women minus nine months (signifying the start of customary marriage) (Walters 2008: Chapter 4).

From a moral demography perspective, the myriad modes of being and belonging in modern Africa affect not only our measurement tools and categories, but also the construal through which decisions were taken and demographic action took place. As described above, Johnson-Hanks' definition of 'construal' is 'the actor's interpretation of, and engagement with, the conjuncture in the form of demographically relevant action'. Interpretation and engagement are determined by predispositions and 'these predispositions are the product of our past experiences, which took place in a social world of people who themselves had similarly structured predispositions' (Johnson-Hanks 2007: 15–16). In thinking about twentieth-century African society, with its growing missionary church, it is not certain that we can talk about 'structured predispositions'. We might instead talk of re-structured dispositions or, better still, continuous making and unmaking of dispositions, for both local people and for the missionaries, through whose eyes we are reading of change. Keeping track of that re-structuring must underlie the use and interpretation of church records for historical demography in the region if censoring and compositional effects are to be accurately processed.

Conclusion/Reflection

After spending the evening stamping marriage certificates, I sat the next morning outside Mua church watching the wedding parties mount the steps. The brides were dressed in white, wearing veils and carrying bright bunches of plastic flowers. Their Catholic marriage was a rite of passage in their lives and an important signifier of their identity as modern women, yet they were not the only marker or the only identity. While I watched, I remembered earlier interactions at Mua: a missionary describing the privilege of being present at important transitional moments in people's lives and another missionary teaching the Chewa *mwambo* (moral code) to modern Chewa medical students. The passion and care with which White Father missionaries followed their converts and documented their lives bode well for historical demography, but we have seen here how that passion changed over time, and the shifts in recording (e.g. through personnel change, expansion of the population or the increasing employment of parish clerks) affect the quality of data in ways that must be accounted for in analysis. The fact that priests at Mua (and at FENZA and Bujora)[9] are now presenting back to local people their own customs, traditions and codes of honour, having spent much of the early to mid twentieth century working hard to intervene and change those moral codes, shows that hegemonic effects are by no means linear. Rather, negotiation between priests and people about faith, morality, modernity and its expression through family organization and sexual practice were myriad and reciprocal in twentieth-century Africa.

Undoubtedly, the church affected the way in which people managed their reproductive and family lives, and certainly this means that parish register data are unrepresentative of wider, non-Christian populations. In turn, the ways in which being, becoming and belonging were conceptualized both by local people and by their priests and missionaries – and the ways in which those conceptualizations changed over time – lead to compositional and censoring effects in the parish registers. African parish registers cannot be used for demographic reconstruction without acknowledging and exploring these effects and relationships. Family reconstitution alone will not yield accurate results. A willingness to go beyond reconstitution into the messy realm of qualitative analysis, and beyond demography into the anthropology of religion and family, and the patience to collect not only demographic events but also markers of presence and 'religiosity'[10] will however yield something richer than a simple reconstruction of demographic rates. It will permit an understanding of how construal shifts over the *longue durée*, how hegemonic models feed and grow in the context of colonialism, modernization and an expanding church, and the impact on how people organize and manage their reproductive lives.

Acknowledgements

The Counting Souls Project was funded by a Wellcome Trust research fellowship [WT095724/Z/11/Z] held at the London School of Hygiene and Tropical Medicine. The Mwanza Historical Demographic Database was funded by a Ph.D. scholarship from the Economic and Social Research Council held at the Cambridge Group for the History of Population and Social Structure, University of Cambridge. The author would like to thank the following authorities for permission to access the parish register data: Bishop Emmanuel Kanyama (Dedza Diocese, Malawi); Bishop Fanuel Emmanuel Magangani (Mzuzu Diocese, Malawi); Archbishop Anthony Mayala and Archbishop Jude Thadaeus Ruwa'ichi (Mwanza Archdiocese, Tanzania); Bishop John Baptist Kaggwa and Vicar General Monsignor Joseph Kato Ssempungu (Masaka Diocese, Uganda); Archbishop Ignatius Chama and Judicial Vicar Father Christian Muselela (Kasama Archdiocese, Zambia).

Sarah Walters is Associate Professor in the Faculty of Epidemiology and Population Health at the London School of Hygiene and Tropical Medicine, where she teaches demography. She directs the Counting Souls Project on the history of fertility and religious change in twentieth-century Africa.

Notes

1. The Counting Souls Project is a Wellcome Trust-funded research programme based at the London School of Hygiene and Tropical Medicine, [WT095724/Z/11/Z]. The objective is to reconstruct the demographic histories of nine Catholic parishes in East and Central Africa.
2. The White Fathers are so-called because of the white robes they originally wore when they were founded in Algiers in the nineteenth century. The society is now officially called the Missionaries of Africa, but they are still colloquially known as the White Fathers, and that is how they are referred to throughout this chapter.

3. The Tanzanian parish data (from Bukumbi, Bugando, Kome Island and Kagunguli) were earlier inputted into the Mwanza Historical Demographic Database, as featured in figures in this chapter. The registers in all parishes remain in use today.
4. Likoma was not eventually included in the Counting Souls database.
5. See, for example, Mua Parish diary, 1 January 1952: 'We now have 6,140 baptised Christians, 1,579 families; 639 of these are broken marriages. Only 2,100 of our 3,324 adults are allowed to receive the sacraments; 2/5ths of our parishioners never receive communion. Out of a total of 2,516 children and youngsters, 750 are illegitimate, from adulterous liaisons'.
6. Many of these baptisms in danger of death were conducted in clinics and health posts, and not always with the patient's knowledge or consent. They are usually but not always identified with the letters 'i.a.m – in articulo mortis'. Later, a separate register was established for the baptism of those in danger of death, making them easier to identify and exclude from analysis.
7. See also Chilubula diary, 1 September 1907.
8. Indeed, the mission at Mua tried repeatedly to abolish the *nyau* and the *gule wamkulu*, and made representation to the colonial authorities to that end. In October 1946, the District Commissioner ordered the people of Mua: 'when you want to dance your nyau, do it in one place, in a place where there is no school of the mission, in a place where there are no Christians, when you want to dance go far far, kutali uko! Kutalindithu! [that is far! Very far!]' (translated by Fr. Claude Boucher).
9. The Faith and Encounter Cultural Centre (FENZA) in Lusaka, Zambia and the Sukuma Museum at Bujora, Mwanza, Tanzania are research centres, archives and museums of local culture founded by the White Fathers, similar to the Kungoni Centre for Culture and Art and the Kafukufuku research centre at Mua.
10. Church attendance and payment of tithes, missionary notes on character, etc.

References

Austen, R.A. 1968. *Northwest Tanzania under German and British Rule: Colonial Policy and Tribal Politics, 1889–1939*. New Haven: Yale University Press.

Baker, E.C. 1931. *Report on the Administrative and Social Conditions on Ukerewe*. Dar es Salaam: Tanzanian National Archives.

Bledsoe, C.H., and F. Banja. 2002. *Contingent Lives: Fertility, Time, and Aging in West Africa*. Chicago: University of Chicago Press.

Boucher, C., G.J. Morgan and A. van de Arjen. 2012. *When Animals Sing and Spirits Dance. Gule Wamkulu: The Great Dance of the Chewa People of Malawi*. Oxford: Kungoni Centre of Culture and Art.

Brass, W. 1968. *The Demography of Tropical Africa*. Princeton: Princeton University Press.

Briggs, P., and M.-A. Bartlett. 2010. *Malawi*, 5th edn. Chalfont St Peter: Bradt Travel Guides.

Burridge, W. 1966. *Destiny Africa: Cardinal Lavigerie and the Making of the White Fathers*. London: G. Chapman.

Ceillier, J.-C. 2008. *Histoire des Missionnaires D'afrique (Pères Blancs): De la Fondation par Mgr Lavigerie à la Mort du Fondateur (1868–1892)*. Paris: Karthala.

Clement, D. 1977. 'The Research Committee at Bujora', *Tanganyika Notes and Records* 75: 81–82.

Colwell, S. 2000. 'Vision and Revision: Demography, Maternal and Child Health Development, and the Representation of Native Women in Colonial Tanganyika'. unpublished Ph.D. thesis. Urbana: University of Illinois.

Comaroff, J., and J.L. Comaroff. 1991. *Of Revelation and Revolution*. Chicago: University of Chicago Press.

Cory, H. 1953. *Sukuma Law and Custom*. London: Published for the International African Institute by Oxford University Press.

Del Panta, L., R. Rettaroli and P.-A. Rosental. 2006. 'Methods of Historical Demography', in G. Caselli et al. (eds), *Demography: Analysis and Synthesis: A Treatise in Population*. Oxford: Elsevier, pp. 597–618.

Feltz, G. 1990. 'Catholic Missions, Mentalities and Quantitative History in Burundi 1990–1962', in B. Fetter (ed.), *Demography from Scanty Evidence*. Boulder, CO: Lynne Rienner, pp. 113–132.

Fleury, M., and L. Henry. 1956. *Des Registres Paroissiaux à L'histoire de la Population: Manuel de Dépouillement et D'exploitation de L'état Civil Ancien*. Paris: Institut National D'Études Démographiques.

Garvey, B. 1994. *Bembaland Church: Religious and Social Change in South Central Africa, 1891–1964*. Leiden: E.J. Brill.

Goody, J. 1976. *Production and Reproduction: A Comparative Study of the Domestic Domain*. Cambridge: Cambridge University Press.

Grondin, E. 1995. *Kisa Cha Wanawake Wanne Wa Kimasai: Miongoni Mwa Wairaqw*. Peramiho: Peramiho Printing Press.

Hastings, A. 1974. *Christian Marriage in Africa: Being a Report Commissioned by the Archbishops of Cape Town, Central Africa, Kenya, Tanzania and Uganda*. London: Society for Promoting Christian Knowledge.

———. 1979. *A History of African Christianity, 1950–1975*. Cambridge: Cambridge University Press.

———. 1990. *Modern Catholicism: Vatican II and after*. Oxford: Oxford University Press.

———. 1996. *The Church in Africa, 1450–1950*. Oxford: Clarendon Press.

Hinfelaar, H.F. 1994. *Bemba-Speaking Women of Zambia in a Century of Religious Change (1892–1992)*. Leiden: E.J. Brill.

———. 2004. *History of the Catholic Church in Zambia*. Lusaka: Bookworld Publishers.

Hodgson, D.L. 2005. *The Church of Women: Gendered Encounters between Maasai and Missionaries*. Bloomington: Indiana University Press.

Hunt, N.R. 1988. '"Le Bébé en Brousse": European Women, African Birth Spacing and Colonial Intervention in Breast-Feeding in the Belgian Congo', *International Journal of African Historical Studies* 21(3): 401–32.

———. 1991. 'Noise over Camouflaged Polygamy, Colonial Morality Taxation, and a Woman-Naming Crisis in Belgian Africa', *Journal of African History* 32(3): 471–94.

———. 1999. *A Colonial Lexicon of Birth Ritual, Medicalization, and Mobility in the Congo*. Durham, NC: Duke University Press.

Iliffe, J. 1979. *A Modern History of Tanganyika*. Cambridge: Cambridge University Press.

Isichei, E.A. 1995. *A History of Christianity in Africa: From Antiquity to the Present*. London: Society for Promoting Christian Knowledge.

Johnson-Hanks, J. 2004. 'Uncertainty and the Second Space: Modern Birth Timing and the Dilemma of Education', *European Journal of Population* 20: 351–73.

———. 2006. *Uncertain Honor: Modern Motherhood in an African Crisis*. Chicago: University of Chicago Press.

———. 2007. 'What Kind of Theory for Anthropological Demography?', *Demographic Research* 16(1): 1–26.

Kachipila, H. 2006. 'The Revival of "Nyau" and Changing Gender Relations in Early Colonial Central Malawi', *Journal of Religion in Africa* 36(3/4): 319–45.

Knodel, F.J. 1979. 'From Natural Fertility to Family Limitation: The Onset of Fertility Transition in a Sample of German Villages', *Demography* 16(4): 493–531.

Kreager, P. 2011. 'The Challenge of Compositional Demography', *Asian Population Studies* 7(2): 85–88.

Kuczynski, R.R. 1948. *Demographic Survey of the British Colonial Empire*, 3 vols. Oxford: Oxford University Press.

Larsson, B. 1991. *Conversion to Greater Freedom?: Women, Church and Social Change in North-Western Tanzania under Colonial Rule*. Stockholm: Almqvist and Wiksell.

Laslett, P. 1977. *Family Life and Illicit Love in Earlier Generations: Essays in Historical Sociology*. Cambridge: Cambridge University Press.

Linden, I., and J. Linden. 1974. *Catholics, Peasants and Chewa Resistance in Nyasaland, 1889–1939*. London: Heinemann.

Nolan, F. 2008. 'Les Débuts de la Mission de Bukumbi au Sud du Lac Victoria (dans la Tanzanie Actuelle) 1883–1912', *Histoire, Monde et Cultures Religieuses* 4(8): 11–38.

———. 2012. *The White Fathers in Colonial Africa (1919–1939)*. Nairobi: Paulines Publications.

Notkola, V. 2000. 'Mortality Transition in the Ovamboland Region of Namibia, 1930–1990', *Population Studies* 54: 153–167.

Notkola, V., and H. Siiskonen. 2000. *Fertility, Mortality and Migration in Subsaharan Africa: The Case of Ovamboland in North Namibia, 1925–90*. Basingstoke: Macmillan.

Page, H.J., and R.J. Lesthaeghe (eds). 1981. *Child-Spacing in Tropical Africa: Traditions and Change*. New York: Academic Press.

Peel, J.D.Y., and T. Falola. 2005. *Christianity and Social Change in Africa: Essays in Honor of J.D.Y. Peel*. Durham, NC: Carolina Academic Press.

Raum, O.F. 1972. 'The Chaga of North-Eastern Tanzania', in A. Molnos (ed.), *Cultural Source Materials for Population Planning in East Africa. Vol. 2. Innovations and Communication*. Nairobi: East African Publishing House, pp. 68–80.

Roura, M. et al. 2009a. 'Scaling up Stigma? The Effects of Antiretroviral Roll-out on Stigma and HIV Testing. Early Evidence from Rural Tanzania', *Sexually Transmitted Infections* 85(4): 308–12.

———. 2009b. '"Just Like Fever": A Qualitative Study on the Impact of Antiretroviral Provision on the Normalisation of HIV in Rural Tanzania and Its Implications for Prevention', *BMC International Health and Human Rights* 9(22): 9–22.

Ruggles, S. 1992. 'Migration, Marriage, and Mortality: Correcting Sources of Bias in English Family Reconstitutions', *Population Studies* 46(3): 507–22.

Sayer, A. 2000. 'Moral Economy and Political Economy', *Studies in Political Economy* 61: 79–104.

Schoenmaeckers, R. 1981. 'The Child-Spacing Tradition and the Postpartum Taboo in Tropical Africa: Anthropological Evidence', in H.J. Page and R. Lesthaeghe (eds), *Child-Spacing in Tropical Africa: Traditions and Change*. New York: Academic Press, pp. 25–71.

Shorter, A. 2006. *The Cross and Flag in Africa: The 'White Fathers' during the Colonial Scramble (1892–1914)*. Maryknoll, NY: Orbis Books.

Smythe, K.R. 1999. '"Child of the Clan" or "Child of the Priests": Life Stories of Two Fipa Catholic Sisters (Regarding the Consequences of Christian Conversion and Assimilation in Twentieth-Century Tanzania)', *Journal of Religious History* 23(1): 92–107.

———. 2006. *Fipa Families: Reproduction and Catholic Evangelization in Nkansi, Ufipa, 1880–1960*. Portsmouth, NH: Heinemann.

Summers, C. 1991. 'Intimate Colonialism: The Imperial Production of Reproduction in Uganda, 1907–1925', *Signs* 16(4): 787–807.

Sundkler, B., and C. Steed. 2000. *A History of the Church in Africa*. Cambridge: Cambridge University Press.

Szreter, S., H. Sholkamy and A. Dharmalingam. 2004. *Categories and Contexts: Anthropological and Historical Studies in Critical Demography*. Oxford: Oxford University Press.

Tanner, R.E.S. 1969. 'Christianity in Usukuma, Part 3: The Christian Who Does Not Practise', *African Ecclesiastical Review* 11: 284–93.

Van Breugel, J.W.M. and M. Ott. 2001. *Chewa Traditional Religion*. Blantyre: Christian Literature Association in Malawi.

Van de Walle, E. 1988. 'Birthspacing and Abstinence in Sub-Saharan Africa', *International Family Planning Perspectives* 14(1): 25–26.

Varkevisser, C. 1973. 'The Sukuma of Northern Tanzania', in A. Molnos (ed.), *Cultural Source Materials for Population Planning in East Africa. Vol. 3: Beliefs and Practices*. Nairobi: East African Publishing House, pp.234–48.

Vaughan, M. 1983. 'Which Family?: Problems in the Reconstruction of the History of the Family as an Economic and Cultural Unit', *Journal of African History* 24(2): 275–83.

Waliggo, J.M. 1976. 'The Catholic Church in the Buddu Province of Buganda, 1879–1925', unpublished Ph.D. thesis. Cambridge: University of Cambridge.

Walters, S. 2008. 'Fertility, Mortality and Marriage in Northwest Tanzania, 1920–1970: A Demographic Study Using Parish Registers', unpublished Ph.D. thesis. Cambridge: University of Cambridge.

———. 2016. 'Counting Souls: Towards a Historical Demography of Africa'. *Demographic Research* 34(3): 63–108.

Walters, S., S. Helleringer and B. Masquelier. 2013. 'Report on the Likoma Island Anglican Parish Registers', unpublished manuscript, available on request.

Wilson, M. 1957. *Rituals of Kinship among the Nyakyusa*. London: Published for the International African Institute by the Oxford University Press.

Wrigley, E.A. 1966. 'Family Reconstitution', in D.E.C. Eversley, Peter Laslett and E.A. Wrigley (eds), *An Introduction to English Historical Demography*. New York: Weidenfeld and Nicolson, 96–159.

Wrigley, E.A., and R.S. Schofield. 1973. 'Nominal Record Linkage by Computer and the Logic of Family Reconstitution', in E.A. Wrigley (ed.), *Identifying People in the Past*. London: Arnold, pp. 64–101.

———. 1989. *The Population History of England 1541–1871: A Reconstruction*. Cambridge: Cambridge University Press.

Wrigley, E.A., R.S. Davies, J.E. Oeppen and R.S. Schofield. 1997. *English Population History from Family Reconstitution, 1580–1837*. Cambridge: Cambridge University Press.

Yeager, R. 1989. *Tanzania: An African Experiment*, 2nd edn. Boulder: Westview Press.

Chapter 3

Between the Central Laws of Moscow and Local Particularity

The Reproduction of Subgroups in the South of Tajikistan

Sophie Roche and Sophie Hohmann

Introduction

The Soviet Union was at once a political unity and a cultural disunity. Much of the Communist Party's investment was intended to produce a new kind of human being, essentially a 'homo sovieticus'.[1] However, despite its planned economy, cultural revolutions and union-wide demographic policies, the Soviet Union never achieved this outcome, at least not in all of its intended dimensions. Comparative analysis of the many outcomes of its policies has to date concentrated on the level of the Soviet republics or on ethnicity – both identities that in some areas were introduced by the Soviets themselves and that have been questioned seriously regarding their capacity to capture group dynamics on the ground. In this chapter we suggest using the concept of subgroups for analysing demographic aspects of this history.

By subgroups we understand groups that are transgenerational, inclusive of both genders, and use nuptiality, fertility and mortality strategically to maintain and reproduce group identities. The concept, applied in a Central Asian context, refers to groups that do not use ethnic markers, and even less national ones, to negotiate identities as a means towards a common objective, namely, group reproduction. Tajikistan has been remarked repeatedly for the existence of such groups, and especially for their limited recourse to national identity as a focus of solidarity. While this situation is gradually changing, demographic developments tell us much about how these groups have used nuptiality, fertility and to some extent even mortality and migration to maintain groupness against the efforts of, first, Soviet modernization and, second, national homogenization. The focus here will chiefly be on the interplay of marriage, reproduction and population displacements.

In the following we begin with a short historical overview that situates Tajikistan within the broader context of the Soviet Union and its fertility history. We highlight the role of women not only because they were a strong pillar of the communists' concept of modernity, but because in the Tajik context, the role of women best demonstrates the tension between central laws (mostly produced in Moscow) and the production and reproduction of groups at the local level. The role of siblings is crucial, as we shall demonstrate. After comparing fertility in Tajikistan and Russia, we focus on two groups in a district in southern Tajikistan, Khatlon, from a former kolkhoz near Shahrituz where mountaineers from the Qarategin valley were relocated in from 1947 to 1953. As groups articulate themselves at their borders, we approach demographic change and its meanings through a comparison of neighbouring subgroups. Against this background, we then discuss how these subgroups contributed to specific fertility developments that resisted both Soviet modernization and nationalizing efforts.

A Short Historical Overview of Tajikistan

The demographic history of Tajikistan reflects the political conditions that have shaped the region of Central Asia throughout the last century.[2] The small Central Asian republic of Tajikistan was cut out of the former Emirate of Bukhara in the process of nation-building under the Soviet Union, becoming its outer border until the Afghan–Soviet War of the 1980s. From 1929 onwards, it was considered one of the Soviet Socialist Republics (SSRs). Soviet policy was characteristically shaped by top-down relations between the political centre in Moscow and the several republics dependent on this centre. Family laws, gender politics, the planned economy, educational structures and so forth were designed in Moscow as all-Union projects. In the course of this policy, the Tajik language was created (Rzehak 2001) and Tajik culture became part of a folkloristic celebration of difference – a result of turning culture into a Soviet political project (Baldauf 2007).

One of the last republics to come under full Soviet control, Tajikistan remained at the periphery of the Soviet project and was the most distinctive republic in demographic terms. Until the socialist revolution that implemented increased control of the Bukharan Emirate, fertility in Central Asia seems to have been rather low with high infant mortality due to epidemics (typhus, cholera, parasites, etc.) afflicting local populations (Khan and Ghai 1979; Jones and Grupp 1987; Islamov 1988). The population increased considerably after the establishment of the Soviet Union, influenced by introduction of its healthcare system (Krader 1971; Islamov 1988; Bushkov 1993). Lublin (1991: 37) states that throughout the 1960s and 1970s, the total population of the three Central Asian republics – Uzbekistan, Tajikistan and Turkmenistan – grew 'at least three times faster than they had during the previous two decades'. The Tajiks are said to have had the highest fertility rate in the Soviet Union, with an average family size of 6.6 members per family, many families having seven or more children (which was the case for only one per cent of Russians) (Lublin 1991: 46). Although Soviet family politics entered the privacy of families to a certain degree, the family was not included in the ideology of women's liberation. This forced many women to participate in the production process, yet continue to bear the full burden of the household (including childcare in some areas, at least until the 1960s).

The role of women in Central Asia has long been a political subject. The Bolsheviks' 'liberation' campaign of the 1920s marked the beginning of an aggressive gender politics. Over more than four decades of struggle with Soviet gender concepts, Central Asian women experienced changes that profoundly penetrated all domains of everyday life.[3] Even if these changes were very heterogeneous and varied among ethnic groups, among nations and urban or rural areas, they did introduce common features and shared experiences. For instance, school education became obligatory for all children – girls and boys alike – and women were expected to participate fully in industrial and agricultural production.

While the Bolshevik movement was primarily urban, from 1928 onwards the industrial revolution was carried into rural areas. The collectivization of agriculture and mechanization of farming were introduced in five-year plans. This campaign affected the family heavily as an economic unit (farmer family – *khojagi dehqoni*) in remote rural areas of Tajikistan. Although collectivization arrived almost a decade later than in Russia, the tremendous changes affected women similarly. Women were forced to work on the collective farms while at the same time taking care of their children, the household and the production of domestic products such as bread and butter. The burden on women in the early Soviet period is today remembered by many elderly women as 'the black days in which we had to raise our children'.[4] Doctors were responsible for defining the health of workers and restricting women from taking leave to care for ill children. As elderly women emphasized, many children succumbed in consequence due to lack of care. Reproductive patterns in this period were marked by high infant mortality and early infertility.

This approach to health reflects the patronage system maintained by the Soviet state in the field of medicine. A particular relationship between the state and doctors was established that redefined individual relations between doctors and patients into a patron–client relationship (Solomon 1990). One consequence was that, despite the development of medical technology, treatment in the healthcare system remained selective and ideologically driven. In their role as state agents, doctors could specify people's ages in remote rural areas, a prerequisite for marriage and legal maturity. They also had the power to attest pregnancies, and often accorded maternal leave so late that the women would work until the very birth.

Stalin's first attack on the family took the form of collectivization programmes, with the aim of destroying the farmers' extended families. The farm family had long maintained a certain independence compared to industry by owning land and cattle and using hired labour. Collectivization aimed to reshape the family as an economic unit. It is believed that at least one-eighth, but possibly even one-sixth of the peasant households – that is, about 25 million peasants – were wiped out during Stalin's purges, which persecuted not only the so-called *kulak*, but also his entire family, including children (Harwin 1996: 14). Following the quotas that Stalin set for each republic, arbitrary mass persecution reached its peak in 1937 and 1938 (Werth 2009: 335). However, while the persecution of *kulaks* succeeded in changing land ownership patterns, the social configuration of communities was not destroyed by this campaign. In some regions, such as in Tajikistan's mountainous areas, entire villages fled to other regions, reorganizing themselves in a safer area. While Creed (1998: 129), in his research on Bulgaria, found a fertility transition to low fertility within one generation during the period of collectivization, this was not the case in Tajikistan. There collectivization initially had some impact on fertility, but after the Second World War (the 'Great Patriotic War'), the fertility rate steadily increased.[5] Evidently Tajikistan's population reacted differently to Stalin's radical modernization measures.

At the end of the 1940s, large-scale relocation campaigns affected the mountainous population of Tajikistan (Abdulaev 2002; Loy 2005; Ferrando 2011). Complete villages were forced to resettle in areas where agriculture was more successful, such as the south of Tajikistan. People were moved by helicopter and truck, and literally dropped in uninhabited forests and different environmental conditions. Forests had to be cleared in the south of Tajikistan in order to make space for intensive and extensive cotton cultivation. The group that we will deal with below, people from the village Qandow, were left in the forest of Shahrituz and had to clear it first in order to build houses and lay out fields. The different climatic conditions between the mountains and plains were difficult for elders and children to bear, and many died as a result. These villagers were integrated into agricultural administrative units, 'the brigades within a Kolkhoz'. One consequence was that the village communities maintained their internal hierarchy and practices[6] rather than being modernized.[7]

Roy (2000) has emphasized that this administrative practice in fact reproduced traditional communities. However, the continuity of kinship ties and village communities by no means guaranteed their cohesion, as Ferrando (2011) has demonstrated in his research on groups resettled to the Ferghana Valley. Small communities (or brigades) nonetheless succeeded in maintaining their internal hierarchies and cultural practices, thus reproducing group identities (Dudoignon 1994; Dudoignon and Noak 2013). The groupness that was produced and reproduced at this level was not regional, but focused on a much smaller village context. This reflects the communities they had lived in back in the mountains, where different villages lived in competition and established ritual practices different from each other.[8] During the Soviet period, the social mobility of any community member necessarily went through its internal group hierarchy, which came to be linked directly to the political centre. The leader of the community became the head of the brigade, Kolkhoz or Sovkhoz, who could then move on to become a regional leader and eventually belong to the political elite in the capital,

Dushanbe. Success thus depended on the communities' approval and on the network of individuals originating from one's village (comparable to Kyrgyzstan (Ismailbekova 2011)).

Recognition of Motherhood

Demographers have repeatedly emphasized the role of state politics in regulating fertility in European as in the global south (e.g. van de Walle and Knodel 1980; Singh and Casterline 1985). For the Soviet Union, we see similarly the state's family politics as having had a considerable impact in shaping family planning. Of particular interest is the differing impact that laws – generally designed in Moscow – have had on local groups in the Muslim periphery.

During the Great Patriotic War (1941–45), 27 million people perished in the Soviet Union (Winter 1992; Harwin 1996: 19). Whole villages were emptied of men. Hence, one of Stalin's main demographic concerns was to raise fertility in order to meet the supply of men needed to fight the war and keep the economy going. Even fourteen years after the war, women outnumbered men by 20 million. This led to the implementation in 1944 of stricter laws against abortion and the relaxation of laws for illegitimate children, whose upbringing until the age of twelve was taken over by the state. The state also introduced different kinds of incentives to benefit children. The law of 1944, for instance, introduced a one-time payment at the birth of each child (Harwin 1996: 19–23).[9] However, fertility continued to decrease in the European parts of the Soviet Union while increasing in the southern tier.

The leading institutions of the time were thus more concerned about the sharp decline in fertility in the European parts of the Soviet Union than about high fertility rates in the southern republics. While the Soviet Union far into the 1970s implemented laws to counteract decreasing fertility in the Slavic republics, these laws, when applied to the whole of the Soviet Union, failed to have their intended impact, namely: (1) improving the living standard of the poorest families; and (2) easing the burden of working mothers. The laws did not increase numbers of children in medium-sized families; rather, they encouraged 'high-parity families to produce even more children' (Jones and Grupp 1987: 270). More concretely, Barbieri et al. (1995) have shown that the central laws of Moscow had a very different effect in Uzbekistan, suggesting that subgroups follow an autonomous path of development despite common laws.

By the 1960s, fertility differences had become so important that political concerns were raised. In the army, Russian native speakers had already become a minority, a serious concern to the whole structure of the Soviet Union in which Slavic people held leading positions. The demographic conference in Tashkent in 1965 became a first effort to discuss the fertility situation in the Muslim periphery; however, concrete implementation of family planning in the south was perceived as discriminatory (Weber and Goodman 1981).[10] The aim of the conference was 'to construct a socialist population policy supported by scientific arguments which were tenable on the international scene ... However, discussion of fertility differences in the several Soviet republics was blurred by continuing concern about declining fertility differences in European populations' (Barbieri et al. 1996: 71). Only in the 1970s were these discussions translated into family planning. A more radical programme started in the 1980s with a sterilization campaign in the peripheral southern republics (reportedly, Uzbekistan). Quotas of births per every hundred women were established and doctors were urged to sterilize women without their knowledge after the second or third child – a procedure never officially discussed. Once again we see doctors employed as state workers actively engaged in shaping the demography of communities in the interests of the state.

Demographic discussion within the USSR was driven by ethnic categories. While statistics of ethnic or national groups differed in every census, the principle of approaching Soviet society through this classification remained constant and was politically motivated (Mazur 1967; Arel 2002). Arel remarks, for instance, that in the Tajik census of 1989, no less than forty 'unrecognized group names' were recoded as 'Tajik' (2002: 816). Efforts to separate populations along religious lines have turned out to be as unproductive for the study of groups as have ethnic classifications (cf. Mühlfried and Sokolovskiy 2011). Mazur (1967), for example, has shown that differences in child-woman ratios within Muslim groups were larger than between groups classified as Orthodox Christian and Muslim; the Muslim Tatars have long followed a Slavic Russian pattern of fertility, while the southern tier has maintained higher levels. The call by Agadjanian and Makarova (2003) to pay more attention to nuanced differences and to 'situate demographic trends fully and soundly within the context of the recent dramatic political and socio-economic changes' thus needs to be taken seriously.

Early Soviet policy, as we have noted, enjoined liberation for women while increasing the burden of their responsibilities to the family and society. By the 1960s, conditions for women began to adjust and their workload could become more manageable. As one woman explained, women with several small children could stay at home 'because the salary of one household member was enough to feed the family'. Nonetheless, the administrative strategy that situated women between their traditional roles and their labour force contribution to the kolkhoz continued to create problems (Harris 2004; Kamp 2006). While in European Russia women's full integration into the economy was accompanied by a substantial fertility decline, Tajikistan had made it to the top of the list of all Soviet republics with 37.4 births per 1,000 population (Kuniansky 1981: 39) – a phenomenon observed with anxiety by the authorities.

By the 1970s, these demographic developments thus appeared to require a new approach. Female labour participation was even higher in rural areas than in urban centres, including in Tajikistan (Kuniansky 1981: 26).[11] The authorities concluded that when too many women participate fully in the labour market, they are likely to neglect private plots and the survival of families. A new politics was therefore implemented to try to break with the conflict generated by the double effort to increase fertility and labour participation simultaneously. Motherhood received political recognition through financial incentives distributed to mothers. 'We were having children in order to get a Jiguli', a Tajik woman explained, as having as many children meant they would be given medals; with ten surviving children, they would receive a car (Jiguli). To understand this policy, we have to go back to Russia. As Jones and Grupp (1987) have emphasized, demographic policy during the Soviet era was Russia-oriented (also see Blum 1994; Barbieri et al. 1995). In Tajikistan, the position of women had only partly changed under Soviet laws as women remained 'bearers of tradition' within the communities (Tett 1995). Despite their participation in Kolkhoz labour, women's status depended on successful reproduction. Even if we may question the effect of payments on fertility, women in interviews did emphasize that payments were recognition by the state of the difficulties of motherhood. (Men saw this differently, claiming that payments did not influence family planning.)[12] Further sons were a source of wealth and social security. In many villages we found families with eight sons occupying important positions such as village leader, international organization leader, owners of village shops, etc. These families were considered wealthy compared to those who lacked sons. Central Asian society remained based on virilocal residence patterns where the youngest son takes over the compound of his parents and cares for them.

The symbolic valuation of motherhood thus appears to have been a central factor in increasing fertility far into the 1980s, with a peak in 1987 for Tajikistan (see Figure 3.1). Jones and Grupp (1987: 15–22) argue that fertility increase reflects several factors, notably the well-developed healthcare system, a decrease in local conflicts and warfare, as well as the pronatalist politics of the Soviet state. While the politics of labour and family planning were centralized, local outcomes could vary considerably, not merely because of differing recourse to reproductive technologies, but reflecting community concepts and cultural understandings of motherhood and children. Figure 3.1 shows the Total Fertility Rate (TFR) of Russia and Tajikistan compared. We see the peak in the late 1970s compared to Russia, whose fertility continues to decrease in the same period and under the same politics (Blum 1987).

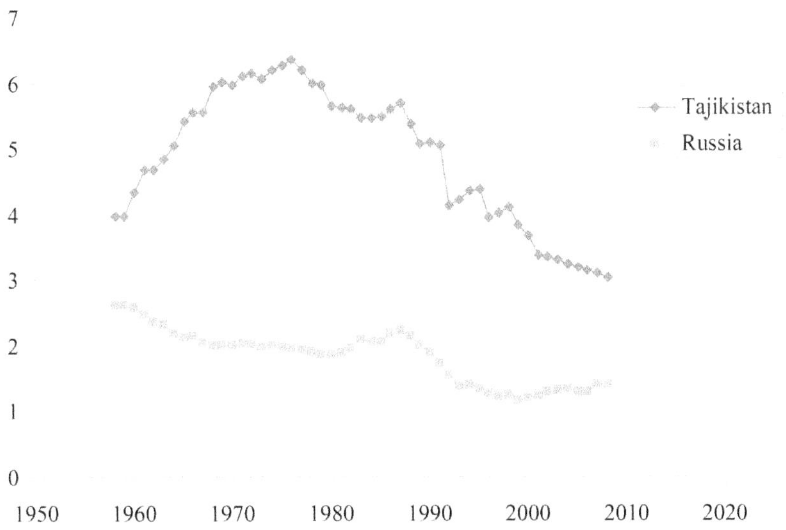

FIGURE 3.1 Total Fertility Rates in Russia and Tajikistan, 1958–2010

How was and is Fertility Regulated?

Concerning cultural and social factors, we have seen that politics influenced the status of motherhood and honoured families with many children. Centralized policy-making also ensured that the costs of bringing up children were low. While collectivization (1920s and 1930s) and the Second World War are remembered as 'black days' by mothers, by the 1960s, kolkhoz communities provided free education, gender-based workloads, socialized children into the community, and secured every member with a (decent) income and a place in the community when they reached adulthood.

The high mortality levels of the 1930s (due particularly to a severe famine in 1933) led to the identification of population growth as 'an ideological issue . . . regarded as an indicator of the country's well-being' (Barbieri et al. 1996: 70). Since abortion had become the principal method of family planning, it was banned in 1936, with the implementation of pronatalist measures. These laws were only reversed after Stalin's death, and abortion became legal again in 1955. Some women explained that they did use contraception secretly, expecting their husband to reject family planning. Some women used herbs to regulate fertility, yet we do not know to what degree these were used and about their success (Harris 2002). Most commonly, abortion was and still is used as a method of family planning by ending a given pregnancy. Although abortion had already been legalized in 1920, the law never developed the same dynamic in the south as it did in Russia (Harwin 1996: 8). The abortion rate rose rapidly in the north towards the end of the 1920s: '18–20 women of every 100 who attended maternity clinics were asking for a termination, with poverty as a chief reason' (Harwin 1996: 9). While the rate was much lower in Tajikistan (see Figure 3.2), abortion remained the primary way of controlling fertility even after the Soviet period, increasingly joined by the IUD.[13] Turner (1993: 141) gives an abortion rate for Tajikistan of 43.5 per 1,000 women. From the 1980s onwards, active fertility prevention was effected by doctors through forced sterilization.

The Ethnographic Research Setting

Most approaches take countries or ethnic groups as the unit of reference for demographic estimates. As we have seen, the

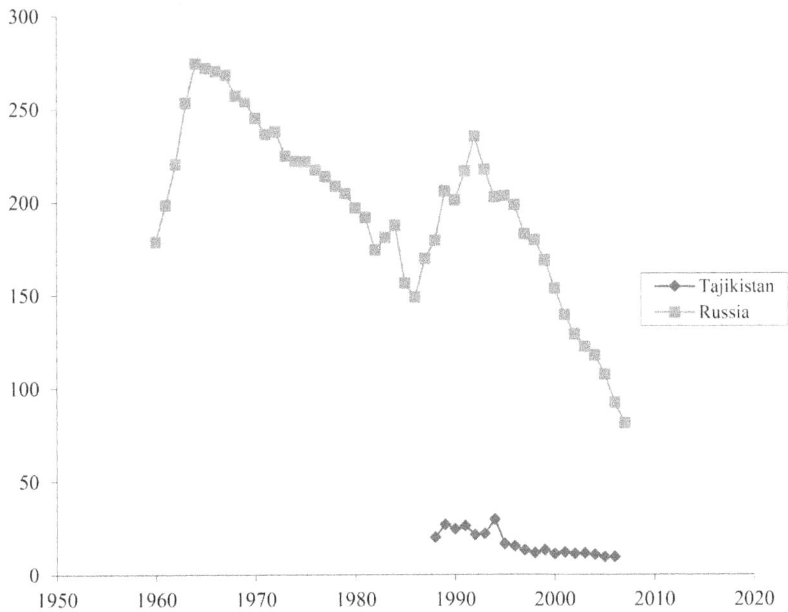

FIGURE 3.2 Number of Abortions per Hundred Live Births

motivations behind these categories were driven by the state's claims to control, particularly in the Soviet era. Tajiks were identified as an 'ethnic group' entitled to their own national territory, while Samarkand and Bukhara, the cultural centres in which Persian speakers (Tajiks) had primarily lived, were nonetheless integrated into Uzbekistan. Subsequently, researchers have come to argue that Tajiks, stripped of their cultural centres, did not develop a national identity, while mountain villages simply did not share any kind of national identity.

Roy has suggested that kolkhoz communities were in fact the major subunits providing peoples' identities (cf. Dudoignon and Noak 2013). A kolkhoz usually includes several villages and kin groups. Contrary to the theoretical assumption of cultural homogeneity, many if not the majority reflect a variety of identities (Kılavuz 2009; Ferrando 2011). Communities were inclusive in that the celebration of minor differences between groups was done on equal terms – all villagers were invited indiscriminately to participate in life cycle rituals. Differences in rituals marked regional identities, ethnic identities, religious convictions and so forth. Beyond these micro-identities, the Kolkhoz community grew together through its common participation in labour and because children attended the same schools.

In the following we will concentrate on the kolkhoz known as Leninobod Uchastka and the subgroups within it. One of these groups is the Qandowi, who were relocated between 1949 and 1953 from the mountainous areas to the southern plains for cotton cultivation in Shahrituz. Among the people in Shahrituz, they were referred to as 'Kyrgyz' because they had been resettled from an area in which most inhabitants are Kyrgyz. Although they were Tajik speakers (and most were bilingual or trilingual), they did not mix with local groups either within the kolkhoz or with local residents. They called themselves 'Qandowi' and thus used a territorial term (that is, their village of origin) to refer to their subgroup as it was maintained and reproduced over several decades.

In so doing, the Qandowi and other subgroups did not conform to the Marxist-Leninist concept of ethnicity that expected ethnic groups to evolve naturally into a nation. It is beyond the scope of this chapter to engage in the discussion of ethnic categorization at the regional level: suffice to say that, since the first census of the Bolshevik era in December 1926 until the 1989 census, the categories employed have served the interest of political power (Abashin 1999, 2007) rather than reflecting area-specific group formation processes for which language and even kinship (for Tajiks and Uzbeks) were less important than economic niches, educational levels, rituals, religious descent and place of residence.

With the end of the Soviet Union, Tajikistan experienced increasing political tensions that eventually led to civil war. The war started in the capital, Dushanbe, in 1991 as a power struggle between religious-democratic and communist forces and economic interest groups. It then moved south and later into all regions. The civil war uncovered solidarity groups (*mahallgaroi*), which were accorded regional labels and expressed political interests. From 1992 onwards, various such groups had formed and were roaming through the country. Put very simply, kolkhoz structures were seen as the basis for the recruitment of these groups, together with political networks (Ro'i 2000; Kılavuz 2009). A peace agreement was successfully signed in 1997. What is important for the present discussion is that the war was the decisive moment in which group divisions were activated and became visible (Roche 2014). In other words, the experience of civil war forced people to take sides and uncovered fundamental group attachments. When pro-state militias reached Shahrituz, the Qandowi fled to the Afghan border along with other groups of the Leninobod Uchastka that had also been relocated, like their neighbours the Kanishbegi. In other words, when the immediate need to take sides arose, they fled as a group, thus affirming their identification with a demographic marker – migration that had brought them together in Shahrituz in the first place. The local inhabitants (Mestni, Uzbek, etc.) did not leave, or only did so for a short period. After the Qandowi and Kanishbegi left, the remaining groups plundered their houses and took literally everything that was not unmovable.

When local commanders called back the 'Kyrgyz' as 'Turkic brothers', some of the Qandowi went back. However, they were identified as Tajik from Qarategin and hence as enemies. All the men were killed and the women were taken away. This is how they learned the ethnic lesson in a violent context that fixed identities politically. The civil war and postwar politics forced people to become exclusive in their choice of identification. Further, subgroup identities such as 'Qandowi' or 'Kanishbegi' gradually merged into political categories. These categories used regions such as Qarategin, Kulob, Leninobod and Pamir to give a single identity to clusters of subgroups. Today these classifications continue to play a central role in power distribution, while at the same time being strongly countered by a state ideology that constructs a supposedly unified Tajik identity against Turkic (Kyrgyz or Uzbek) and other non-Tajik groups (Mestni, Arab, Russian, etc.).

The civil war experience shows that the Qandowi acted as a group. While sociopolitical circumstances identify the Qandowi as a group, we wish to test to what degree they are a subgroup in the sense outlined at the beginning of this chapter. We will test, first, to what degree the Qandowi intermarried with neighbouring subgroups within the Kolkhoz and outside; second, whether their fertility behaviour differs from other subgroups; and, third, we will analyse the factors responsible for maintaining their distinct group identity. These data together indicate what strategies the Qandowi used to reproduce as a subgroup, at the same time resisting Soviet modernization (despite successful female participation in the market economy and high literacy among women) and homogenization (as members of a national republic, the Tajik nation-state).

The Dataset

For statistical analysis, we use the micro-census taken in 2006 and 2007 during an ethnographic fieldwork conducted by Roche. The data were collected among a group in the south of Tajikistan (Leninobod Uchastka). As noted above, the Leninobod Uchastka is a subunit of the kolkhoz and a community of people from different areas of Tajikistan. The material was assembled on the basis of genealogies, thus including people who do not live in this defined territory. However, within a given area, all households (61 in all) have been systematically visited and registered. While for the first part we only use household information for the Leninobod Uchastka, in the second part we will use the whole dataset, including those who married out of the Leninobod Uchastka. This is necessary to construct a sample that – even if limited – is large enough for statistical analysis. We begin by noting sex ratios and then proceed to ethnic composition, marriage and fertility.

The sex ratio calculated in Table 3.1 includes all living members who live or have lived within the respective households. The result is lower than the demographic norm of 105 and lower than the ratio of 104 as identified in prewar Tajikistan (Hohmann, Roche and Garenne 2010). The sex ratio changed during the civil war to over 106 and despite local variations (as for the Qandowi) has since remained high at the national level. This is probably due to the high migration rate, many men being temporarily or permanently away in Russia or elsewhere for work (Laruelle 2013).

The ethnic composition of the sample in Figure 3.3 reflects the situation of the south. Since the forced relocation campaigns, the area has become a mix of various groups, most of them using emic terms that refer to their place of origin rather than to ethnic or national identifications. This self-identification distinguishes each group from others with whom the same space is shared (i.e. a

TABLE 3.1 Sex Ratios in Leninobod Uchastka

	Leninobod Uchastka	
	All	2007
Men	310	244
Women	300	247
Ratio	103.3	98.8

Source: Micro-census conducted by Roche, 2006–2007

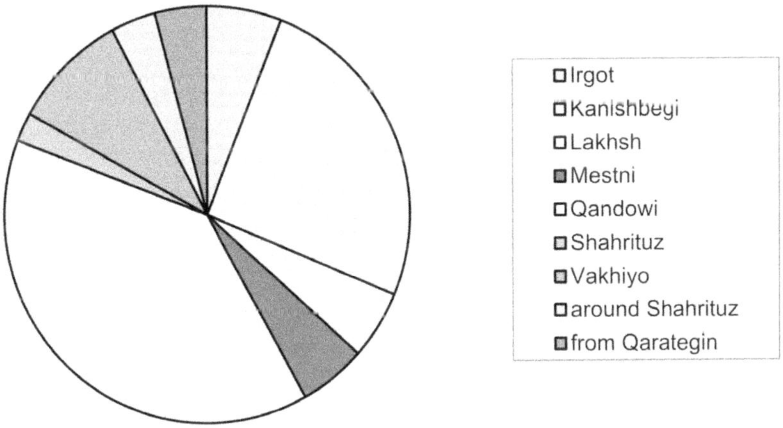

FIGURE 3.3 Ethnic Composition of Census, Leninobod Uchastka

Kolkhoz). In the following we will see to what degree these self-reported identity groups are distinctive demographic subgroups. The categories employed in these statistics do not match those claimed by the state, reflecting instead the specificity of the area.

We use two of the subgroups within the Leninobod Uchastka in order to identify common and different strategies of group reproduction. The following tables show the degree of intermarriage with neighbouring groups and those they consider to be from the 'same' group.

Of the 127 people, 47.2 per cent marry within those groups they consider the same, namely 'Qandowi'. About 40 per cent marry outsiders. This is a very high percentage, which reflects less the importance of exogamy than that of regional identities that are prioritized in defining marriage alliances. Twenty-five persons, that is, half of those in the category 'other', come from Leninobod Uchastka, but are not identified by a specific regional or ethnic marker. In sum, 85 (60 + 25) out of 127 marry within their own group and within their own residential area.

The Kanishbegi, who are another important group within the Leninobod Uchastka, use similar categories to describe marriage partners, showing the same majority marrying within subgroups they consider the same.

Figure 3.4 compares the two subgroups' marriage behaviour. The Qandowi tend to have a larger range of ages at first marriage compared to the Kanishbegi, who clearly favour earlier marriage at ages 20 and under.

TABLE 3.2 Intermarriage of Qandowi in Leninobod Uchastka

Qandowi married to:	Number of people	Relative percentages
other	17	13.4
Dushanbe	1	0.79
Gharmi*	1	0.79
Irgoti*	2	1.57
Jailghan	1	0.79
Jillikul	2	1.57
Jirgatol	1	0.79
Kanishbegi*	2	1.57
Kobodiyon	3	2.36
Komsomolobod	1	0.79
Kulobi*	1	0.79
Kurghan Tepe	1	0.79
Kyrgyz*	6	4.72
Kyrgyzstan	2	1.57
Lakhsh	8	6.3
Leninobod	1	0.79
Muk	1	0.79
Qandowi*	60	47.2
Shahritus	11	8.66
Tatar*	1	0.79
Tojikobod	1	0.79
Vakhiyo*	3	2.36
	127	100

* Refers to a previous regional or ethnic identities rather than to contemporary residence localities

Source: Micro-census conducted by Roche, 2006–2007

TABLE 3.3 Total Qandowi Marriages

	Marriage totals	Marriages by %
Qandowi	60	47.24
Outside	50	39.37
Other	17	13.39
Total	127	100

Source: Micro-census conducted by Roche, 2006–2007

We now turn to comparison of fertility behaviour between these subgroups. If the Kanishbegi favour early marriage, we can expect them to have slightly more children than the Qandowi. Figures 3.5–3.7 include the Qandowi and the Kanishbegi, as well as two other subgroups of the Leninobod Uchastka, for comparison.

TABLE 3.4 Total Kanishbegi Marriages by Own and Other Subgroups

	Number of people	Relative percentages
Other	24	28.92
Kanishbegi*	31	38.55
Faizobod*	1	1.205
Jirgatol*	1	1.205
Kobodiyon*	1	1.205
Qandow*	2	2.41
Russian	1	1.205
Shahritus	3	3.614
Tojikobod*	2	2.41
Uzbek	1	1.205
Vakhiyo*	5	6.024
Other	10	12.05
	82	100

* Refers to a previous regional or ethnic identities rather than to contemporary residence localities
Source: Micro-census conducted by Roche, 2006–2007

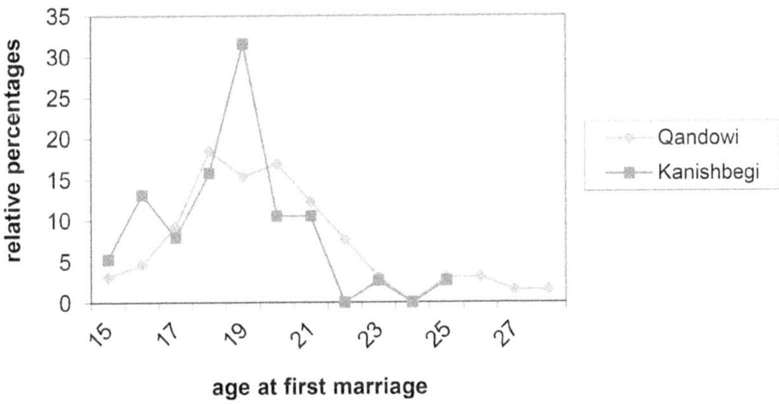

FIGURE 3.4 Age at First Marriage Compared, Women Only

Figure 3.5 shows the absolute number of children born to women in 2007. This serves a heuristic purpose, indicating simply that there has been a broad convergence of reproductive patterns from the 1960s. (Note, however, that a fertility decline cannot be identified accurately from this graph, as most women have not yet completed their fertile period.) The principal fact of interest here is solely that the Qandowi have a slightly lower fertility than the Kanishbegi in the 1970s, but the subgroups all seem to converge on one pattern

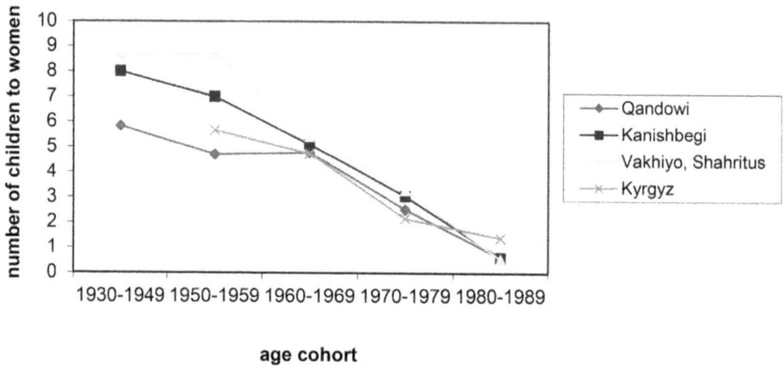

FIGURE 3.5 Numbers of Children Born to Women, by Age Cohort

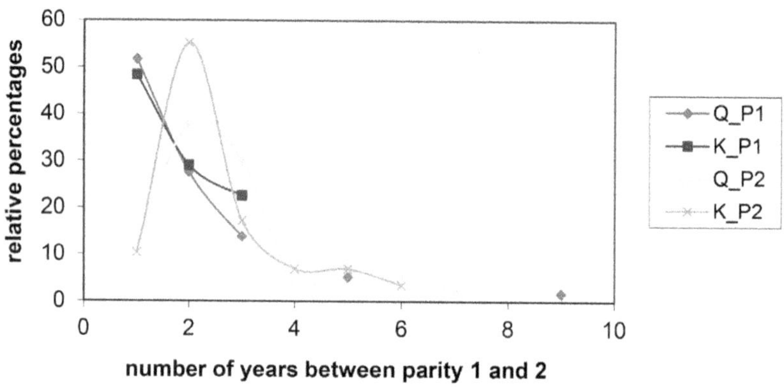

FIGURE 3.6 Parity (P1 and P2) Compared, Qandowi (Q) and Kanishbegi (K), Women Only

in the 1980s – with some exception for the Kyrgyz. While fertility between the 1930s and 1950s appears more distinctive between subgroups, these data need to be treated with caution, on two counts: first, because of the small sample; and, second, because political arrangements may motivate some groups more than others to omit children.

Figures 3.6 and 3.7 compare parity among the Qandowi and the Kanishbegi. The results tell us that women in both groups start their fertility history within the first year of marriage (an observation also true for the whole of the Soviet Union) and that it is at higher-order parities that the groups differ. The second child for the Kanishbegi in over 50 per cent of the cases comes after the next two years, while

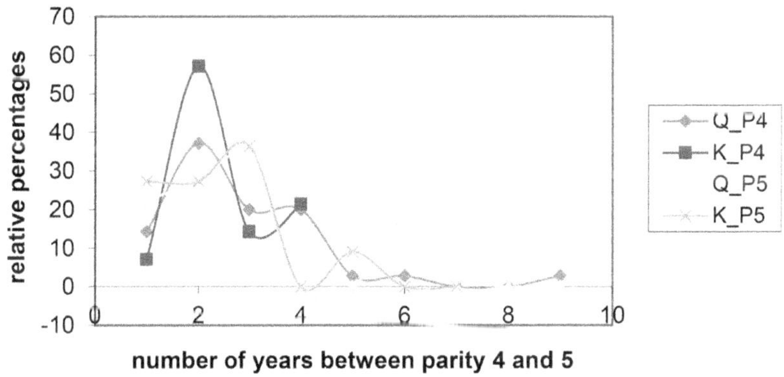

FIGURE 3.7 Parity (P4 and P5) Compared, Qandowi (Q) and Kanishbegi (K), Women Only

for the Qanishbegi, it is after two to three years. Parity 4 continues in the same scheme for the Kanishbegi, who have their third child again after two years, while the Qandowi will take two to four years. Most interesting is the change at parity 5 in which, for both groups, the two-year gap changes into a three-year gap.

These figures confirm the claims of young women that a family with four children is one they regard as optimal and suggest that intentional strategies are used to postpone the birth of the fifth child as much as possible. Postponing strategies seem to start as early as the third child for the Qandowi, while this is less the case for the Kanishbegi.

Discussion: Strategies to Reproduce Groups

In the preceding pages we have identified in the micro-census the different terms that people use to distinguish themselves from neighbouring subgroups. On the basis of these emic concepts of groupness, we have tested to what degree subgroups differ in terms of their nuptiality and fertility histories. We now wish to discuss the qualitative strategies that people use to reproduce as groups, and argue that such strategies are crucial to understanding the larger divide that separates demographic developments in the north of the former Soviet Union from the south.

Let us start by taking regional and ethnic identities as a way in which people relate to their own community. People with origins from predominantly Tajik mountain areas (Vakhiyo, Kanishbeg) have more children than those from mixed areas (whether these are considered as Tajik and Kyrgyz, or under the more specific locational Qandow, Lakhsh and Irgot identities). They also have higher fertility than local people (Mestni). The crude birth rate of 5.4 for Leninobod Uchastka is slightly lower than the findings of Turner (1993), who identifies a TFR of 5.9 lifetime births per women among ethnic Tajiks. Tajik fertility as a mechanism of subgroup reproduction rests, first, on how kin groups organize the marriage of their children; second, on territoriality; and, third and more particularly, on the dynamics of siblingship.

Kinship and Marriage

Tajiks follow patrilineal descent and use the term *avlod* to refer to the minimal lineages that form the basis of their society. The term *avlod* is of Arab origin and refers simply to a 'succession of sons'. In other words, Tajik do not have a complex tribal, lineage or clan system when compared to their Kyrgyz neighbours. While kinship closely follows male descent, the identity of different kin groups amongst the Tajik comes chiefly from the locations people live in (Samarkandi, Qandowi, Kanishbegi, etc.). We can thus speak of a Tajik kin system as composed of small groups that may share language (or dialect), ritual practices and classificatory features, but that draw their commonness from cohabitation, shared occupations and intermarriage. We call subgroups those people who prioritize marriage amongst each other, who claim relationship (mostly some kind of kin relation, which they are often unable to specify), use sibling relationships to adapt to changing political and economic conditions, share a dialect and ritual practices, and cohabit (see also the Introduction in this volume, p. 2). These subgroup identities are self-identifications based on residence rather than ethnic belonging. For instance, the Qandowis, although using this self-identification (i.e. their village of origin before 1947), had begun after only one generation to distinguish themselves from the 'mountaineers' living in and around the village of Qandow.

Marriage is virilocal, women moving to their husbands' home, yet they do not change their *avlod*. Women remain completely dependent on their brothers (for healthcare, conflict resolution, etc.) throughout their lives until their own sons are old enough to care for them. Marriage between the children of siblings (i.e. between the children of two brothers, and between the children of two sisters – but not brother and brother) are allowed and accepted as much as marriage to an external (i.e. non-Tajik) group. This openness of marriage rules has allowed Tajik subgroups to adapt to the arrangements of peoples with whom they have been cohabiting over the centuries. Consequently, we find slightly different cultural practices depending on the adjacent groups with which they co-reside; in Bukhara these are Uzbeks (Finke and Sancak 2012), while in Tajikistan they are mainly Uzbeks and Kyrgyz.

The Qandowi of Leninobod Uchastka, for instance, have kept close contact and even intermarried with the Kyrgyz from Jirgatol (a mountainous district in the east of the country). In the context of such kinship and marriage practices, we might expect groups to dissolve after a few generations into neighbouring majority groups. This, however, is not the case. The marriage rules allow simultaneously for adaptation and protection. For example, marriage between the children of two sisters is used to reunite the kin group where geographical distance had previously separated members due to forced relocations and war. The practice of siblings' children marriage is found in early Islam and has long been referred to as an Islamic practice intended to keep family wealth within the group. The practice has been maintained by the Tajiks, despite the fact that this traditional economic function does not hold for the Tajiks under Soviet law. Indeed, if property consolidation was the main issue, then the destruction of family farms during the collectivization of the 1930s would have meant the end of Tajik kinship. Instead, they reconstituted subgroups at other places and used strategies of marriage to maintain their distinct identities. Siblings are at the base of people's descent histories, which may cover large distances, migration and extend over several centuries. What Conte and Walentowitz (2009) have identified as *nasab* (genealogy, transgenerational relationship, *sajara* in Central Asia) in the Middle East to some degree also captures the centrality of siblingship in Tajikistan. *Nasab* in Islam is a masculine concept of descent, which, however, overshadows the centrality of sisters and brothers and the strategies of sisters who have been married to far-distant places; these women continue to initiate more marital links between the place to which they moved on marriage and their parents' place of residence, as well as maintaining the dependence of sisters on their brothers.

The micro-census of 2006/2007 shows how groups continue to understand themselves as distinct. This can be seen in nuptial behaviour and to some extent in the number of children and in parity. Thus, while, on the one hand, groups differ in their nuptial and fertility history, on the other hand, they have adjusted on the whole to what we have earlier called 'a Soviet life course' (Roche and Hohmann 2011). By this we mean that during the Soviet period, schooling was associated with rising age at first marriage, leading to a clear bulge around nineteen years – as is also evident in the even higher percentages displayed by the Kanishbegi (see Figure 3.5). Since Perestroika, nuptial strategies have become more plural and different among the groups, young women getting married earlier, and more women aged above twenty years finding partners.

The Dynamics of Sibling Sets

Table 3.2 shows that more than 85 out of 127 people marry within the group, yet we may wonder why 42 others nonetheless marry externally. Looking at how fathers and mothers choose their children's partner provides necessary clues. The eldest son inherits his father's title and replaces him after his death in most family decisions. However, it is the youngest son who usually stays with his parents, while all other male siblings and their families move out of the family compound after having lived for some years within it. There are, moreover, important patterns characterizing marriage within groups. A sample of eleven youngest and thirteen eldest brothers of thirteen families shows the following results: of the thirteen eldest sons, three married relatives from their mother's side, and five relatives from their father's side; of the eleven youngest sons, four married relatives from the father's side and one from the mother's side. This does not include daughters, who were often exchanged among sisters (i.e. their mothers). In many cases among Qandowi mothers who experienced forced relocation, their eldest sons were married to a relative of the mother.

The eldest son, as the favourite of the mother, is urged to marry as his parents wish. He will later replace the father and take decisions over his siblings. In this sense, the eldest son has the responsibility for reproducing his father's group's interests. The efforts of mothers to marry their eldest son to their own relatives speaks for their active investment in linking that son to their *avlod*, which is in cultural terms the most effective increase of social security for a Tajik woman. The daughter-in-law who will look after her in old age is then a close relative and is more likely to be close to her emotionally.[14] Even if the parents live with the youngest son, the eldest son and his family will keep close relationships with the parents and whenever possible reside nearby. The youngest son has the least choice in conjugal life as his wife will be responsible for practical old age care of the elderly parents. He also needs to reproduce through sons, if necessary through a second wife. Any additional successful sons can only increase the extended family's economic fortunes and social status. While this pattern of inheritance might lead us to assume that most investment should be in the youngest son, this is usually not the case. While the youngest has care responsibility, he will rely on his eldest brother for financial support – and this depends on the eldest brother's emotional tie to his mother. Elderly fathers who lack networks are able to benefit from these arrangements, as the wider social (or kin) group can put pressure on the sons to care for him. He is less vulnerable than his wife, whose kin group may be far distant.

Against the background of these strategies, we can understand why Tajik marriage rules have helped to maintain subgroups while simultaneously allowing them to integrate into a given kolkhoz unit. Statistically we may find a great variation of emic ethnic categories within such units. However, considering the strategy of using children to integrate and reproduce subgroups enables us to understand how a kolkhoz is structured by subgroup adaptations to changing economic, political and social changes.[15] Fertility variation is an important index of this adaptation since it depends more on a son's status within the family than on his ethnic identity. Middle sons may marry outside the group and be happy if their offspring are 'only' daughters, yet eldest and youngest sons cannot. While this can differ amongst families, it is a more widespread pattern among Tajiks.

Sibling marriages result not only from their parents' reproductive decisions, but also incorporate the group's strategy of survival. Sibling marriages are, more generally, indicators of fertility transition. Parents educate their sons as a way of maximizing their security. They do so by emphasizing different educational careers as well as allocating them to specific partners. For instance, parents try to have one son educated in religious knowledge, one in a secular domain (university education and the opportunity to get a state-paid job) and others to be economically productive (trade, construction worker, artisan or work migration). They do not allow all sons the same choice, but keep the eldest and best educated near them (the largest expenses are on this son), while the youngest remains within their household (entailing the lowest level of expenses) to look after them in old age.[16] Middle sons remain relatively free in their educational career as well as in their choice of partner – here we find different strategies, with some families being very strict in choosing the partner and others less so. Within these strategies, middle sons are sometimes more successful and sometimes less so, but without directly affecting their parents' security interests.

The youngest and eldest sons live under the strictest control of parents to the extent that a mother may actually hinder her son from having any intercourse with his wife – i.e. in order to avoid childbearing (this from an interview with a youngest son who lives in Russia, but married a woman back home to provide a household help to his mother). While this is not a standard pattern, Figure 3.8 demonstrates the degree of family control over reproduction. Middle sons are the freest both in terms of choosing partners and in family size. As a mother told me, her eldest son could live with three daughters (without necessarily taking another wife to produce sons),[17] but she could not accept this from her youngest, and so forced him to take a second wife (as the first could have no more children after their two daughters).

Figure 3.8 shows how the dynamics of siblings and their marriages are key to understanding the demographic trajectory of recent Tajik fertility history. While the fertility of middle sons changes most radically along with socioeconomic and political changes, that of eldest and youngest sons appears more resistant to change. Here again the cultural practice of keeping eldest and youngest sons close to the family impacts directly on fertility behaviour. Middle sons, in having the most flexible situation, come to have a fertility history that reflects more general patterns of fertility decline in Central Asia. In other words, they behave as fertility transition theory expects them to do, reducing the size of their families along with socioeconomic changes. As mothers' security depends on the eldest and youngest sons, the changes in these children's fertility histories carry more risk both to their mothers and to the continuity of the subgroup.

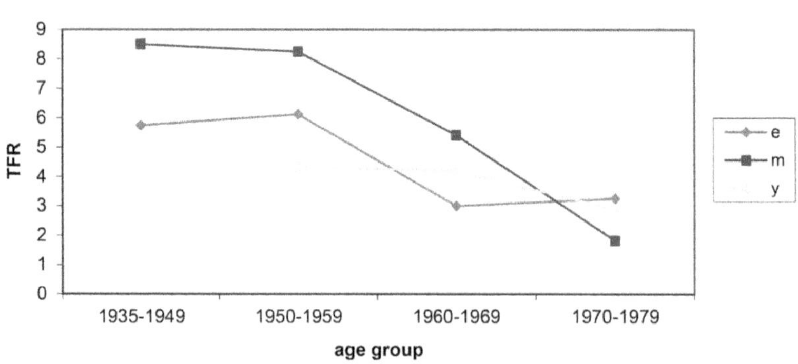

FIGURE 3.8 Total Number of Children to Eldest, Middle and Youngest Sons

While, in all, eldest and youngest siblings may have fewer surviving children than their middle brothers, their parents will make sure that they do not fall below a certain level and will make especially sure that there are male descents.

The study of siblingship and fertility history proves that subgroups can resist demographic changes, and maintain and reproduce themselves by strategically managing sets of siblings. In this way parents can increase their security by making sure that their group is reproduced through male children, while integrating into society by intermarrying middle sons with neighbouring groups. While in practice this model is less rigid than the overall statistical patterns might suggest, ethnographic research clearly supports and explains the statistical trends (Roche 2014).

Between the Laws of Moscow and Local Particularity

Some demographers of the 1980s have tried to capture the opposition between centralized Soviet policies and local variations, their models employing culture (reduced to ethnicity and religion) as a variable or filter rather than as a contextual factor that allows groups to adapt to political, social and economic changes without dissolving. Instead, demographers link high fertility to other factors lying outside the family: an improved healthcare system, a decrease in local conflicts and warfare, and people's responses to the pronatalist politics of the Soviet state. Jones and Grupp (1987: 15–22), for example, use the idea of a 'cultural filter' that integrates only those elements of modernization that are compatible with patriarchal family values. This argument is analogous to other discussions that attempt to identify causal links between Islam and high fertility, an approach trenchantly critiqued by Obermeyer (1992), and rejected statistically by Mazur (1967).[18]

For a long time, demographic developments were viewed in the USSR in economic and military terms, and high fertility was considered a positive marker. It was expected that the family as a factory of cultural production would change along with modernization (i.e. large families giving way gradually to nuclear families). Where this did not happen, abortion would be used to regulate in either direction, its prohibition serving to increase fertility, while implementation would tend to limit fertility not only directly but also via increases in female participation on the labour market. The state approached demographic questions through radical methods in which doctors, for example, would decide the age of a woman and the stage of her pregnancy. Later, doctors were co-opted by the state in a fertility limitation campaign, notably in 1996 in Uzbekistan. Following quotas set by the state, doctors would sterilize women after the second or third child, sometimes without telling the person concerned. If a doctor refused, he or she risked his or her job.[19] Such approaches to family planning, whether supporting or forbidding abortion, forced sterilization, etc., show that medicalization of the female body, not the family as social body, has been the focus of attention and change. Michel Foucault (1997, 2007) has suggested the notion of 'biopower' to capture objectification of the body through political power. Examination of biopolitics reveals which institutions and groups inscribe social processes in individual human bodies for the purpose of better controlling society and groups within it.

While centralized politics were expected to produce one people ('homo sovieticus') differentiated only in some folkloristic traditions, the demographic material presented here indicates different outcomes and thus poses several questions. Obviously, many people in the southern tier did not follow all developments in the same way, despite a similar medicalization of motherhood (i.e. birth in hospitals, uniform techniques and medical treatment all over the Soviet Union, and doctors as collaborators of the state). Despite access to medical treatment and to education for all Tajiks, and the major involvement of women in the labour force, fertility remained high among certain groups far into the 1980s. In this chapter we have argued that such significant differences in demographic development were possible due to subgroups' strategies to reproduce as a group rather than to assimilate into a national or ethnic macro-group. The main groups in Tajik society have been described previously as patronage networks and clan groups (e.g., Collins 2006; Kılavuz 2009) or ethnoregional groups (e.g., Bushkov 1993; Jean and Mullojanov 2008; Ferrando 2011). However, reliance on ethnicity and networks captures only some aspects of group behaviour (Heathershaw 2009); a network is at best an incomplete guide to group identities and their maintenance, which require analysis of demographic developments.

The focus on siblingship has enabled a new approach to group reproduction within the context of the Soviet Union. While laws and normative rules were similar throughout the republics, local groups in Tajikistan successfully resisted the fertility transition that occurred in the north. While these groups have experienced a transition more recently, this has occurred most radically in the families of middle sons, while eldest and youngest family members remain under parental control. The latter members have fewer children than their middle siblings and a more constant fertility history, as their families remain under the close surveillance of parents who keep fertility independent of external forces.

Acknowledgements

We thank all the persons who supported the fieldwork of Sophie Hohmann (INED, Paris) and Sophie Roche in Tajikistan. This chapter has profited particularly from research undertaken in 2006 and 2007, financed by the Max Planck Institute for Social Anthropology, Halle. We thank Philip Kreager for the opportunity to present the material and his solid support in editing and improving the chapter.

Sophie Roche currently leads the junior research group 'The Demographic Turn in the Junction of Cultures' at the Cluster of Excellence 'Asia and Europe in a Global Context' at the University of Heidelberg. She is the author of *Domesticating Youth: Youth Bulges and their Socio-Political Implications in Tajikistan* (Berghahn Books, 2014).

Sophie Hohmann is Lecturer in the Department of Eurasian Studies at the French Institute for Oriental Studies (INALCO); she is also Associate Researcher at the Centre for Russian, Caucasian and East-European Studies (CERCEC, EHESS/CNRS) in Paris. She holds a Ph.D. in social sciences from the EHESS (School of Advanced Studies in Social Sciences) in Paris.

Notes

1. 'Homo-sovieticus' is a concept articulated at the party level, integrating the state and society (Lefort 1979, 1999, 2008).
2. For an overview of Russian health politics in Turkestan, see Hohmann (2009).
3. Kamp (2006); Northrop (2007). See also Part 3, 'Gender', of the collected volume by Sahadeo and Zanca (2007).
4. For more information on this period in Tajikistan, see Roche (2014).
5. According to Turner (1993: 141), the TFR for Tajikistan rose from 3.8 births per woman in 1959 to 6.3 in 1976.

6. In the era between the first forced relocation campaigns in 1925/1926 and 1941, about 48,700 farmers' households (*dehqon*) were moved to the southern Vakhsh valley (Ro'i 2000: note 4).
7. In other words, the destruction of large family networks and development of nuclear families in which both partners participate in labour production.
8. Even today, each village is proud of reproducing its own tradition in which differences serve as markers of group identity.
9. According Harwin (1996: 40), child benefits were 50 rubles for the first and 100 rubles for the second and third children. Moreover, Jones and Grupp (1987: 276) add that nonworking mothers received 30 rubles each for the birth of their first, second and third children. Moreover, new birth payments were introduced into the southern territories in 1983: for the fourth child, the family received a one-time payment of 65 rubles, and for the fifth child, 85 rubles. Monthly payments of 4 rubles per child were given to the family after the birth of the fourth child, which became 6 rubles after the birth of the fifth child; these payments went on until a child attained the age of five years (Jones and Grupp 1987: 273).
10. See the discussion on the 25th and the 26th Party Congress in 1976 and 1981, respectively. Earlier discussion that treated 'Slavic' and 'Muslim' populations in opposition to each other was perceived as discriminatory in the latter Congress, and measures taken to regulate fertility eventually varied little among the regions (Weber and Goodman 1981).
11. However, this may have been due to the fact that women remained members of their kolkhoz even if they only participated in it seasonally or for a few hours per week.
12. Jones and Grupp (1987: 275) mention that, depending on the economic value of the payments, the support given could be quite substantial for the families concerned. Extremely poor families considered them a welcome supplement, but they did not provide an incentive to women who were employed and sufficiently well-off.
13. Turner (1993: 142) remarks that the lowest proportion of women practising fertility control is among Tajiks (14–18 per cent).
14. In one family, a sister emphasized that her eldest brother had been forced by his mother to marry a Tajik on the basis that he must reproduce for the Tajik group. The family referred to themselves as Qandowi and the brother produced nine children, of which five died. The sister, in contrast, married outside the group, divorced three times and eventually lived with a Mestni.
15. This argument of integration through difference has been developed as a general theory by Günther Schlee (2001, 2008).
16. In cases where the youngest son married externally, for instance, to a local Uzbek, he moved out of the parental house and another brother accepted the parents' choice that he stay.

17. After a university education, the eldest son remained in the capital, Dushanbe, and thus broke with the tradition of staying close to the mother. However, he continued to care for the parents and remained the head of the siblings – no decision would be taken without him.
18. For a discussion on Islam and demography, see also Harris (2002).
19. This information was collected by Sophie Hohmann in Uzbekistan during a field study in 2004.

References

Abashin, S.N. 1999. 'Statistika kak instrument etnografi cheskogo issledovaniya: Uzbekskaya sem'ya v XX v' ['Statistics as a Means of Ethnographic Research: The Uzbek Family in the Twentieth Century'], *Etnografi cheskoe Obozrenie* 1: 3–16.

———. 2007. *Die Sartenproblematik in der russischen Geschichtsschreibung des 19. und des ersten Viertels des 20. Jahrhunderts*. Berlin: Klaus Schwarz.

Abdulaev, R.A. 2002. 'Reshenie problemy bezhentsev i vynuzhdennykh pereselentsev Tadzhikistana 90gg. XX v' ['Solving the Problem of Refugees and Internally Displaced Persons from Tajikistan in the 1990s'], *Vestnik universiteta* 3: 16–42.

Agadjanian, V., and E. Makarova 2003, 'Former Soviet Modernization to Post-Soviet Transformation: Understanding Marriage and Fertility Dynamics in Uzbekistan', *Development and Change* 34(3): 447–73.

Arel, D. 2002. 'Language Categories in Censuses: Backward- or Forward-Looking?', in D.I. Kertzer and D. Arel (eds), *Census and Identity: The Politics of Race, Ethnicity and Language in National Censuses*. Cambridge: Cambridge University Press, pp. 92–120.

Baldauf, I. 2007. 'Tradition, Revolution, Adaptation: Die kulturelle Sowjetisierung Zentralasiens', in M. Sapper, V. Weichsel and A. Huterer (eds), *Machtmosaik Zentralasien*. Berlin: Bundeszentrale für politische Bildung, pp. 99–120.

Barbieri, M., A. Blum, E. Dolgikh and A. Ergashev 1995. *La transition de fécondité en Ouzbékistan*, Dossiers et recherches 44. Paris: INED, Tachkent : Comité ouzbek de la prévision et de la statistique; Moscow: Département de démographie de l'Institut de la prévision économique.

———. 1996. 'Nuptiality, Fertility, Use of Contraception, and Family Policies in Uzbekistan', *Population Studies* 50: 69–88.

Blum, A. 1987. 'La transition démographique dans les républiques orientales d'URSS', *Population* 2: 337–58.

———. 1994. *Naître, vivre et mourir en URSS 1917–1991*. Paris: Plon.

Bushkov, V.I. 1993. 'Tadschikistan vor dem Bürgerkrieg: Eine traditionelle Gesellschaft in der Krise', *Berichte des Bundesinstituts für Orientwissenschafliche und Internationale Studien* 26, Cologne: Das Institut.

Bushkov, V.I., and D.V. Mikul'skij. 1996. *Anatomiya grazhdanskoy voyny v Tadzhikistane (ethno-sotsial'nye Protsessy i politicheskaya bor'ba 1992–1995).* [*Anatomy of the Civil War in Tajikistan (Ethno-social Processes and Political Struggle 1992–1995)*]. Moscow: Institut ethnologii i antropologii RAN; Institute Prakticheskogo Vostokovedeniya.

Collins, K. 2006. *Clan Politics and Regime Transition in Central Asia.* Cambridge: Cambridge University Press.

Conte, E., and S. Walentowitz 2009. 'Kinship Matters: Tribals, Cousins, and Citizens in Southwest Asia and Beyond. *Études rurales* 184: 217–48.

Creed, G.W. 1998. *Domesticating Revolution: From Socialist Reform to Ambivalent Transition in a Bulgarian Village.* Pennsylvania: Pennsylvania State University Press.

Dudoignon, S.A. 1994. 'Une segmentation peut en cacher une autre: Régionalismes et clivage politico-économiques au Tadjikistan', *Cahier d'Études sur la Méditerranée Orientale et le Monde Turco-Iranien* 18: 73–130.

Dudoignon, S.A., and C. Noak (eds). 2013. *Allah's Kolkhozes: Migration, De-Stalinisation, Privatisation and the Revivals of Rural Islam in the Soviet Realm (1950s–2000s).* Berlin: Klaus Schwarz.

Ferrando, O. 2011. 'Soviet Population Transfers and Interethnic Relations in Tajikistan. Assessing the Concept of Ethnicity', *Central Asian Survey* 30(1): 39–52.

Finke, P., and M. Sancak 2012. 'To Be an Uzbek or Not to Be a Tajik? Ethnicity and Locality in the Bukhara Oasis', *Zeitschrift für Ethnologie* 137(1): 47–70.

Foucault, M. 1997. *Il faut défendre la société.* Paris: Gallimard.

———. 2007. *Naissance de la biopolitique.* Paris: Gallimard.

Harris, C. 2002. 'Muslim Views on Population: The Case of Tajikistan', in J. Meuleman (ed.), *Islam in the Era of Globalization: Muslim Attitudes towards Modernity and Identity.* London: Routledge, pp. 211–22.

———. 2004. *Control and Subversion: Gender Relations in Tajikistan.* London: Pluto Press.

Harwin, J. 1996. *Children of the Russian State: 1917–1995.* Aldershot: Avebury.

Heathershaw, J. 2009. *Post-conflict Tajikistan: The Politics of Peacebuilding and the Emergence of Legitimate Order.* London: Routledge.

Hohmann, S. 2009. 'La médecine moderne au Turkestan russe: Un outil au service de la politique coloniale', *Cahiers d'Asie Centrale* 17/18: 319–51.

Hohmann, S., S. Roche and M. Garenne 2010. 'The Changing Sex Ratios at Birth during the Civil War in Tajikistan: 1992–1997', *Journal of Biosocial Science* 42(6): 773–86.

Islamov, S.I. 1988. 'Divorce in Tajikistan', *Soviet Union Sociological Studies* 6: 108–10.

Ismailbekova, A. 2011. 'The Native Son in Rural Kyrgyzstan: Democracy, Kinship, and Patronage', Ph.D. dissertation. Halle-Wittenberg: Martin-Luther-University of Halle-Wittenberg.

Jean, I., and P. Mullojanov 2008. *Reflecting on Peace Practice Project: Conflict and PeaceBuilding in Tajikistan*. Cambridge: Collaborative Learning Projects.

Jones, E., and F. Grupp 1987. *Modernization, Value Change and Fertility in the Soviet Union: Soviet and East European Studies*. Cambridge: Cambridge University Press.

Kamp. M. 2006. *The New Woman in Uzbekistan: Islam, Modernity, and Unveiling under Communism*. Seattle: University of Washington Press.

Khan, A.R., and D. Ghai. 1979. *Collective Agriculture and Rural Development in Soviet Central Asia*. London: Macmillan.

Kılavuz, I.T. 2009. 'The Role of Networks in Tajikistan's Civil War: Network Activation and Violence Specialists', *Nationalities Papers* 37(5): 693–717.

Krader, L. 1971. *Peoples of Central Asia*. Bloomington: Indiana University Press.

Kuniansky, A.S. 1981. 'Fertility and Labor Force in USSR. Theories and Models', Ph.D dissertation. Houston: University of Houston.

Laruelle, M. 2013. *Migration and Social Upheaval as the Face of Globalization in Central Asia*. Leiden: Brill.

Lefort, C. 1979, 'Le stalinisme sans Staline', in C. Lefort (ed.), *Éléments d'une critique de la bureaucratie*. Paris: Gallimard, pp. 155–235.

———. 1999. *La complication: Retour sur le communisme*. Paris: Fayard.

———. 2008 [1981]. *L'invention démocratique*. Paris: Fayard.

Loy, T. 2005. *Jaghnob 1970: Erinnerungen an eine Zwangsumsiedlung in der Tadschikischen SSR*. Wiesbaden: Reichert.

Lublin, N. 1991. 'Implications of Ethnic and Demographic Trends', in W. Fierman (ed.), *Soviet Central Asia: The Failed Transformation*. Oxford: Westview, pp. 36–61.

Mazur, P. 1967. 'Fertility among Ethnic Groups in the U.S.S.R.', *Demography* 4: 172–95.

Mühlfried, F., and S. Sokolovskiy 2011. *Exploring the Edge of Empire: Soviet Era Anthropology in the Caucasus and Central Asia*. Berlin: Lit.

Northrop, D. 2007. 'The Limits of Liberation: Gender, Revolution, and the Veil in Everyday Life in Soviet Uzbekistan', in J. Sahadeo and R. Zanca (eds), *Everyday Life in Central Asia. Past and Present*. Bloomington: Indiana University Press, pp. 89–102

Obermeyer, C.M. 1992. 'Islam, Women, and Politics: The Demography of Arab Countries', *Population and Development Review* 18: 33–60.

Roche, S. 2014. *Domesticating Youth: The Dynamics of Youth Bulge in Tajikistan*. Oxford: Berghahn Books.

Roche, S., and S. Hohmann 2011. 'Wedding Rituals and the Struggle over National Identities', *Central Asian Survey* 30(1): 113–28.

Ro'i, Y. 2000. *Islam in the Soviet Union: From the Second World War to Gorbachev*. New York: Columbia University Press.

Roy, O. 2000. *The New Central Asia: The Creation of Nations*. London: I.B. Tauris.

Rzehak, L. 2001. *Vom Persischen zum Tadschikischen: Sprachliches Handeln und Sprachplanung in Transoxanien zwischen Tradition, Moderne und Sowjetmacht (1900–1956)*. Wiesbaden: Reichert.

Sahadeo, J., and R. Zanca (eds). 2007. *Everyday Life in Central Asia: Past and Present*. Bloomington: Indiana University Press.

Schlee, G. 2001. 'Einleitung', in A. Horstmann and G. Schlee (eds), *Integration durch Verschiedenheit: Lokale und globale Formen interkultureller Kommunikation*. Bielefeld: Trascript.

———. 2008. *How Enemies are Made: Towards a Theory of Ethnic and Religious Conflicts*. Oxford: Berghahn Books.

Singh, S., and J. Casterline 1985. 'Socioeconomic Determinants', in J. Cleland and J. Hobcraft (eds), *Reproductive Change in Developing Countries*. Oxford: Oxford University Press, pp. 199–222.

Solomon, G.S. 1990. 'The Limits of Government Patronage of Science: Social Hygiene and the Soviet State, 1920–1930', *Social History of Medicine* 12(3): 405–35.

Tett, G. 1995. 'Guardians of the Faith? Gender and Religion in an (ex) Soviet Tajik Village', in C.F. El-Solh and J. Mabro (eds), *Muslim Women's Choices: Religious Belief and Social Reality*. Oxford: Berg, pp. 128–51.

Turner, R. 1993. 'Tajiks Have the Highest Fertility Rates in Newly Independent Central Asia', *Family Planning Perspectives* 35(3): 141–42.

Van de Walle, E., and J. Knodel 1980. 'Europe's Fertility Transition: New Evidence and Lessons for Today's Developing World', *Population Bulletin* 34(6): 3–44.

Weber, C., and A. Goodman 1981. 'The Demographic Policy Debate in the USSR', *Population and Development Review* 7: 279–95.

Werth, N. 2009. *L'ivrogne et la marchande de fleurs, Autopsie d'un meutre de masse 1937–1938*. Paris: Tallandier.

Winter, J.M. 1992. 'War, Family, and Fertility in Twentieth-Century Europe', in J.R. Gills (ed.), *The European Experience of Declining Fertility, 1850–1970: The Quiet Revolution*. Oxford: Blackwell, pp. 291–309.

Chapter 4

FEELING SECURE TO REPRODUCE

ECONOMY, COMMUNITY AND FERTILITY IN SOUTHERN EUROPE

Patrick Heady

Introduction

One of the great merits of ethnographic fieldwork is that it allows us to investigate particular realities, enabling us to achieve a deeper understanding of local developments than could be obtained from statistical data on general trends. This applies to studies of demographic issues as much as to any other theme of anthropological investigation. In-depth studies of special subpopulations can identify the often complex reasons why their demographic behaviour departs from the average pattern for the population as a whole.

But what happens when the demographic behaviour of a special population is not exceptional? For instance, the developments that have happened there might be typical of similar populations in the same country – or even in a wider multinational region. Does this mean that ethnographic methods have nothing useful to tell us? In this chapter I argue that, on the contrary, ethnographic studies of typical demographic developments are particularly valuable. By generating insights that could not be accessed by standardized demographic surveys, they enable us to query the assumptions on which general theories are built, and to identify alternative and possibly more realistic explanations. Implicitly they raise questions about the relationship between interpretive insight and statistical reasoning to which I will return below. First, however, I should like to introduce my own field site and some of the questions that it raised.

The Privatization of Social Life

When I arrived in 1989 to start fieldwork in a valley in Carnia, in northeast Italy, local people told me that life had recently undergone a great change. In the old days (the expression they used was *una volta*), people used to help each other (*a si davasi una man*),[1] but nowadays everyone looked after their own affairs (*ognuno va per conto suo*), the old *allegria*, a word that conveys the idea of publicly shared joyfulness, had disappeared, and even the bars – a locus of all-male sociability – which used to be full every evening were now almost empty (Heady 1999).

This was their way of talking about a shift to private and family-based sociability that occurred between 1960 and 1990 across much of southern Europe. In order to give a more general picture, I will also refer to ethnographic accounts of three other field sites:

— Loizos' (1981: 11–49) description of the Cypriot village of Argaki in the late 1960s and early 1970s, where the traditional pattern of sociability was still largely intact, though some people were starting to opt out;
— the Aragonese village of Belmonte,[2] where Lisón Tolosana (2004: 143–57) reported a transformation that occurred between 1960 and 1975;
— the Andalucian village of Los Olivos, where Collier (1997) discusses the change that took place between her first visit in the mid 1960s and her return in the early 1980s.

The latter two were Spanish field sites where the same ethnographer was present before and after the change took place. There are of course some differences in these accounts, but all would agree that before the transformation, the village bars were the centre of most men's social life, there were rituals that emphasized the unity and distinctness of each particular village, and both men and women paid great attention to the expectations of older people and of the village community as a whole. After the transformation, all these features were much less marked. This decline in intravillage social life was accompanied by some geographical widening of social networks, including marriage ties.

TABLE 4.1 Estimated Fertility Levels, Ovasta and Ovaro (1991)

	Children 0–9	Women 25–34	Children per woman	Source
Ovasta 1991	13	13	*1.00*	Own interviews
Ovaro 1991	174	158	*1.10*	ISTAT census figures

The Onset of Ultra-low Fertility

There was another major change that figured prominently in my early conversations in the valley. Over the previous few years, deaths had greatly outnumbered births – something that local people could hardly fail to notice, given the practice of advertising births with coloured rosettes on household doors and of plastering funeral announcements on walls and local notice boards. The shortfall of births was partly due to a tendency for young adults to leave the valley, but the main reason was the low birth rate amongst the women who remained.

Table 4.1 gives figures for the *comune* of Ovaro and for the village of Ovasta (one of the *frazioni* of Ovaro) on which I concentrated during my fieldwork in Carnia. The table uses the ratio of children aged less than ten to women aged 25–34 inclusive to provide an approximate estimate of the lifetime fertility of local women. The results suggest that the local birth rate during the 1980s had fallen to little more than one child per woman – scarcely more than half the level needed to replace the population in each generation.

Extreme though they may seem, figures like these could have been replicated, at much the same time, in many parts of southern Europe (Frejka and Calot 2001).

Possible Links between Changed Patterns of Social Interaction and Ultra-low Fertility

We thus have two phenomena – a change in social behaviour closely followed by the onset of ultra-low fertility – that occurred together in Carnia and that also seem to have occurred at much the same time in other parts of southern Europe. This raises the question of whether the change in social behaviour helped to cause the fall in fertility – in Carnia itself and also over the region as a whole.

The purpose of this chapter is to examine possible answers to this question by looking simultaneously at two kinds of evidence – ethnographic evidence relating to Carnia and other field sites, and comparative statistical evidence relating to Europe as a whole. The attempt to combine the two kinds of evidence raises a number of methodological questions. Two important issues are, first, whether there are certain phenomena that are best captured by one method rather than the other and, second, how and when the two kinds of data can be validly linked into a single overarching explanatory account. I will return to these questions at the end of the chapter, but in the meantime the following points are worth bearing in mind. Local findings are most likely to be useful if the localities in question are typical in relevant ways – and relevance itself depends on the question being asked and on the theoretical framework that gives each question its point.

Theories of Economy, Sociability and Fertility Levels

From Economy to Social Relationships

Before discussing the possible impact of social changes on fertility levels, there is another question to be asked – namely what precipitated the changes in social interactions described above? As it happens, this is something on which the Carnians themselves have very clear ideas. In their view, social relationships had deteriorated because of *benessere* – the prosperity that had accompanied the shift from agriculture to other occupations, which meant that people no longer had to rely on each other for the practical needs of life.

Until the early 1970s, Ovasta's economy, like that of many other Carnian villages, was based on a combination of seasonal emigration by young and middle-aged men, with small-scale cultivation and dairy farming carried out by women, adolescents and the older men. The village-level production system called for both mutual forbearance and for a substantial amount of active cooperation: formally, in maintaining paths, managing the village woods and the collective dairy; and informally in a readiness to lend each other a hand in the minor emergencies that can arise from changeable mountain weather.

It was a physically and mentally demanding way of life. So when, as a result of Italy's economic progress during the postwar years, well-paid factory and office jobs became available down in the north Italian plain and also, though less plentifully, in Carnia itself, most people took the opportunity to improve their living standards by switching to less strenuous jobs as employees in the new economic sectors. The previous economic system went into gradual decline during the second half of the twentieth century, with a particular crisis occurring during the late 1960s and early 1970s. In Ovaro *comune* a 30 per cent decline in cattle numbers between 1950 and 1970 was followed by a fall of about 40 per cent during the 1970s themselves. In Ovasta the early 1970s saw the end of cheese-making operations by the village dairy as well as the end of seasonal emigration by young men. Between 1961 and 1971, permanent emigration from the valley reduced Ovaro's human population by 21 per cent, continuing at a slower pace during the 1970s and 1980s – and generating a sense of local decline that made the subsequent impact of falling fertility appear particularly severe.

The accounts from the other three field sites agree on the origin of the social changes. In Belmonte and los Olivos, as in Carnia, these changes coincided with a collapse in the local agricultural economy caused by the new possibilities of earning much higher incomes in factory and office work. Argaki was the exception that proved the rule: at the time Loizos was there, agriculture was booming, while the minority who were starting to reject collective sociability were people who had used their education to find nonagricultural work. So in this respect, as well, the Carnian experience appears to correspond to that of rural areas in other parts of southern Europe.

From Social Relationships to Fertility

It is now time to consider the consequences of these shared social changes. Among the various explanations proposed for the European demographic transitions, there are three theoretical approaches that highlight the role of social relationships.

The first approach, advocated by Lesthaeghe and colleagues, relates the decline of fertility to changes in social values as a result of economic change (Lesthaeghe and Wilson 1986). The argument is rooted in a tradition of modernization theory that goes back to Tönnies (1887) and Durkheim (1992 [1888]). The central idea is that agricultural communities are characterized by close social ties to kin and neighbours, and a shared value orientation that emphasizes the physical perpetuation of the community itself. A commitment to at least replacement fertility is part of this overall worldview. Economic modernization loosens these traditional ties, leading to the development of more individualistic values. For people whose values emphasize individual self-determination, parenthood appears as merely one among many possible lifestyle choices – and their pursuit of alternative goals leads to subreplacement fertility.

This argument is consistent with economic developments in southern Europe during the second half of the twentieth century, during which many parts of the region experienced the move out of agriculture and the rise in education levels and service employment, which have been associated with demographic transition in many parts of the world. It is also consistent with the move from collective to privately based social life reported in our field sites – and with some of the things that local people say about the change in social behaviour. Some inhabitants of Los Olivos attribute the change to a newfound tendency to think for themselves (Collier 1997: 3–6), while the Carnian complaint, that everyone now prioritizes their own affairs (which was echoed by other inhabitants of Los Olivos (Collier 1997: 5)), makes the same point in a less appreciative way.

While Lesthaeghe's version of modernization theory draws on psychological theories of individual fulfilment,[3] the 'kin influence theory', proposed by Newson, offers an alternative account of the social and psychological processes involved (Newson et al. 2007; Newson and Richerson 2009). Newson draws on evolutionary theory to suggest that close relatives are likely to encourage potential parents to have more children, whereas nonrelatives are likely to be indifferent – with the result that the closer the contacts between relatives, the more support there is likely to be for profertility social norms. A corollary of this is that the wider the social reference group and the smaller the proportion of close relatives that it contains, the weaker the encouragement for fertility is likely to be. Newson notes that economic development typically widens the spatial range of social interactions (Watkins 1990) and argues that it also increases the range of social contacts in other ways. Given the increased range of social contacts, the predictions for fertility are the same as those produced by Lesthaeghe's theory.

Newson's hypothesis of widening social networks is borne out by the ethnographic data. In Carnia and Belmonte the move out of agriculture was accompanied by a spatial widening of the social field from which marriage partners were chosen. Collier reports that in Los Olivos, people's sense of local identity had changed – from one that opposed their own village to neighbouring villages, to one in which their own village was seen as a source of connections to the region as a whole.

However, although both Lesthaeghe's version of modernization theory and Newson's kin influence theory are consistent with what we know about the direction of social change, they face a common difficulty when it comes to linking these social changes to the changes in fertility that have occurred in southern Europe. The problem is that, although the social relationships highlighted by these theories have changed in the required direction, the changes have not been very great when viewed in comparative terms.

In Carnia, the inhabitants of Ovasta may well be more individualistic than they once were, but many still live in three-generation households (Heady 1999: 28), suggesting that the traditional extended-family model remains strong. Similarly, although the geographical range of Ovasta's marriage field had extended, local ties remained extremely important: in 1991, everyone living in Ovasta had either been born into an Ovastan family or had married into one.

Statistics tell the same story. Even after the social changes, comparative survey data shows that people in the south of Europe interact with their relatives far more than people in the north (Murphy 2008; Kohli et al. 2010). The same is true of other indicators of attachment to, or individualistic detachment from, traditional family values – such as divorce rates, births to unmarried mothers (Billari and Kohler 2004) and the tendency to live alone (Gruber and Heady 2010a). This picture of rather limited change is confirmed by Italian statistics on residential patterns in the second half of the twentieth century. Although the proportion of couples living *with* the parents of one partner has sharply declined, this change has been almost balanced by a corresponding increase in the proportion of couples living *near to* the parents of one or other partner (Viazzo and Zanotelli 2010: 75). In terms of a continuum from individualism to familism, southern Europe remains a good deal nearer the familistic end than do the countries of northwest Europe.

Given this moderate decline in commitment to family ties, both Lesthaeghe's and Newson's theories would predict a moderate decline in the birth rate, but not the exceptionally deep declines that actually occurred. By the end of the twentieth century, southern European birth rates had fallen so much that fertility was lower in the statistically familistic south than in the statistically more individualistic countries of northern Europe (Billari and Kohler 2004). It was in an attempt to explain this paradox that Dalla Zuanna (2001) put forward the third theory that I want to consider here.

Dalla Zuanna argued that the concern in traditionally familistic societies was not simply with the number of children that could be brought into the world, but with meeting the ideals of successful parenthood. These ideals involve producing children, but also caring for them and providing for their future – and in modern economic conditions, according to Dalla Zuanna, this can best be done by restricting the number of children in order to provide both high material living standards and a good professional education. Meeting these standards is important not just for personal wellbeing, but also because of their impact on the family's social status. To use the well-known term from Mediterranean anthropology, it is a question of the family's honour and, although Dalla Zuanna himself does not describe the social processes concerned, involves being judged by one's neighbours and social equals. Krause's (2005) ethnography of parenthood in Tuscany in the mid 1990s documents the intense pressures on young mothers to meet the appropriate standards.[4]

Despite this ethnographic support, Dalla Zuanna's argument does face some difficulties. In particular there is no real explanation of why, if materially competitive familism is severely limiting fertility now, it did not have such a major effect before. Nevertheless, the argument has been well received because it seems to many readers (including the present author) to capture something important about southern European attitudes to parenthood. It is also interesting because it suggests that, even in the past, social attitudes were not simply and straightforwardly pro-fertility – but rather that there were a number of potentially opposed attitudes to fertility, which might be affected by economic change in different ways.

To sum up this stage of the discussion: we have three existing theories that all say something useful about the connection between social relationships and fertility, but none of which is complete. In the next section I will draw on ethnographic data to provide a fuller description of the conflicting social pressures that encouraged and discouraged fertility in Mediterranean Europe before the main impact of economic change.

Fertility and Social Pressure in Traditional Mediterranean Society

At one level, these were indeed societies that encouraged fertility. Parenthood was the mark of successful adulthood, and seeing one's children married and parents themselves was the sign that one had completed a satisfactory life (Loizos 1981). This held not just for individuals and families but also for the community as a whole. In many parts of southern Europe, annual rituals celebrated the renewal of village life through the coming of age of new cohorts – and marked their readiness to start courtship. In Carnia itself, another ritual placed the collectivity of village adults in a quasi-parental relationship to all the village children (Heady 2003). So at the level of official ideas and rituals, the members of these societies espoused the value of fertility and encouraged each other to pursue it – just as Lesthaeghe and Newson would expect.

But this is only part of the picture. A *leitmotif* of Mediterranean anthropology has been the contrast between two levels of social reality – an overt level of unity and cooperation and a covert level of conflict and rivalry (Loizos 1981; Heady 1999; Just 2000), much of which is pursued by way of social pressure and the politics of reputation (Bailey 1971). Reproductive matters are a particular focus of this sense of envious rivalry. Families scheme against each other to arrange the best marriages for their own children, and women feel that their own success as lovers, and later as mothers, is threatened by the spiritual power of other women's envy and by the social consequences of spiteful gossip (Cole 1991: 114–24; Stewart 1991: 232–37; Heady 1999: 78–81).

All in all, it could be said that while everyone is in favour of fertility in general, when it comes to particulars, they favour their own fertility and discourage the family-building efforts of their neighbours and rivals. This is quite a long way from the picture painted by Lesthaeghe and Newson, but it is still some way from the materialistic familism posited by Dalla Zuanna. The question for theorists, but also for local people themselves, is how to handle the tensions surrounding reproduction so that they do not disrupt the social life of the community as a whole.

One way in which this can be done is by emphasizing the aspects of life in which the villagers do share common interests – for instance, in practical economic cooperation or in the staging of religious and secular rituals that themselves call for active commitment and cooperation. Another way is by segregating the – usually male – sphere of public sociability from the private sphere in which both men and women see themselves as members of a particular family, pursuing its own interests in opposition to the manoeuvres of rival families. Readers will recognize in this some of the main features of the traditional pattern of sociability described at the start of this chapter.

Another way is to place controls on the pattern of marriage and reproduction, ensuring that it conforms to socially acceptable rules. This can involve the formation of the couple: births outside marriage were strongly disapproved in most Mediterranean societies. It can also involve the provision of an adequate material base – as when, in Los Olivos, the parents of a new couple would invite the village as a whole to inspect the new home and furnishings they had provided. More subjectively, it could involve the sense of inner security felt by a young couple who knew that they could meet the required standards and so be sure of support from the community at large. At the same time, the possession of wealth and the consciousness of a certain inner toughness might also enable young couples to feel, at least partially, independent of the pressure of local opinion.

In these respects, traditional arrangements do come close to Dalla Zuanna's and Krause's depiction of competitive materialistc familism – placing it in the context of a dialectic of rivalry and mutual support. In the next section I will look more closely at some of the underlying principles involved.

A Theory of Fertility and Social Pressure

A full account of the impact of social pressure on fertility needs to take account of three things: the need for psychological security; the sources of psychological threat; and the sources of psychological support. This section will tackle these three points in turn.

Feeling Secure to Reproduce

One source of insight into the psychological preconditions for motherhood is provided by the images of family life that mothers-to-be seek out for themselves. In this connection it is worth citing a recent study of the images presented in Spanish magazines for mothers-to-be. Fernandez (2013) describes one of the images thus:

> This image is the classic representation of the nuclear family as a perfect image of wellness, happiness, beauty, health, success, security, affection and protection. This image have [*sic*] also some aspects related to life course (age, purchasing power, couple conventions, etc.). And aspects of the links and their importance in the conduct or happiness of people: love, attachment, protection, security, etc.

Similar images could probably be found in comparable magazines all over the world. And since no one forces women to buy magazines of this kind, it is likely that the imagery corresponds to what the editorial team have found makes their magazine attractive to potential purchasers – by reflecting the emotional needs of mothers-to-be. If so, three key points stand out: the life of the new nuclear family is represented as good in itself; they have the economic means to support it; and the mother can feel free from outside threats. Condensing the message still further, the mother can be sure that her parenthood will be welcomed and that she has the material and psychological resources to manage, even if it is not.

This need for security creates the possibility for women's fertility choices to be open to social influence. There are also theoretical reasons why we should expect this to be so. Newson cites one of them when setting out the basis of the 'kin influence' theory. Newson's argument is rooted in evolutionary theory. Her starting point is Boyd and Richerson's (2005) argument that, because culture is central to human adaptation, we as a species have evolved to learn from other people as well as from experience. This is the evolutionary basis of our susceptibility to influence and it underlies social as well as technical learning. This openness to influence is adaptive for individuals because without it, they could not participate effectively in the human division of labour.

Newson's argument is that a general susceptibility to influence would also apply to decisions affecting fertility. A second approach from evolutionary theory focuses specifically on reproduction. Hrdy (2009) notes that humans are 'cooperative breeders', inasmuch as mothers depend on the cooperation of many other individuals in rearing and providing for their young. She also notes that cooperative breeding is not just about cooperation – a good deal of competition and coercion goes on as well. The competition is for social positions that provide the opportunity of reproduction, while the coercion is often necessary to ensure that the individuals assigned the role of helping actually do provide the required help. This is not to deny that genuine altruism also plays a role, but that role is only one part of a more complex story (Hrdy 2009: 175–208).

Within the context of this overall story, there is an important difference between Newson and Hrdy regarding the extent of encouragement one expects from close relatives. Newson argues, in line with the early writing of Hamilton (1963), that close kin will assist each other to reproduce (in this context by encouragement and positive social pressure). This is the basis of her argument that a high proportion of relatives in the social network will have a positive influence on fertility. However, a later article by Hamilton[5] on 'selfishness and spite in an evolutionary model' (1970) suggests that this need not be the case. The key point of this article – which is consistent with much of the evidence that Hrdy presents – is that, within an ongoing group interaction, the long-term reproductive success ('inclusive fitness') of any individual depends on ensuring that the members of the group to whom she is most closely related (including of course herself) have the highest chances of reproduction. This can be achieved in two ways: by helping those to whom she is most closely related, but also by obstructing those to whom she is less closely related (which is what Hamilton (1970) means by 'selfishness and spite', and what in our context would be active discouragement and negative social pressure). For selfishness and spite to make evolutionary sense, it is not necessary for the victims to be unrelated to the aggressor – they simply have to be less closely related than the people she is trying to benefit. As such, kin-dense networks offer no automatic protection against selfish and spiteful discouragement of the kinds documented in Mediterranean ethnography.

The coercion in animal species of cooperative breeders – both in competition for the right to breed and in ensuring that helpers actually do deliver – is frequently very brutal. This is where the human openness to influence (stressed by Boyd, Richerson and Newson) comes in. In human societies, physical coercion, although not totally absent, generally remains in the background. Humans can obtain similar results using language and other subtle signals to convey emotional pressure and rewards. This is surely the source of some of the key features of the ethnographic reports cited above: pressure and disapproval to discourage rival families from reproducing, and respect, good fellowship and public celebrations as rewards for those who play their parts fully in the cooperative economic activity that underlies the reproductive success of the community as a whole.

Within this general framework, we can understand the varying levels of reproductive conflict by looking at the practical situation – the degree to which, simply by reproducing, different members of the same community are competing for the same limited pool of resources. And we also need to consider the practical and social resources on which individuals and the community at large can draw to soften the resulting conflicts.

The Source of Threat: Endogamy and the Intensity of Reproductive Conflict

Children in traditional Mediterranean societies were generally fed, clothed and looked after by their own parents and other close relatives – and therefore provided no immediate drain on the resources of the rest of the community. However, over the long term, they did provide a threat in that, by growing up and remaining in the same community, they would compete with the children of other families for the use of the community's common resources. These might include common pastures and other items that were formally designated as collective property. Yet, these are not the only – or even the most important – resources for which the village's future inhabitants will be competing. To understand what is at stake, we need to consider the implications of local marriage patterns. Several Mediterranean village ethnographies provide systematic information about the geographical origin of marriage partners (e.g. Christian 1989: 41; Ott 1993: 51; Heady 1999: 131; Just 2000: 110–12). Until the last few decades, the results showed a characteristic pattern. Though kin ties extended very widely (even to other continents), local endogamy ensured that the ties between co-villagers were particularly dense.

Endogamy gives a particular meaning to relationships of reproduction. We can start by considering marriage. Each marriage redistributes property between the families of the bride and groom – either at the time or at the death of the older generation – and so the marriage market can be seen as a kind of game in which parents effectively stake a certain amount of property on each of their children in the hope that they will obtain partners with matching or better property endowments. In this game each actual marriage represents a disappointment for the other potential partners of the bride and groom, making it a zero-sum game. The effect of endogamy is that both winners and losers come from the same small community, maximizing the tensions involved.

What is true of marriage is also true of giving birth. In an endogamous community, each birth reduces other families' prospects of receiving large marriage settlements when their own children marry. This happens in two ways. If the child is a girl, then her future dowry will reduce the wealth that her family is able to settle on its other children. At the same time, she represents additional competition for other parents, in their attempts to marry their daughters to the sons of wealthy families. If we switch the words 'son' and 'daughter', the same argument applies to the birth of boys.

In these circumstances, it is not surprising that – as reported in many ethnographies – marriages become the object of competitive manoeuvring or that young mothers feel oppressed by a sense of the envious hostility of other women. On the positive side, public opinion provides a powerful incentive to behave as responsible parents, providing one's children with the necessary capital to make good marriages when the time comes. Either way, the net effect of these pressures would be to keep the birth rate below what it would otherwise have been.

Given the pressures that local endogamy gives rise to, one might wonder why any communities would adopt this approach to residence and marriage. However, although it would be a mistake to attribute any form of social behaviour entirely to ecological and economic factors, there are good reasons why people in agricultural communities might choose to remain near their parental home and marry partners from the same community. The importance of inheritance as a way of transmitting land and agricultural buildings provides a strong reason for continuing to live near one's parents. If both men and women inherit land, a local marriage provides a way of building a more substantial family landholding. Even if this is not the case, a local marriage will provide a connection to another local family that would be a valuable source of both practical and social support. So there is nothing irrational about endogamous marriage, but that does not stop it being a major source of intracommunity competition and psychological pressure.

Psychological Support: Cooperation as a Source of Protective Social Capital

Nevertheless, birth rates in traditional Mediterranean societies were well above replacement level, so people must have had some sources of psychological strength to set against the pressures of mutual discouragement. The argument of this section is that much of this strength was provided by traditional relationships of production.

Production, unlike reproduction, is not a zero-sum game. There are many ways in which members of an endogamous community can cooperate to raise their mutual welfare. At the whole-village level, this can be done by sharing in the joint work of maintaining the collective capital of the village (common lands, dairies, school buildings, roads and docks). Groups of families and neighbours can join together in work rotas or share the task of herding each other's animals. People can also help each other out in emergencies – bad weather, illness or temporary financial difficulties – resulting in a higher overall level of economic wellbeing than if people did not cooperate in these ways. As a byproduct of these practical benefits, effective cooperation can also generate a strong sense of mutual goodwill.

This is a repeated theme in Mediterranean ethnography. Writing about village society in Kabylia, on the southern shore of the Mediterranean, Bourdieu (2013: 58–59, 75–77) points out that sociability and work were understood as a single set of self-reinforcing relationships. Patron–client relationships are understood in the same way, in that mutually beneficial practical arrangements both underpin and depend on corresponding social relationships of god-parenthood and so on. (For a famous account, see Campbell (1964) on the relationship between Greek shepherds and urban patrons.) In describing Belmonte before its transformation, Lisón Tolosana (2004: 143–49) argues that the community was held together by a sense of honour that was essentially based on economic dealings: self-reliance to the extent that was possible, not skimping on work or payment, a readiness to provide help in case of genuine need, and a readiness to take on public duties if one was in a position to do so were the characteristics of an honourable man. Meeting these standards was a basis for personal respect – and mutual respect was a source of social cohesion and an implicit guarantee for the continuance of the system of cooperation.

So when the Carnians attributed the collapse of local social life to the ending of mutual economic help, their sense of loss was founded in sentiments that would be recognized throughout the Mediterranean. The mutual goodwill and the sense of self-worth that mutual assistance had provided were important sources of psychological strength. But how exactly did they limit the discouragement of fertility?

There are several ways in which this could have happened. One way would be by enhancing the social capital of individual families. The contributions that young couples and their relatives had made to the welfare of other members of the community could be treated as a form of social capital, protecting them from excessive demands from other members of the community – including demands that they meet higher material preconditions for having children. Another possibility would be by enhancing the social capital of the community as a whole. If people felt that they were themselves protected and supported by an effective village community, they might be more likely to pay attention to the pro-fertility messages implicit in village rituals of annual renewal. A third possibility is that the general atmosphere of goodwill generated by successful cooperation softens the more negative messages arising from rivalry for limited resources, and so diminishes the sense of pressure.

Further research[6] would be needed to establish that mechanisms like these were actually in operation, but there is nothing in them that contradicts what we know about attitudes in the societies in question. They would not remove the downward pressure on fertility resulting from competition for limited resources, but they could have created a space for the development of an implicit compromise that permitted replacement level fertility.

Implications of this Theoretical Model: Predictions and Results

Summary of the Model

To sum up, the key points of the model are:

1. parents, particularly mothers, need to feel approval, or at least that they have the support necessary to withstand disapproval;
2. disapproval of fertility is sharpest where each family's offspring will later be competing for access to the same local resources, including collective property and the marriage market. The underlying disapproval of fertility is therefore greatest in populations where people live where they were born and marriage is locally endogamous;
3. the psychological self-assurance and social support needed to resist this derives from the goodwill generated from local economic cooperation.

Implications for Traditional Society and the Process of Modernization

In this model, everything depends on the balance between points 2 and 3 above. If the disapproval resulting from the competition for fixed resources is high, then the psychological support resulting from cooperative production will also have to be high if the result is to be above-replacement fertility. A combination of this kind would generate something like the system of social pressures that used to be characteristic of Mediterranean societies. We could call this a high-pressure system.

But it would also be possible to have a low-pressure system. In such a system, competition for local resources would be low – either because people moved a good deal or because employment did not depend on a finite amount of local land. As a result, there would be little need for families to discourage each other's fertility, and so the need for psychological support would also be low. In such a system, people might or might not cooperate economically, but their capacity to reproduce would not depend on the mutual goodwill that this cooperation generated. Something like this, with relatively high geographical mobility and a good deal of economic individualism, seems to have been characteristic of northwest Europe in preindustrial times (MacFarlane 1978).

But how might either system react to the move from agriculture to an industrial and service economy (i.e. to what is often referred to as a modern economy)?

The ethnographic examples suggest that local economic cooperation would rapidly decline, leading to a collapse in the psychological support that it provided. This would have little impact on a low-pressure system, since mutual cooperation would already be low. But in a high-pressure system, the result would be to remove the protection against the powerful forces discouraging fertility. The outcome would depend on the impact of modernization on the level of mutual discouragement.

One effect of the switch from agriculture to other forms of employment is to lessen people's dependence on the highly local resource of agricultural land – and hence the competition over who will gain access to it. Since this competition is at the base of the discouragement of fertility, it should also lead to a decline in the intensity of mutual discouragement. However, competition and mutual discouragement would probably not disappear altogether since land is not the only local resource for which people might compete. Housing would remain an important asset and so would positional goods such as social and political roles carrying particular prestige. Last but not least, there would be competition for jobs in the new nonagricultural economic sectors. Though capital and jobs in these sectors would be relatively mobile (at least compared to agricultural land), it still makes sense to think of a finite quantity of local employment opportunities and to compete for access to them.

By having children themselves or discouraging other potential parents, people would be competing for their children's access to these resources in two or three decades' time. Would it make sense to view this competitively? The answer could be 'yes', but only if the children were likely to remain in the same local area when they grew up. Generational continuity and local endogamy are defining characteristics of high-pressure systems – but, as we saw earlier, one of the early consequences of modernization is an increase in geographical mobility.

The crucial question is how much spatial mobility increases. If it increases to the level typical of low-pressure systems, then there will be little reason for mutual fertility discouragement. In that case the net effect of the collapse of competition and mutual discouragement on the one hand, and the collapse of cooperation and mutual psychological support on the other would be to convert a high-pressure system to a low-pressure system. Since pro- and anti-fertility pressures had been reduced to much the same extent, the new system would probably be close to equilibrium with approximately replacement-level fertility.

But if spatial mobility in the former high-pressure system remained lower than in a typical low-pressure system, it would mean that it still made sense for potential parents to compete over their children's future access to local resources. In this case, some downward pressure on fertility would remain. In that situation the result of the collapse of cooperation and mutual psychological support would be a fall in fertility – probably some way below replacement level.

Statistical Evaluation

Can these predictions be tested against statistical evidence? Not surprisingly, there are few if any statistical measures for the patterns of community interaction discussed in the ethnographic literature, but some things can be measured on the basis of data in comparative social surveys, local demographic statistics and a comparative network study called KASS, on which we in the Max Planck Institute at Halle worked together with anthropological colleagues in several European countries.[7] Among the variables that can be measured are the extent of interaction with close relatives, local endogamy and the spatial concentration of relatives, and local fertility rates.

Fieldwork for the KASS study was carried out between 2005 and 2007 in nineteen field sites spread between eight European countries: Sweden, France, Germany, Austria, Italy, Croatia, Poland and Russia. In each country the field sites included at least one urban and one rural locality. The fieldwork involved a combination of qualitative ethnographic methods and fixed-format network interviews with small but representative samples of local people, using a specially developed computerized questionnaire known as the Kinship Network Questionnaire (KNQ). An average of thirty network interviews were carried out in each field site, focusing on informants' knowledge of, and interactions with, their relatives, and also collecting a good deal of background information about the informants and other members of their networks. Figure 4.1 is based on these interviews, while Figure 4.2 is based on official statistics for the same local areas.

The figures are scatter-plots in which each point is labelled by the first letter of the country's English-language name, and the type of area is indicated by the icon concerned: for rural areas a circle with a white centre, for urban localities a black dot of the same size, and for two small-town locations a circle containing a cross. The icons are grouped into three columns labelled by European macro-region. The

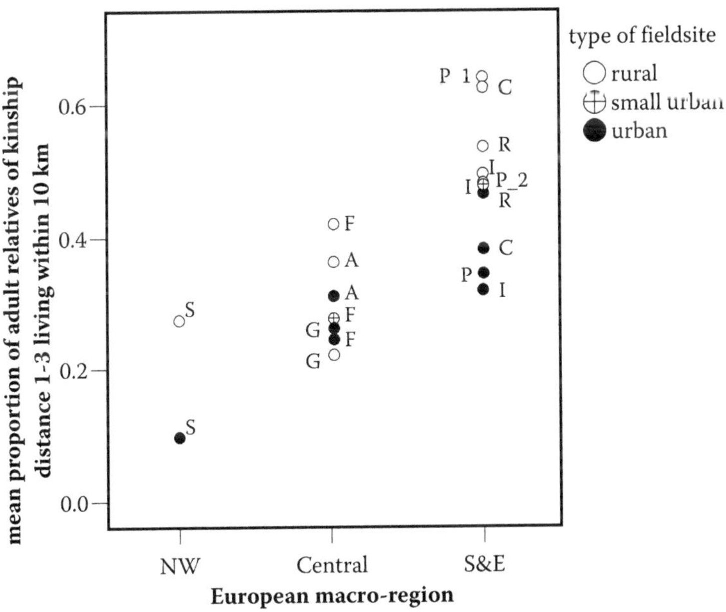

FIGURE 4.1 Spatial Concentration of Relatives by Macro-Region and Area Type

Description: *Fieldsite location.* The letter by each icon indicates the country in which the fieldsite is located: Sweden (S), France (F), Germany (G), Austria (A), Italy (I), Croatia (C), Poland (P) and Russia (R).

macro-regions are not of equal size, but the grouping – into 'north-western', 'central' and 'southern and eastern' Europe – corresponds to differences in contemporary statistics on household composition (Heady, Gruber and Ou, 2010a: 42–43), as well as reflecting the geographical groupings proposed by Laslett (1983) and differences in national kinship terminologies (Schlee and Heady 2010).

Figure 4.1 records the clustering of kinship networks in each of the nineteen field localities. The measure of clustering, which is given on the vertical axis, is the proportion of close adult relatives who live within 10 kilometres of the informants' current homes. 'Close' is defined as 'within three kinship steps': the first step includes parents, siblings and adult children; the second step includes uncles, aunts, nephews, nieces, grandparents and in-laws; and the third step includes first cousins, in-laws' partners, and great-uncles and aunts. Highly clustered networks reflect a tendency for adults to remain close to their childhood homes and to marry partners from the same local area – the characteristics that we would expect on theoretical grounds to be associated with a 'high-pressure' system of demographic influences.

As we might expect from the earlier discussion of Mediterranean endogamy, the three Italian field sites report high levels of kinship clustering. It is interesting to note that comparable levels are reported from the other field sites in the southern and eastern macro-region, suggesting that local continuity and a degree of endogamy are equally characteristic of eastern Europe. For the purposes of this discussion, it is unfortunate that KASS did not happen to cover either Spain or Greece, two of the classical countries of Mediterranean ethnography. However, by combining KASS data with data from other surveys, it is possible to reach some conclusions about these countries as well. A number of comparative surveys have found that social interaction and mutual assistance between family members is more frequent in southern Europe (including Greece and Spain) than in the north. Well-known discussions of this data include Reher (1998), as well as the articles by Murphy (2008), and Kohli et al. (2010) mentioned earlier. It is also the case that analyses of the KNQ data demonstrate that more clustered networks lead to higher levels of mutual help between relatives (Gruber and Heady 2010b). So, by combining these two sets of findings, we can conclude that Spain and Greece are almost certain to be among the countries with high levels of local endogamy and kinship clustering.

Figure 4.1's findings for the other macro-regions are also in line with expectations. The Swedish field sites (the only ones from northwest Europe) show very little kinship clustering, indicating equally low levels of local continuity and endogamy. The geographically intermediate field sites in the central macro-region display intermediate levels of kinship clustering. This would be consistent with a gradual rise in the intensity of local and kinship ties as one travels from northwest Europe to the south and east, but an alternative possibility is that there are successive step-like differences between distinct macro-regions. The stepwise view would be consistent with the levels of family interaction reported by Kohli et al. (2010) in their comparative study, and also with the finding of Schlee and Heady (2010) that the differences in recorded behaviour correspond to distinct patterns of kinship terminology.

From the viewpoint of our model, the important point is that the distinction between the three macro-regions corresponds to a distinction between three successive levels of local continuity and endogamy, and hence three distinct levels of negative pressure on fertility. In order to counteract this and thus achieve replacement fertility or better, local communities in different parts of Europe would have required the social support generated by corresponding levels of cooperation, leading to different overall systems of demographic influence. There would have been a low-pressure system (with low endogamy and low cooperation) in the northwest; a middling-pressure system (with intermediate levels of both endogamy and cooperation) in the central macro-region; and a high-pressure system (with high levels of both endogamy and cooperation) in the south and east.

This brings us to the crucial set of predictions – those regarding the impact of economic 'modernization' on local birth rates. Our data do not let us compare rural communities before and after they abandoned agriculture, but since most of our rural field sites still contain active farming communities, we can obtain a similar effect by comparing them with urban areas in the same country. (The assumption underlying this substitution is that in one crucial respect, the economic structure of modern urban areas is likely to resemble that of rural areas after they have abandoned agriculture, namely that neither offer much scope for mutual economic assistance between people in the same local area.)

Looking again at Figure 4.1 and comparing the rural field sites with the urban areas, we see that – as we would expect – local endogamy is more common in rural areas. But it is not much more common, which shows that an underlying preference for local continuity and endogamy (and therefore the pressures that they generate) can survive the transition from a rural to an urban way of life. This means that the competitive downward pressure on urban fertility is likely to be lowest in the northwest macro-region, middling in the central region, and highest in the south and east. In the absence of the positive emotional support generated by economic cooperation, the differences in competitive pressure would be transmitted directly to fertility behaviour, leading to a sharp downward gradient in urban fertility levels from an approximately replacement level in the northwest to a very low level in the south and east.

The data shown in Figure 4.2 test the validity of this prediction. The field sites in the three macro-regional columns are the same as those in Figure 4.1. The vertical axis gives a measure of fertility for the local statistical district that most closely corresponds to the field site concerned. Ideally we would have used official figures for the Total Fertility Rate, but since these are not generally provided for local districts we have calculated our own approximate

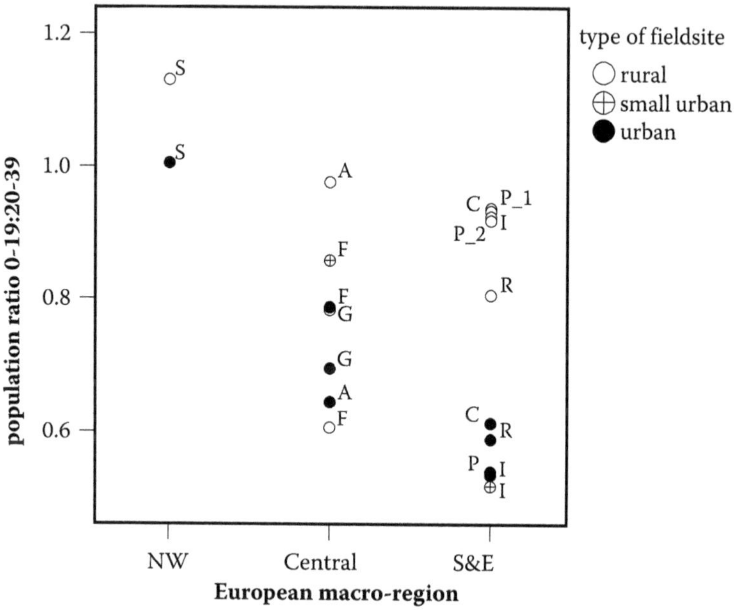

FIGURE 4.2 Population Ratios 0–19 Years: 20–39 Years, According to Local Official Statistics

Description: *Fieldsite location*. The letter by each icon indicates the country in which the fieldsite is located: Sweden (S), France (F), Germany (G), Austria (A), Italy (I), Croatia (C), Poland (P) and Russia (R).

fertility indicator. This is the ratio of the total population (male and female) aged 0–19 inclusive to the total population aged 20–39. Though the measure is a little crude, population ratios equal or greater than one will usually indicate replacement-level fertility or above, while ratios below one would correspond to subreplacement fertility.

As expected, urban fertility is highest in the single urban field site located in the northwestern macro-region – a suburb of Stockholm with a population ratio of about 1.0. The urban sites in the central macro-region have below-replacement fertility with population ratios between 0.6 and 0.8. Finally the figures for the urban field sites in southern and eastern Europe – with population ratios ranging from just above to some way below 0.6 – show the lowest fertility levels of all, both absolutely and in comparison with the values for the corresponding rural areas. These results confirm the theoretical prediction that the fall in fertility as a result of changing from an agricultural to a more urban way of life is likely to be greatest in areas with high levels of local continuity and endogamy.

Overall, the statistical findings are consistent with the theoretical model of social pressure and fertility developed in previous sections of this chapter.

Concluding Discussion

To conclude, I would like to discuss how the argument developed here might connect to wider debates about the relationship between anthropology and demography. In a recent review article, Johnson-Hanks (2008) argued that anthropologists should engage more directly with the substantive processes of demography – and, in particular, with the causes and consequences of different rates of fertility and mortality. She felt that a sustained anthropological look at the bundle of interconnected changes known as the 'demographic transition' would benefit both demography and anthropology. Demography would benefit from in-depth anthropological investigation of the concepts it uses, particularly the concept of modernization that, though central to demographic theories of transition, is often vaguely theorized and superficially measured. Anthropology would benefit from the opportunity of using quantitative data to demonstrate that important social phenomena have holistic aspects that cannot be reduced to questions of individual motivation. Both disciplines would benefit from a critical evaluation of theories of rationality – either as an innate human propensity or as a learned form of internalized self-discipline encouraged by modern bureaucratic systems.

The present study clearly follows a similar, though not identical, agenda, so it is worth asking how far its findings meet Johnson-Hanks' expectations. It also offers an opportunity to assess some of the methodological issues that arise when one attempts to combine these very different disciplinary perspectives in practice. I will start by considering some methodological points.

The first point concerns complexity. When one tries to combine different perspectives in the same chapter, there is simply more to say than there would be if one stuck to a single disciplinary or theoretical point of view. This leads to presentational problems – important points, both of theory and of evidence, have to be condensed in order to fit the argument into the space of a single chapter. I have tried to indicate where I have done this, but this is a practical rather than an ideal solution. It remains the case that several points deserve a fuller treatment.

There is also the question of what to leave out altogether. By focusing on psychological pressure, and the economic and social factors that determine its intensity, I do not mean to imply that these social pressures are the only thing that determines fertility decisions – or to deny the potential importance of changing tradeoffs between fertility and other desirable goods, of the practical help provided by relatives and neighbours, or of the role of social networks in transmitting information about contraception or about new possibilities of social behaviour. But what I *am* claiming is that the social-influence story told in this chapter hangs together logically and does enough to explain both the ethnographic and the statistical data to be worth presenting in its own right. If this presentation is found to be convincing, it would make sense to ask how the social influence explanation might be integrated with these other possible approaches and, indeed, with background data about changing mortality levels and contraceptive techniques, but all these things would be topics for later chapters. The priority here is to make a case for the social influence approach.

The complexity involved in an interdisciplinary approach is not just a matter of presentation – it is also a matter of formulating the triple connection between ethnography, theory and demographic statistics in the first place. There are many possible ways of linking the three domains, and the challenge is to pick out the most fruitful.[8]

The easiest link to make is that between the theory and the statistical data. Once the theory is clear, the choice of relevant data is comparatively simple. Statistical analysis can invalidate or confirm a theoretical prediction – and both outcomes can play a helpful role. By showing that the fall of southern European fertility was greater than predicted by the first versions of modernization and kin influence theory considered here, statistical data showed that the theories were not validated as they stood, and so opened the way to the search for new theoretical formulations. The confirmation of some predictions of the model developed here provides some justification for continuing to work with it.

However, although this testing function is vital, statistical data by itself rarely suggests new insights. Linking statistics with ethnography can be fruitful in this respect, as in the opening section of this chapter. In that case it was important not just that statistics about low fertility could be linked to a description of social change in one field site, but also that similar ethnographies of social change were available for sites in other lower-fertility countries. As with any kind of evidence, ethnographic findings are more valuable if they can be replicated.

But the link that produces most new insight is the one between theory and ethnographic data. In the present study the crucial turning point was the demonstration that none of the three initial theories of social interaction and fertility provided an adequate analysis of the conflicting pressures described in ethnographic accounts of pretransformation agricultural communities. This provided the stimulus for the development of an alternative model – in which, again, ethnographic data was very helpful in identifying possible causal mechanisms. As we have seen, these hypothetical causal mechanisms turned out to be consistent with the available statistical data.

This is, I think, the way in which Johnson-Hanks hoped that ethnographic and demographic approaches would interact, so the final step is to look again at the findings this interaction has produced. As a start, we can look at how the new model modifies the conclusions of the three theories with which we started.

Two central elements of Newson's kin influence hypothesis carry through to the new model. These are the openness of potential parents to social influence and the tendency of people to exercise that influence in a way that promotes the fertility chances of their own close relatives. However, because one of the main ways in which this is done is by discouraging the fertility of less-close relatives, the conclusion that kin-dense social networks will promote overall fertility is not supported.

As we have seen, Dalla Zuanna's and Krause's argument is that very low Italian fertility reflects parents' competitive concern to protect family reputation by providing children with high material living standards. This fits into the new model, since an insistence on high material standards is one of the ways in which local public opinion can discourage fertility. The greater prevalence of this pressure in southern Europe than further north is explained by the continuing tendency for southern Europeans to stay close to their childhood homes and marry endogamously, thus placing children in competition for the same local resources to a greater extent than is true in northern Europe.

Lesthaeghe's modernization theory argument that increased individualism has led to lower fertility is also confirmed, but not in the way that standard modernization theory would predict. If this chapter's model is right, fertility does not decline because individualist adults prioritize other goals over parenthood. The reason suggested by the new model is that by staying away from local cooperative activity, individualists undermine the climate of mutually supportive goodwill to which cooperation gives rise, and thus deprive potential parents of psychological support from the local community.

The model is not meant as a complete theory of human decision-making or even of all fertility-related decision making, but even so, it is worth considering some of its general properties. Perhaps the most important is that although individuals and couples make their own fertility choices, these do not simply reflect their own autonomous preferences. The preferences that actually matter also take into account the climate of local opinion: will another child be welcomed? And if, as seems almost inevitable, it is unwelcome to at least some people, do potential parents have enough psychological support to withstand the resulting resentment? By taking account of the objective conditions that intensify or diminish both resentment and support, it is possible to predict variations in birth rates.

The fact that effective fertility preferences are not exogenously given but are modified by social pressure and psychological support means that the system as a whole has certain properties that may not be deducible from the attitudes of the individuals within it. This has implications for the research strategy that we choose. Ordinary survey methods, which collect data on individual attitudes and circumstances, are not likely to be enough. They need to be complemented by methods that can capture what is happening at a community level. This is one of the things that make ethnographic fieldwork so valuable, but the point is not restricted to qualitative methods. In order to test the resulting insights, we need quantitative methods that treat communities themselves as units of analysis. This idea underlay the design of the KASS project, which enabled us to generate the results displayed in Figures 4.1 and 4.2. The deeper lesson may be that if we are to combine the insights generated by ethnographic and demographic methods, we may need to rethink the way we apply the methods themselves.

Acknowledgements

I would like to thank colleagues for commenting on earlier versions of the ideas presented here. I am particularly grateful to Nancy Konvalinka and Marysia Galbraith for ongoing discussions of these themes, and to Rebecca Sear and Lesley Newson for introducing me to evolutionary theories of fertility. Astrid Bochow and Philip Kreager have been constructively critical editors. Nevertheless, the responsibility for the views expressed here is mine alone. I thank Campus Verlag for permission to reproduce Figures 4.1 and 4.2.

Patrick Heady coordinates a research project on 'kinship, universals and variation' at the Max Planck Institute for Social Anthropology, Halle. He obtained a Ph.D. from LSE in 1996 based on fieldwork in the Italian Alps. Between 2004 and 2008, he coordinated an EU-funded research project on 'kinship and social security' in Europe.

Notes

1. Most people in Carnia speak both Italian and Friulian. This expression is Friulian; the others are Italian.
2. Lisón Tolosana (2004) does not name the village, but from the context it appears to be Belmonte de los Caballeros, the subject of his earlier (1966) ethnography.
3. Since his 1986 paper with Wilson, Lesthaeghe has considerably elaborated his approach to fertility change in modern society, including discussion of the relevance of Maslow's psychological theory of motivation and personality (Lesthaeghe 2014).
4. Paxson's (2005) ethnography of parenthood in Athens makes a similar point when she notes that a major reason for restricting fertility to one child was a concern to be a good parent to the child one did have.
5. Hamilton's original articles are very technical. They are reproduced in Hamilton (1996) along with introductory commentaries by the author, which make the issues much easier for nonspecialists to grasp.
6. This research could be ethnographic, based on the impressions gathered in conversations and participant observation. But it could also – in principle at least – be quantitative. Within a single community, young couples' fertility could be correlated with the extent of help that they and their relatives had offered to other members of the community, and with their participation in collective activities, to see whether or not there was a statistical relationship. The overall fertility levels of different communities could be correlated with the extent of participation in informal helping relationships, formal economic cooperation and collective ritual performances.
7. KASS was largely financed by a grant from the European Union's Sixth Framework research programme. The results are published in three volumes: Grandits (2010); Heady and Kohli (2010); and Heady and Schweitzer (2010).

8. As an illustration of the difficulty in deciding which links to emphasize, it may be worth noting that this is not the first time I have written about the theme of this chapter. Heady (2007), Heady, Gruber and Ou (2010b) and Heady (2011 and 2012) draw on much the same data to make the case that changes in local social interactions have contributed to the decline of fertility in southern Europe, but formulate the argument in different ways.

References

Bailey, F. (ed.). 1971 *Gifts and Poison: The Politics of Reputation*. Oxford: Basil Blackwell.

Billari, F., and H. Kohler. 2004. 'Patterns of Low and Lowest Low Fertility in Europe'. *Population Studies* 58: 161–76.

Bourdieu, P. 2013. *Algerian Sketches*. Cambridge: Polity Press.

Boyd, R., and P. Richerson. 2005. *The Origin and Evolution of Cultures*. Oxford: Oxford University Press.

Campbell, J. 1964. *Honour, Family and Patronage: A Study of Institutions and Moral Values in a Greek Mountain Community*. Oxford: Oxford University Press.

Christian, W. 1989. *Person and God in a Spanish Valley*. Princeton: Princeton University Press.

Cole, S. 1991. *Women of the Praia: Work and Lives in a Portuguese Coastal Community*. Princeton: Princeton University Press.

Collier, J. 1997. *From Duty to Desire: Remaking Families in a Spanish Village*. Princeton: Princeton University Press.

Dalla Zuanna, G. 2001. 'The Banquet of Aeolus: A Familistic Interpretation of Italy's Lowest Low Fertility'. *Demographic Research* 4(5): 133–62.

Durkheim, E. 1992 [1888]. 'Suicide and Fertility: A Study in Moral Statistics'. Translated H. Sutcliffe, Introduction J Simons. *European Journal of Population* 8: 175–97.

Fernandez, S. 2013 'Re-building Links: Images of Motherhood'. Paper presented at American Anthropological Association annual meeting, Chicago, November 2013, session on 'Life Course and Family Formation: Parenthood, Work and Care-Giving in "Late-Forming" Families in Europe and the Caribbean'.

Frejka, T., and Calot, G. 2001. 'Cohort Reproductive Patterns in Low-Fertility Countries', *Population and Development Review* 27(1): 103–32.

Grandits, H. (ed.). 2010. *Family, Kinship and State in Contemporary Europe*, vol. 1, *The Century of Welfare: Eight Countries*. Frankfurt: Campus Verlag.

Gruber S., and P. Heady. 2010a. 'Kinship in Transformation – Measures and Models', in H. Grandits (ed.), *Family, Kinship and State in Contemporary Europe*, vol. 1, *The Century of Welfare: Eight Countries*. Frankfurt: Campus Verlag, pp. 363–90.

———. 2010b. 'Domestic Help', in P Heady and M. Kohli (eds), *Family, Kinship and State in Contemporary Europe*, vol. 3, *Perspectives on Theory and Policy*. Frankfurt: Campus Verlag, pp. 83–125.

Hamilton, W. 1963. 'The Evolution of Altruistic Behaviour', *American Naturalist* 97: 354–56.

———. 1970. 'Selfish and Spiteful Behaviour in an Evolutionary Model', *Nature* 228: 1218–20.

———. 1996. *Narrow Roads of Gene Land, the Collected Papers of W D Hamilton*, vol. 1, *Evolution of Social Behaviour*. Oxford: Oxford University Press.

Heady, P. 1999. *The Hard People: Rivalry, Sympathy and Social Structure in an Alpine Valley*. Amsterdam: Harwood Academic.

———. 2003. 'Conscripts and Christians: Representing Kinship and Affinity in the Carnian Alps', *Journal of the Royal Anthropological Institute* (NS) 9: 77–95.

———. 2007. 'Fertility as a Process of Social Exchange', *Demographic Research* 17: 465–96.

———. 2011. 'Relatives and Neighbours: A Generalised Influence Perspective on European Fertility'. Paper presented at the SSHA Conference, Boston, session on 'Kinship and Fertility: New Approaches to Demographic Change'.

———. 2012. 'The Implicit Contracts of European Kinship: Gender, Generation and Society', in N. Konvalinka (ed.), *Modos y Maneras de Hacer Familia: las Familias Tardías, una Modalidad Emergente*. Madrid: Biblioteca Nueva, pp. 33–52.

Heady, P., S. Gruber and Z. Ou. 2010a.'Family, Kindred and Marriage', in P. Heady and M. Kohli (eds), *Family, Kinship and State in Contemporary Europe*, vol. 3, *Perspectives on Theory and Policy*. Frankfurt: Campus Verlag, pp. 31–69.

———. 2010b. 'Birth Rates, Values and Social Patterns', in P. Heady and M. Kohli (eds), *Family, Kinship and State in Contemporary Europe*, vol. 3, *Perspectives on Theory and Policy*. Frankfurt: Campus Verlag, pp 203–24.

Heady, P., and M. Kohli (eds). 2010. *Family, Kinship and State in Contemporary Europe*, vol. 3, *Perspectives on Theory and Policy*. Frankfurt: Campus Verlag.

Heady, P., and P. Schweitzer (eds). 2010. *Family, Kinship and State in Contemporary Europe*, vol. 2, *The View from Below: Nineteen Localities*. Frankfurt: Campus Verlag.

Hrdy, S. 2009. *Mothers and Others: The Evolutionary Origins of Mutual Understanding*. Cambridge, MA: Harvard University Press.

Johnson-Hanks, J. 2008 'Demographic Transitions and Modernity', *Annual Review of Anthropology* 37: 301–15.

Just, R. 2000. *A Greek Island Cosmos*. Oxford: James Curry.

Kohli, M., M. Albertini and H. Künemund. 2010. 'Linkages among Adult Family Generations: Evidence from Comparative Survey Research', in P. Heady and M. Kohli (eds), *Family, Kinship and State in Contemporary*

Europe, vol. 3, *Perspectives on Theory and Policy*. Frankfurt: Campus Verlag, pp. 225–48.

Krause, E. 2005. '"Toys and Perfumes": Imploding Italy's Population Paradox and Motherly Myths', in C. Douglass (ed.), *Barren States: The Population 'Implosion' in Europe*. Oxford: Berg, pp. 159–82.

Laslett, P. 1983. 'Family and Household as Work Group and Kin Group: Areas of Traditional Europe Compared', in R. Wall, J. Robin and P. Laslett (eds), *Family Forms in Historic Europe*. Cambridge: Cambridge University Press, pp. 513–563.

Lesthaeghe, R. 2014. 'The Second Demographic Transition: A Concise View of its Development', *Proceedings of the National Academy of Sciences*, PNAS 2014 111 (51): 18112–15.

Lesthaeghe, R., and C. Wilson. 1986. 'Modes of Production, Secularisation, and the Pace of Fertility Decline in Western Europe, 1870–1930', in A. Coale and S. Watkins (eds), *The Decline of Fertility in Europe*. Princeton: Princeton University Press, pp. 261–292.

Lisón Tolosana, C. 1966 *Belmonte de los Caballeros*. Oxford: Oxford University Press.

———. 2004. *Invitación a la Antropología Cultural de España*. Madrid: AKAL.

Loizos, P. 1981. *The Heart Grown Bitter: A Chronicle of Cypriot War Refugees*. Cambridge: Cambridge University Press.

MacFarlane, A. 1978. *The Origin of English Individualism: The Family, Property and Social Transition*. Oxford: Basil Blackwell.

Murphy, M. 2008. 'Variations in Kinship Networks across Geographic and Social Space', *Population and Development Review* 34: 19–49.

Newson, L., and P. Richerson. 2009. 'Why Do People Become Modern: A Darwinian Mechanism', *Population and Development Review* 35(1): 117–58.

Newson, L., T. Postmes, S.E.G. Lea, P. Webley, P.J. Richerson and R. McElreath. 2007. 'Influences on Communication about Reproduction: The Cultural Evolution of Low Fertility', *Evolution and Human Behavior* 28(3): 199–210.

Ott, S. 1993. *The Circle of Mountains: A Basque Shepherding Community*. Reno: University of Nevada Press.

Paxson, H. 2005. 'Underfertility's Challenge to Family and Gender Relations in Urban Greece', in C Douglass (ed.), *Barren States: The Population 'Implosion' in Europe*. Oxford: Berg, pp. 137–58.

Reher, D. 1998. 'Family Ties in Western Europe: Persistent Contrasts', *Population and Development Review* 24(2): 203–34.

Schlee, G., and P. Heady. 2010. 'Terminology and Practice: European Kinship in a Worldwide Perspective', in P. Heady and M. Kohli (eds), *Family, Kinship and State in Contemporary Europe*, vol. 3, *Perspectives on Theory and Policy*. Frankfurt: Campus Verlag, pp. 347–74.

Stewart, C. 1991. *Demons and the Devil: Moral Imagination in Modern Greek Culture*. Princeton: Princeton University Press.

Tönnies, F. 1887. *Gemeinschaft und Gesellschaft*. Leipzig: Fues's Verlag.

Viazzo, P., and F. Zanotelli. 2010. 'Welfare as a Moral Obligation: Changing Patterns of Family Support in Italy and the Mediterranean', in H. Grandits (ed.), *Family, Kinship and State in Contemporary Europe*, vol. 1, *Eight Countries*. Frankfurt: Campus Verlag, pp. 47–92.

Watkins, S. 1990. 'From Local to National: The Transformation of Demographic Regimes in Western Europe, 1870–1960', *Population and Development Review* 16: 241–72.

Chapter 5

Ambivalent Men

Male Dilemmas and Fertility Control in Senegal

Sara Randall, Nathalie Mondain and Alioune Diagne

Introduction

Despite substantial progress in economic development, advances in education and significant declines in child mortality over the last two decades, fertility remains high in francophone West Africa. In Senegal the use of modern contraception is quite low (10 per cent of all women), although over 90 per cent women and 93 per cent men know of at least one modern contraceptive method and most know of several (Agence Nationale de la Statistique et de la Démographie 2012). The barriers to fertility decline and greater uptake of contraception are unclear and important questions remain. Is demand for modern contraception low because people do not want to control their fertility, because they distrust the available methods or because they face various barriers to access? To what extent is culturally determined pronatalism still a major part of people's mindsets and what role does religion play in influencing both reproductive intentions and behaviour? Gender is a crucial dimension in addressing these questions. In what ways do men and women differ in their attitudes to fertility control and available methods, and how are these negotiated and managed? Do men pose a barrier to women's desire to control fertility or is this an oversimplified perspective of gendered roles in relation to fertility and fertility control? In considering male roles and influences on reproductive decision-making, is the couple the appropriate unit of analysis?

Demographic and Health Surveys (DHS) now collect much data from men allowing analyses of determinants of male reproductive behaviour, attitudes and practice around contraception, fertility preferences, unmet need and male roles in the demographic transition, with further focus on the role of the couple, their characteristics, agreements, disagreements, consistencies, inconsistencies and communication (Ezeh 1993; Becker 1996; Bankole and Singh 1998; Hulton and Falkingham 1996; Dodoo 1998; Andro and Hertrich 2002; Benefo and Pillai 2005; DeRose and Ezeh 2005; Takyi and Dodoo 2005; Kulczycki 2008). Despite this plethora of survey data, much research into the role and contribution of men and gender relations to reproductive behaviour has incorporated qualitative or ethnographic approaches that move away from the somewhat ethnocentric assumptions about communication, power and influence implicit in questionnaires (Bawah et al. 1999; Wolff et al. 2000; Castro 2001; Agadjanian 2002, 2005; Bawah 2002; Hollos and Larsen 2004; Sargent 2007; Izugbara and Ezeh 2010). Questionnaires limit the opportunity for respondents to express uncertainty and dilemmas, and they constrain possible analyses to the categories and conceptual frameworks originally used to construct the questions (Hulton and Falkingham 1996; Timaeus and Moultrie 2008). In contrast, qualitative methods encourage respondents to express worries and indecision. They allow researchers to identify and then pursue inconsistencies. More generally, they facilitate a nuanced understanding of how people talk and think about fertility control and contraception, and the associations they make spontaneously. Such data give a more nuanced understanding of the diversity of factors influencing decisions or nondecisions.

We begin to answer the questions outlined above through analysing empirical qualitative data on men's beliefs and behaviours around reproduction, fertility control and contraceptive use in a small Senegalese town in the early stages of fertility transition. In examining men's attitudes to fertility control and contraception, and men's representations of their roles in reproductive decision-making, we interpret their statements whilst considering how gender-based differences in the acceptability of fertility control under different circumstances are mediated and moulded by socially accepted gender roles, and the extent to which individuals have the agency to negotiate. We demonstrate the pitfalls of pre-classifying responses into analytic categories before really hearing what people are saying. Throughout we remain aware that in-depth interviews can be seen by respondents as public declarations and that, for men in particular, the social importance of being observed and heard to agree with socially acceptable norms and religious values by the interviewers may inhibit some from expressing what they really think, because such opinions might be criticized by others or even seen as blasphemous ideas.

Men, Fertility Control and Family Planning in Sub-Saharan Africa

Until the 1990s the role of men in both fertility and fertility control was largely ignored in demographic research (Greene and Biddlecom 2000). However, the role of male sexual behaviour in the emerging HIV epidemic, alongside the change of policy direction as a result of the Cairo Population Conference in 1994 towards reproductive rights and reproductive health, led to a burgeoning of research on men's role in reproductive decision-making in the late 1990s (Pinelli 2001).

Studies on male roles in fertility behaviour fall into three main themes, with DHS data constituting a major source of evidence. Investigations into the causes of the considerable unmet need for contraception among women showed that a key factor in many contexts was male opposition to fertility control – or at least female perception of male opposition – leading to research on male fertility preferences and male attitudes to fertility control. Bankole and Singh (1998) established that, with the exception of West Africa, male family size preferences and fertility intentions did not differ as much as expected from women's, although much of the agreement occurred because in pronatalist contexts, both partners wanted more children. The focus on fertility preferences was largely determined by available DHS data, an approach somewhat undermined by Agadjanian's (2002) insights from qualitative research in Maputo, which demonstrate clearly that, at an individual level, fertility preferences may be very labile and, even when expressed, they are not necessarily goals to which individuals aspire. Nevertheless, because in some contexts stated male preferences do differ from those of women, both at aggregate and at couple levels, the nature of these differences and their role in determining fertility behaviour has been investigated (Dodoo et al.

1997; Casterline et al. 2001), from which spousal communication emerged as a key issue.

DHS spousal communication data cover whether both members of a partnership know the other's fertility preferences and attitudes to contraception, as well as documenting whether these issues have been discussed within the couple. Direct spousal communication is usually associated with increased use of contraception. Where spousal communication about fertility is low (primarily in West Africa and Pakistan), there is evidence that proxy reporting by women on their husbands' attitudes is rather unreliable (Dodoo 1998; Wolff et al. 2000; Casterline et al. 2001; Andro and Hertrich 2002; Bawah 2002; Maharaj and Cleland 2005; Kulczycki 2008).

The third line of research examines the role of power in couples' relationships and at a wider societal level as a factor inhibiting women from pursuing contraceptive behaviour that would seem logical in terms of their expressed desires (Dodoo et al. 1997; Blanc 2001; Castro 2001; DeRose and Ezeh 2005; Avogo and Agadjanian 2008; Kulczycki 2008; Izugbara and Ezeh 2010).

There is increasing evidence that survey-based conceptualizations of fertility strategies framed around either wanting more children, or wanting to stop or space are too limited and do not take into account the substantial economic, domestic and other uncertainties that many people in poor populations face (Smith 2004; Johnson-Hanks 2005; Osei 2009; Towriss 2014) or the possibility that many individuals do not hold strong fertility preferences that guide behaviour (Agadjanian 2002; Gribaldo et al. 2009). Collecting survey data on couples makes an implicit assumption that couple communication is critical. Although important in many contexts, couple communication remains fairly uncommon in West Africa (Andro and Hertrich 2002), where qualitative studies show that it may be necessary to look beyond the couple for wider influences on male and female reproductive decision-making related to the gender system (Mason 1997). This includes: peer and family pressure, the social importance of demonstrating fertility for young women (Smith 2004; Izugbara and Ezeh 2010), the role of rumours and fears (Castle 2003; Foley 2007; Osei 2009), and the general role of male social networks (Agadjanian 2002, 2005).

More qualitative research is needed on men's role in fertility behaviour and use of family planning in diverse higher fertility contexts (Andro and Hertrich 2002). The questions used in survey approaches generally assume that men and women either approve or disapprove of contraception per se and allow little room for expressing either ambivalence or acceptability of some methods but not others. Although unmet need for contraception usually refers to spacing and limiting of childbirth, needs for postponing and avoiding are rarely identified. Understanding the diversity of sexual relationships and partnerships and the extent to which male attitudes to contraception differ according to both the nature of the partnership and the reproductive context may tell us more about male attitudes and the social and religious factors that influence men's reproductive behaviour than do questions about the general acceptability of fertility control or about couple communication.

The Context of Gender Relationships in Senegal and in the Small Town

Our case study focuses on a small town of around 18,000 inhabitants in 2010, whence considerable male out-migration to Italy has occurred since the late 1980s. The town is on a main arterial road in Louga region with quite good general infrastructure. International migration has contributed to a high standard of material living for families with migrants. However, migration has resulted more in visible investment in conspicuous material goods and impressive villas than in local investment in services and generating employment (Riccio 2006; Diop 2008). It has impacted not only on the material wellbeing of families and households but also on residential patterns. Many absent migrant men continue to play a major role in day-to-day household life through mobile phone contact. The small town is situated in the Wolof heartland of Senegal and the majority of the population are Wolof or are heavily influenced by Wolof language and culture.

Much of the literature on gender relationships in Sub-Saharan Africa is centred on women's roles and status in the society, and male roles are often inferred from such studies. According to Dial: 'In Senegal, tradition and then the Muslim culture have perpetuated a system of inequality and sexual domination which are justified by their "nature", tradition and religion' (our translation: Dial 2008: 15). In particular, Wolof social norms determine that the head of the household is male (usually the oldest male) and that women are subject to his authority. According to Pezeril (2007), for followers of the Mouride brotherhood, a woman's maternal role is idealized and sacred, and her principal task in life is to bring up her children properly; submission to her husband is an essential contribution to this maternal success. Women's subordinate position is reinforced by patrilocal norms whereby the new wife moves to her husband's family home, often co-residing with her in-laws and co-wives. These social norms also impose considerable obligations on men, the most important of which is the provision of economic support: a married man is expected to be financially responsible for his wife and children, and to house, clothe and feed them (Antoine and Djire 1998; Antoine 2002; Antoine and Dial 2005). These strongly felt social obligations and the impossibility of fulfilling them are leading many men to either postpone marriage or to migrate (Mondain et al. 2012a). There are also strong religious obligations on men. Publicly, they are expected to be good Muslims, go to the mosque, fast and abstain from alcohol. Men should also show respect for their parents and support them in old age.

Within marriages, these powerful Wolof social norms structure the relations within the couple. However, marital relationships are also being shaken up by broader social changes related to economic crisis, urbanization, increases in female schooling and international migration, all of which are contributing to modifications of the family and intergenerational relationships that were at the core of the social organization of most African societies (Vignikin 2007).

The largely Wolof community in the small town study site epitomizes these Wolof patriarchal and patrilocal social and cultural norms. Many people adhere to the Mouride or Tidjan brotherhoods, where men and women's roles are precisely circumscribed, the latter in the domestic sphere and reproduction (Pezeril 2007), and the former as family support and bread winners. The geographical proximity to Touba, the Senegalese city which is a destination for pilgrims, is visible through the number of mosques, and Koranic schools, and local male discourse is full of moralistic and religious overtones. This context is thus likely to reinforce hierarchical social relationships favouring men and the elderly, these relationships being particularly easy to maintain as the extended families live together in large compounds. However, as shown by Perry (2005) for rural Wolof, the knock-on economic changes wrought by free market reform mean that whereas female subjugation is usually maintained, at least in public, rural Wolof women are developing considerable autonomy through new economic participation in trade, and in private they are challenging aspects of patriarchal domination. Pezeril's (2007) reflection on her research among the Baay Faal (a subgroup of Mourides) also emphasizes recent transformations in women's domestic and public autonomy, and their increasing participation in public political, economic and religious life.

Because both religion and tradition play critical roles in the Senegalese political, economic and social spheres, in this case both Islam (Kaag 2011) and Wolof cultural values will have an important influence on sexual and family planning behaviour (Dial 2008). The Mouride and Tidjani brotherhoods are also extremely active among migration networks (Navarra and Salis 2011), so it is likely that they strongly influence individuals involved in transnational relationships by transmitting core values of morality, including what is acceptable regarding marital and sexual behaviours. It is, however, difficult to disentangle religious obligations from tradition as both concur to create a system of unequal gender relationships characterized by male domination. In particular, Wolof cultural values expect a wife to be patient and obey her husband whilst satisfying him sexually; the fulfilment of these roles will provide her children with 'Baraka', necessary for her own reputation and thus her old-age security (Dial 2008). In general, religious authorities and Wolof cultural traditions advocate abstinence until marriage, faithfulness between spouses and if abstinence and/or faithfulness is not possible, then plural marriage (i.e. polygamy) (Diop 1985).

Appropriate public appearance is very important and takes two major forms. It is difficult for men or women to challenge publicly the accepted norms and value of male dominance or the important values of Islam. Furthermore, proper public presentation and appearance is a significant social value: being well dressed, having a modern house, investing in material goods and being seen to provide well for one's family. This importance of appearances has ramifications for our research because the interviews, although undertaken in private, seem to have been interpreted by some men as a public statement. Thus, we hypothesize that men often felt obliged to demonstrate their authority over their wives and other women through what they said in interviews, and that justifications of their statements and behaviour had to be couched in the locally accepted doctrines of Islam. In general, women seemed to be less bound by these social norms and used their interviews as a forum to express emotions and dilemmas about aspects of their social life and its constraints. Increasingly, urban Senegalese girls and women are becoming academically and economically successful and, despite the patriarchal values, the context is far from the extensive oppression of women on many fronts described recently for northern Nigeria (Izugbara and Ezeh 2010). Most women in the small town have considerable freedom of movement and carry on their own economic activities. Male dominance is largely expressed in the domestic arena and through public discourse. This appears clearly in recent analysis of women's interviews from the same community, highlighting women's increasing weariness with absent husbands and the pressure and control exercised by their families-in-law; the fact that women both expressed this and some had even initiated divorce, as seen elsewhere in Senegal (Tall and Tandian 2010), is symptomatic of ongoing transformation of gender relationships (Mondain et al. 2012b).

Contraception and the Acceptability of Fertility Control

In terms of family planning activities, discussions with medical personnel and with a women's information network established that, at the time of the fieldwork in 2007, condoms were widely available in shops, stalls and pharmacies, and a range of contraceptive methods (pill, IUD, injection) were available at a subsidized rate for married women at the health centre. Local access to contraception for unmarried, divorced and widowed women was less clear, although there was easy transport to the more anonymous city environments in Dakar or St Louis. Local statistics obtained from the chief medical officer suggested that around 9 per cent married women of reproductive age in the town were using some form of modern contraception supplied through the clinic in 2007.

In order to understand the gendered nature of what is acceptable in terms of fertility control, how it can be and is discussed by both men and women, and how men negotiate and justify their reproductive roles in this northern Senegalese population, it is essential to first disentangle different dimensions of fertility control and marital contexts (Figure 5.1).

A first stage considers whether fertility control of any sort is acceptable to men of different ages and situations and, if acceptable, whether this is in all, or only some, dimensions of postponing, spacing, limiting and avoiding births; the second stage identifies different sorts of fertility control and the contexts in which they can occur. Postponing refers here to avoiding pregnancy before childbearing has started, either before marriage or in the early years of marriage, usually with the expectation that one day childbearing will happen. For a variety of reasons, individuals who already

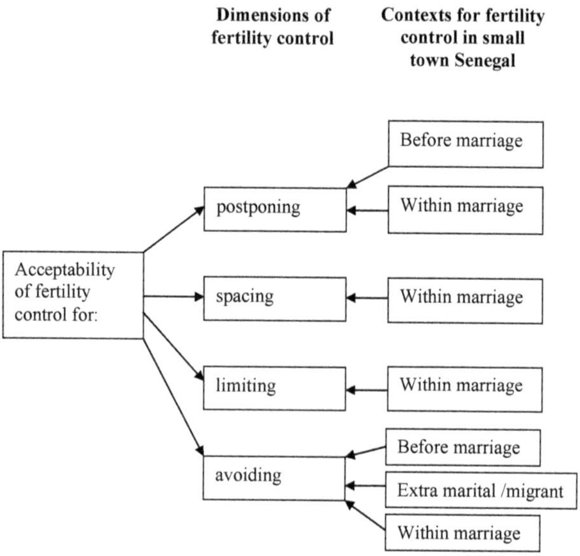

FIGURE 5.1 Dimensions and Contexts of Fertility Control

have children may want to avoid births at different stages in their reproductive lifetimes (Timaeus and Moultrie 2008). Limiting refers to the intention to have no further births. In Senegal, where premarital births are quite frequent (but few women experience more than one), spacing and limiting strategies occur primarily within marriage. Both postponement and avoidance can be premarital and avoidance can also be extramarital. We contend that both men and women may approve of some dimensions and contexts of fertility control whilst having very strong opinions about the unacceptability of others. Approval of contraceptive use may also be related to attitudes towards the acceptability of sexual activity in that context.

Methods

Qualitative data were collected in 2007 in the small town following up a larger qualitative study undertaken in 1999 in the same town (and also in a village and Dakar), thus providing an element of time depth to examine transformations over a period of rapid social change (see Randall and LeGrand 2003 for details of the 1999 sample selection; see also LeGrand et al. 2003). The earlier research focused on reproductive strategies and showed that migration to Italy was having a major impact on marriage dynamics in the small town; this finding stimulated the 2007 study to investigate the consequences of this adult male migration on family and household dynamics of those left behind. To this end, four Senegalese postgraduate sociology students undertook eighty-four in-depth qualitative interviews with adult men and women of all ages. Ethics approval was obtained from the University College London ethics committee.

In each of the town's six administrative neighbourhoods, six men and six women, stratified by age, were selected at random and interviewed by same-sex researchers. All interviews were undertaken in Wolof and translated and transcribed in French immediately for rapid feedback on both the quality of the interview and specific themes and topics. During the translation process, there was much team discussion about appropriate translations of key Wolof terms. Respondents were encouraged to talk about their personal experiences of growing up and their experience as adults, of education, professional life, family in the past and present, and of having marriage and children. Along with a focus on migration decision-making and the impact of other people's migration on individuals, households and more generally in the town, most interviews covered family building strategies, ideal family size, and attitudes towards fertility control and contraception; these topics often emerged spontaneously.

All interviews were entered into an N6 database, where they were coded by authors into predefined and emergent themes. They were analysed by identifying key themes, reading and rereading material coded under those and related topics, and then developing and testing hypotheses about associations between the themes and different discourses associated with each theme. Quotations from interviews are used here to illustrate points made by several respondents, unless stated otherwise. Where possible, we present quite long extracts to demonstrate the context in which statements were made and in response to which questions or stimuli; quotations are selected in order to show how respondents argue their points, the sorts of evidence they use and the associations they make; notably, almost all statements reflect aspects of male–female power relationships.

Men's Attitudes to Fertility Control

Given this overall context of gendered roles and expectations, local interpretation of Islam, migration and modernity, we use our data to analyse which dimensions and contexts outlined in Figure 5.1 are acceptable for fertility control to men, their different types of response, and the factors that influence or determine these responses. Key overlapping themes that emerge are: the importance of religion and, more particularly, of understanding what is permitted in Senegalese interpretations of Islam; the health and integrity of women's bodies; understanding how different forms of contraception work and their influence on the body; and gender roles and power relations. Of these, local understanding of Islamic teaching is a critical dimension of male discourse around the acceptability of fertility control; religion is invoked in most men's statements about reproduction. This is not the case for women.

Male reactions to the idea of fertility control are very heterogeneous and are not consistently related to levels of formal education, participation in the modern economy or migration to Italy. Some of the most conservative men are those with higher education, while some with little or no schooling are in favour of fertility control and small families. Three main sets of male attitudes to fertility control could be identified:

1. fundamentally opposed to the idea of fertility control under any circumstances, invariably invoking religion as the justification;
2. accept the idea of fertility control primarily for birth spacing, justified in terms of health of the mother and child; and
3. fertility control is acceptable.

Islam and economic factors are cross-cutting themes in men's justifications for their attitudes towards fertility control. Senegalese men's economic responsibilities for their womenfolk and children leads economic security to be women's primary expectation from marriage (Antoine and Dial 2005). The pursuit of personal success is largely perceived in economic terms. In order to understand the logic that motivates men's discourse and their actions, we focus on this interplay between religion and economics below.

Opposition to Fertility Control

The largest group of male respondents, encompassing diverse ages, economic situations and education, said they were fundamentally opposed to fertility control. Opposition was couched in arguments that fertility control pitted man against the will of God. Children were considered a gift of God and the more children one has, the more one contributes to the islamic *umha*, the number of Muslims on earth:

> *R.* It's [family planning] a bad thing. It suggests that you are depriving yourself of the good qualities that God had allocated to those who ought to have been born and whom you have stopped from being born They forget that this baby could have saved your life, brought you wealth or God's redemption.
> *I.* But what does family planning really mean to you?
> *R.* Taking pills or other things for perverts or prostitutes. Others use it to reduce births.
> *I.* Do you agree with any of these reasons?
> *R.* With none of them. I agree that we should leave everything to God's decision.
> *Man aged 56: Koranic school, not working, monogamous, 11 children*

> *I.* If your wife wanted to use family planning today what would be your opinion?
> *R.* No, my wife will not use that.
> *I.* Why?
> *R.* Why use family planning? It's as though I weren't a Muslim.
> *Man aged 32: primary education, mechanic, unmarried, no children*

Many men talked about family planning reducing the number of children born, which was seen as an unacceptable challenge to the divine will. This religious justification was backed up by arguments that children were not only a gift from God but also an economic investment for the future – children who will care for parents in their old age. In the current context, where having a son who is a successful migrant to Italy brings previously unimaginable levels of comfort, material goods and financial security for the parents, there is little reason for many people to modify their perspectives of children as investments. Frequent reference to parent–child relationships shows that each generation is seen to have obligations towards the other (Mondain et al. 2012a); this was demonstrated by arguing that if a man's parents had controlled their fertility, then he would not be here today. Interestingly, men saw no contradiction in expressing an ideal number of children whilst totally rejecting fertility control. It seems that such ideal family sizes are not perceived as a personal goal, but as something that can be expressed whilst accepting that God can give more or less and that it is God's will that is paramount:

> I prefer to leave that to God's will despite my own desire to have seven children. *Unmarried man aged 29: secondary schooling*

The rejection of fertility control for these men must be seen within the widespread local understanding that this is Islamic doctrine and that God will always provide the resources necessary for each child.

Acceptance of Fertility Control for Birth Spacing and Health

Everyone (all men and all women) associated short birth intervals (*nef* in Wolof) with potential health problems for both woman and child. *Nef* should be avoided if possible; women who suffer from *nef* are pitied, but there is also an element of shame. Information campaigns targeting both men and women have exploited and reinforced traditional concerns about birth spacing. Whether ideas about health repercussions of short birth spacing are deep-seated from centuries of observations or have largely been recently reinforced by campaigns, men who would never sanction fertility control for limiting births may do so for birth spacing associated with women's health. Both religion and male power are constantly evoked in men's talk around these issues:

> *I.* Does it happen that you say to yourself 'I need so many children'?
> *R.* No. I told you just now that I am Muslim. Children are born through God's will . . .
> *I.* According to you what is family planning?
> *R.* Planning, I've learned about it. I also hear people talking about it, but all that, it's just nonsense.
> *I.* Why?
> *R.* In fact it depends, because planning can be useful if a woman has 'nef', if she has closely spaced births. Even Islam suggests you should use contraception to avoid illness for the mother of children who are born weak or disabled. But if that's not the case I don't agree with family planning
> *I.* And if your wife wanted to use it?
> *R.* If she really needs to, that is she has 'nef' or she has difficult births. In that case yes. But if it's not that then I don't agree.
> *I.* And if, for example, she told you she wanted 4 children?
> *R.* Ahh. My wife would never tell me the number of children she wanted. I am Muslim and it doesn't depend on me or her, that depends on God's will.
> *Unemployed man aged 40: secondary schooling, monogamous, 2 children*

This conversation epitomizes the two dominant themes within male discussions around fertility control in this community: the man both asserts his authority over his wife and demonstrates his public role as a Muslim through emphasizing that neither of them has the right to challenge God's will by having a fixed ideal family size as a target. Whilst making public reference to religion, another respondent describes children as economic objects in which it is risky to invest too much:

> *I.* Are you for or against use of family planning?
> *R.* No I'm not against. I worked for 18 years in a pharmacy. I know why one should use family planning – it's so that you don't accumulate too big a family, because it's good to space births. I entirely agree with planning. Where I am not really convinced it's the idea of having one or two children only. I wouldn't advise that to young people: that's not believing in God. You need at least 4 or 5 children because life doesn't only depend on the good Lord. If you have two kids and then they die what will you do? You could have one child, bring him up well and in good conditions but if he dies what was the point of all your money? That's why I advise you not to depend on that. If you get married it's to have a family. So planning to space children is good but to limit the number of children that's bad. Women shouldn't be forbidden to use planning for spacing but as long as the woman can have children with no problem or risk you shouldn't use it.
> *Aged 63, primary schooling, retired, monogamous, 8 children*

Despite this man's opposition to the idea of 'limiting', he reinforces the idea put forward by Timaeus and Moultrie (2008) that we should look beyond limiting and spacing to avoidance. Reflecting on his wife towards the end of her reproductive years, he says:

> Finally during her last childbirth my wife felt rather weak and she was afraid and came to tell me that 'it would be best if I started to use planning'. I said to her 'of course, go ahead'. I told her that she shouldn't worry about it. She took it for a year and then the midwife told her she could stop.

Such use of contraception to avoid pregnancy because of health problems, albeit having already borne a number of children, is completely acceptable. It is a totally different rationale from the idea of having had enough children and stopping – although the outcome is identical. In this town in 1999, men's opposition to family planning was very entrenched unless their wife's health was at risk; at that time, on being asked about contraception, almost all male respondents spontaneously brought up the issue of woman's (and child) health. There are both religious and economic dimensions here:

everyone knows that Islam sanctions the pursuit of good health at all costs, so a man who states that his wife is using contraception because of health risks of pregnancy will not lose public face. In interviews women were often explicit about their use of health justifications to persuade husbands to let them control fertility. For both men and women, doctors play a critical role: by judging whether a woman's health is at risk and having the authority – acknowledged by local interpretation of acceptable behaviour within Islam – to sanction and provide contraceptive methods. Beyond the religious aspects, economic justifications for maintaining women in good health were related both to their domestic work and avoiding medical bills.

Amongst these men who accept contraception for health, there are, nevertheless, a wide range of attitudes. At one end of the spectrum, there is reluctant necessity:

> *I.* How did you react when she asked your permission to use those methods?
> *R.* At first I didn't agree. I was even opposed to 'planning' because God has programmed a fixed number of children for each of us and in my opinion to stop or limit what has already been programmed it's tantamount to not believing in Him. Only it happened that my wife's health was threatened and under such circumstances one has to agree with those who advise us to use such methods. Even though I was against it I had to accept it because if something happened to her I would be responsible.
> *Aged 53, monogamous, very poor manual labourer, 8 children, 1 dead*

At the other, there is proactive seeking of health:

> *I.* You say that you want lots of children yet your wives use modern contraception. How do you explain that?
> *R.* There's no contradiction. If I suggested to my wives that they use those methods it's just so that they are in good health, that they rest a bit before having another pregnancy. It doesn't mean that they are going to stop having children
> *Aged 44, electrician, some secondary school, 3 wives, 8 children; sent all his wives to get contraception*

Men Who Accept Fertility Control

Those (relatively few) men who accept fertility control for limiting usually couch their acceptance in terms both of economic necessity and of women's health, whilst maintaining their articulation of power over their wives:

> *R.* I am in favour of it and I would have authorised my wife to use it if she had asked me because I think that in certain situations a person really cannot allow himself to have many children. Because it would be difficult. And that could be painful for both the wife and the child. Given the terrible state of employment these days I can easily understand how we have got here . . .
> *I.* Was it useful for you?
> *R.* Yes. If we hadn't used it I would have ended up with more children than I can afford. Life is currently very difficult here.
> *I.* Where did she go for family planning?
> *R.* I don't know. The hospital perhaps? I didn't bother much about that.
> *Aged 51, Koranic + primary school, farmer, 3 children, wife used contraception*

The following man is unusual in that, as well as changing his mind about fertility control, he is not trying to impose anything on his wives:

> *I.* Do you agree with family planning?
> *R.* If life continues to get harder and harder we're going to have to use it soon. Before I was strongly opposed but now I'm basically in favour of it.
> *I.* Do you use it in your family?
> *R.* Even if I don't personally use it my wives have the means to use it without me knowing.
> *I.* But you're not sure?
> *R.* I don't even want to know. All that I ask of our Lord is that he bless those children I already have.
> *I.* But would you have liked to have had more children?
> *R.* Yes, if I had the wherewithal to feed them!
> *Aged 54, primary school, 4 wives (1 dead), many children, unsuccessful migrant in Italy*

Economic constraints are the primary motivation for fertility control for both these respondents, yet both are unwilling to play an active role in the process of obtaining contraception: the first sees his role as just that of giving or refusing permission, while the second does not want to know the details. One could argue that, by distancing themselves from practical contraceptive management, they are therefore distancing themselves from direct responsibility and rendering themselves less vulnerable to public criticism and accusations of sin or of contravening Islamic behaviour.

Amongst our male respondents, the university student cited below was unique in specifically talking about family planning for limiting the number of children because of financial constraints and mentioning neither religion nor health. His subsequent account of discussions with his girlfriend and his awareness that she wants two children demonstrate his intentions to limit family size and his perceptions of a process of communication and negotiation between partners; however, even he still articulates his male authority over her use of contraception:

> *I.* And what about children?
> *R.* I don't want more than 3 [children].
> *I.* Why not?
> *R.* It's what I explained to you just now. Life has become difficult.
> *I.* How would you achieve such a small number of children?
> *R.* It's something we need to manage between us, because I can authorise her to use family planning.
> *Aged 25, unmarried university student*

Most men expect to be the final arbiter of contraceptive use within marriage without wanting to be involved in method choice or logistics. Their descriptions of the process of decision-making are always couched in the vocabulary of male authorization or embargo of their wife's contraceptive use. The forms spousal communication might take and how they would be reported in this context are difficult to envisage, since most men are not interested in the details of family planning methods and where and how they are obtained. This may be partly because of ambivalence about the morality of fertility control and an attempt to distance themselves from behaviour that might be criticized by others in a social context where public appearance is so important

However, interviews with men revealed that, whether men are in favour or not, there is considerable evidence of reluctance to talk about these issues with their wives:

> *I.* You just told me that you want to have lots of children. Do you ever discuss your sexual life or family planning with your wife?
> *R.* I have never done so. A man shouldn't discuss such things with a woman. I'm opposed to planning because you mustn't contravene God's will. It's God himself who gives children to whomsoever he wants. If he decides to give me children I don't see why I should be against it. However I can understand how a sick woman might decide to rest if her doctor advises her to. Ultimately that one can understand, but what women do now is against God's will.

I. So you wouldn't accept your wife using modern contraceptive methods?
R Never ! Unless a doctor asked her to.
Aged 35, Koranic school, mason, 2 children. Currently monogamous

The professed belief that such discussions are inappropriate between man and wife suggests that analysis of survey responses on spousal discussion is unlikely to be very revealing. Body language, overheard conversations and responses to media may be more frequent pathways through which couples communicate their preferences (see Miller at al. (2001) for similar points for Malawi).

Premarital and Extramarital Sex: Contraception, Sin and Morality

The discussions above focus on marital reproduction. Marriage and parenthood are universal aspirations in Senegal and a major aim of marriage is socially sanctioned reproduction (Foley 2007), hence the generalized association of reproductive decision-making within marriage in a context where the most controversial issue would be deciding not to have many children. Yet there is considerable premarital sexual activity. Older men saw premarital pregnancies as a symptom of immorality and an indication of contemporary social problems, although disentangling whether they were condemning premarital sexual activity or pregnancy is difficult. This older unschooled man, whilst accepting family planning for limiting as both compatible with Islamic doctrine and economically sensible, sees contraception as totally unacceptable in a premarital context:

I can't oppose it [family planning] because I know it is a good thing. People say religion is against it but nowhere is it written that you should have children if you can't look after them. Religion does not forbid planning. What it does forbid is that young people who are not yet married use these methods so that they are free to join in debauchery. That is what religion cannot accept. Religion does accept that those people who are legally married plan the number of children they want, bearing in mind their means. If you don't have the resources to have a large family you shouldn't have many children and in order not to have many children you need to use something like those methods.
Aged 61, Koranic school, retired carpenter, 11 children from 2 wives

In contrast, other men condemn family planning both before and within marriage; before marriage it is the sexual activity itself which is morally reprehensible, after marriage the unacceptable behaviour is that of challenging God's will.

> The white people introduced that [contraception] to us and, what is dramatic, it's that young unmarried girls can now do what they want and not get pregnant. That's why we old people, we cannot agree with that, because in our religion we learn that on judgement day the prophet will boast about his people; so why should we want to decrease this people?
> *Aged 65, retired tailor, polygamous 3 wives, 10 living, 6 dead children*

Some men articulated that an important motivation for marriage is to avoid the sin of being sexually active: unable to resist the pressures they chose to marry. This suggests that for them, it is the immorality of premarital sex which makes premarital contraception unacceptable and not the inhibition of pregnancy.

> My reasons [for getting married] were simple: I didn't want to get in the habit of behaving in a morally indecent way
> *Aged 43, primary schooling, married with 4 children*

Men of all ages demonstrate that the morality of using contraception is judged according to context: for some it is not the control of fertility *per se* that they condemn (despite the rhetoric about Islam), but the sexual context in which it is used. Thus unmarried or divorced men may disapprove of contraception within marriage but they are happy to sanction its use for their own sexual activity outside marriage. This is exemplified by a divorced man, aged 44 with secondary education, who, in talking about condoms says :*'Yes! I have already used them because you know, actually I am living a bachelor's life and I can't stop having sex. So in order to be comfortable I use condoms.'*

Yet earlier in his interview he stated:

> Me, I am opposed to planning because if the man and the woman are both healthy I can't see why they should use these methods. . . .
> *I:* If for example you married again would you accept your wife using those methods ?
> *R:* well [a bit embarrassed] we would see . . . that depends if she has health problems, but if she is healthy I wouldn't agree. Because, for me, if I marry it's to create a household and live happily. It's not to create a household and then say that one doesn't want any children.

> Although if the woman has a health problem, that's another issue. I would only accept planning in that case. I can't see any need for a healthy and well person to use planning.

This example of one man's contradictory attitudes towards contraception demonstrates how a long, in-depth interview can occasionally capture those nuances which would remain hidden in most questionnaire based surveys. Many men do not condemn the use of condoms or withdrawal in premarital sexual relations, possibly because premarital pregnancy is seen as a greater moral and economic problem than using a condom.

An additional complication is that condoms are not classified as 'planning' by men in the same way as hormonal methods. This is probably because they are not provided by the medical establishment and no doctor has sanctioned their use, but also perhaps because condoms can be justified in terms of STD prevention and are therefore a legitimate pursuit of health. Men willing to talk about pre-marital condom use did not anticipate any criticism on religious grounds – yet the same men were often wary of admitting the acceptability of hormonal contraception within marriage. Neither men nor women believe that 'planning' (IUD, pill or injectable) is appropriate for pre-marital sex because of worries about harming a woman's future reproductive capacity. Conserving future fertility is a far greater concern than preventing an unplanned premarital pregnancy.

Although condoms were primarily associated with pre-marital sexual activity the following discussion about condoms' acceptability within Islam demonstrates multiple dimensions of morality.

> You know, Islam is not against condom use. Condoms are the simplest of contraceptive methods and our religion accepts them. If your wife is breastfeeding and you want her and you don't want to go out and sin, you can have sex with her using a condom. That protects you and guarantees good health for her.
> *Aged 32, primary school, unmarried, mechanic*

Here condoms protect the man from sin by allowing legitimate sexual relations, whereas protecting his wife from pregnancy whilst breastfeeding appears to be a secondary consideration.

This example is one of a number of double standards. Fertility control here protects the man from sin. Men accept condom use for pre-marital sex because preventing pregnancies in such contexts suppresses the evidence of the socially unacceptable behaviour. Yet many men express strong opposition to fertility control within marriage because marriage is the public stage for reproduction. Sex before or outside marriage is not and should not be for reproduction; because it is for pleasure, either condoms or withdrawal can be used morally to avoid pre-marital pregnancies. For those for whom such sex is totally immoral it is the sexual activity that should be avoided, not the contraception.

Discussion

These Senegalese men are currently caught in a very difficult position between incompatible sets of values and objective economic constraints – made more complicated by the social importance of public appearance. General understanding of local interpretations of Islamic doctrine is that fertility limitation is unacceptable. Publicly, most men need to be seen to conform to this doctrine. Simultaneously there are strong social expectations that men should provide adequate economic support for wives and children, something that is difficult where there is little employment, declining agricultural productivity, and increasing costs of children because of changing educational, health and material expectations. Furthermore, in this patriarchal society, men should be seen to be in control of their wives (Dial, 2008; Foley 2007; Mondain et al. 2012b).

One of our original questions asked whether culturally determined pronatalism remains a major part of people's mindsets? We demonstrate that many men in this community seem to be on the cusp of change. Some gave contradictory attitudes or accounts of their behaviour over the course of the interview; some apparently had very strong feelings about the immorality of fertility control – but then found acceptable exceptions; others admitted that economic constraints had forced them into changing their minds and accepting fertility control. There are strong indications that even those who expressed opposition to contraceptive use may change their minds. We can observe how the 'vital conjunctures' (Johnson-Hanks 2006) they experience are generating social change – a social change that is possible because levels of knowledge about the idea and methods of fertility control are high.

Islamic promotion of the pursuit of health, both directly (in terms of ordering followers to behave in ways that protect and enhance health) and indirectly (in avoiding harmful behavior), strongly mitigates in favour of changing Senegalese attitudes to fertility control

(Musallam 1983, Omran 1992). Our 1999 data had demonstrated clearly how, despite the overt values of male dominance, women exploited what could be seen as the '"health loophole'" to negotiate access to contraception with their husbands. Different thresholds of health problems existed in different contexts and women in each context negotiated within the locally acceptable parameters; life threatening conditions in the village, serious health threats in the small town and trivial conditions such as nausea in pregnancy in Dakar. In both 1999 and 2007 men also cited health as an acceptable justification for fertility control; for them too, the thresholds of justifiable health problems are changing as costs of children and health care costs increase along with economic pressures faced by many households. Thus local interpretations of Islam are both an apparent barrier to fertility decline, but also the vehicle through which it will occur.

These accounts of Senegalese men's attitudes to contraception demonstrate that survey questions such as '"Would you say that you approve or disapprove of couples using a method to avoid getting pregnant?'" may be difficult to answer and that reports of couples' 'discussion about fertility' could be misleading. The context of sexual relations, the type of method and the status of the woman all condition responses. Most men do not have a binary approval or disapproval of contraception: their attitudes depend on the context of sexual relations (pre-marital, marital, extra-marital), whether contraception is to be used for spacing, stopping or avoiding, their own personal situation, and even different contraceptive methods. The validity of fertility preference questions may also be susceptible to the vocabulary used. Although the idea of an ideal number of children was somewhat acceptable, formulating this number as a target was seen as an unacceptable challenge to divine will. Such attitudes are reflected in the 2010 Senegalese DHS where no men in Louga region with fewer than 6 children wanted to limit fertility; countrywide, 20% of men gave a non-numeric answer to the question on ideal family size (ANSD, 2012). Our interviews suggest that a qualitative approach would have demonstrated much more uncertainty in response to these questions with a key problem being that many men have a strong religious opposition to articulating the idea of limitation.

Whether the married couple is an appropriate unit of analysis and whether couple communication means much in this context is another issue. Many men and women believe that sex, reproduction and contraception are not issues to be raised within the couple.

Women's sources of information are other women, female kin, friends, women's associations and professionals. Men learn from the media and from other men. Although some couples discuss reproduction, many men deliberately avoid such conversations because of ambivalence about the whole issue of fertility control, suggesting that, here, explicit couple communication is not necessarily a key element in fertility decline. Although married Senegalese men expect to be the final decision-makers about contraceptive use (women indicate that this is not always the case), many are not interested in the details of contraceptive methods and where and how they are obtained, possibly reflecting this ambivalence. They attempt to distance themselves from the issue through letting moral blame or consequences of modern contraceptive use rest on the woman's shoulders and not theirs.

Should these men be seen as barriers to women's desires to control their fertility? Probably they should not, despite men's pronatalist discourse and apparent opposition to fertility limitation. A major dimension of this opposition is oriented towards ideal family size expressed as a target. It is such language that generates conflict and tensions rather, than the actual fertility control.

This study was limited by its methodology of single in-depth interviews. Although this approach was able to identify ambivalence, contradictions, mind changing and attitudes around reproduction when these were expressed within the single encounter, they remain a fairly structured form of data collection. Many men used the interviews to articulate publically to the interviewer their adherence to a range of socially important values – having authority over one's wife, reproduction within marriage, having a large family, being a proper Senegalese Muslim with the 'correct' values. Such public discourse was less common amongst women in whose accounts the association of fertility control and Islamic doctrine was rarely encountered. For them, male authority was often something to be circumvented, and reproduction was mainly centred on the personal and the practical. Critically, what Muslim Senegalese men think Islamic teachings say about fertility control dictates their parameters of acceptable behavior; this may differ from doctrinal evidence that family planning is acceptable within Islam (Musallam 1983, Sachedina 1990, Omran 1992). In a culture where public face and appearance are extremely important, it is difficult to tease out from interviews the extent to which men just cite religious opposition because they feel that is what they should say – or they are unconvinced by promises of confidentiality and anonymity. Men may also be using the local rhetoric of Islam to serve their own purposes. They want many children, they want to control their wives and to be seen to be in control of their wives, they want the interviewer to believe they are good upright citizens – and Islam is an excellent foil for all of this. In-depth interviews remain artificial situations and although, compared to questionnaires, they allow respondents to play a much greater role in determining what is said and what is important, there remain problems with what is not and what cannot be said (Randall and Koppenhaver 2004).

Ethnographic research undertaken by a man is probably the way forward to addressing many remaining questions. Only through participant observation (Agadjanian 2002) could we learn the extent to which recourse to Islam is just a convenient front to save face and demonstrate respectability, or whether it really is a guiding force of men's reproductive behaviour. Detailed ethnographic work could reveal the extent to which men's talk about control and authority over wives is real or just public face Faced with the resistance of most Senegalese men to gossip with those they don't know (men's focus groups in 1999 were a methodological failure), ethnographic research is the only effective approach to establishing how attitudes are formed, who influences who, and how, and the role of different male social networks in contributing to social change and maintaining or destroying barriers to reproductive change.

Acknowledgements

The original research in 1999 was funded by a Rockefeller grant to Ken Hill and Thomas LeGrand, and the work in Senegal was carried out in collaboration with Cheikh Ibrahima Niang and his team of researchers at the Université Cheikh Anta Diop. The 2007 follow up study in the small town was jointly financed by a Nuffield small grant for social sciences (*'The impacts of out-migration on those left behind: changing family dynamics in small town Senegal')* and an internal grant from the Faculty of Social Sciences of University of Ottawa. Alioune Diagne was awarded a British Academy visiting fellowship (2008) at UCL during which he worked on these data.

Sara Randall was trained in both Anthropology and Demography and works in University College London Anthropology department. She integrates qualitative and quantitative research to research and challenge key demographic and data related issues and paradigms:

health behaviour, reproductive decision making, migration consequences and the nature of key demographic concepts.

Nathalie Mondain is Associate Professor at the School of Sociological and Anthropological Studies, University of Ottawa. Her main research interests are international migration and its effects on the left behind in sub-Saharan Africa; norms surrounding parenthood in different societies; research practices in population and development studies and their relationship to knowledge circulation and behavioural change.

Alioune Diagne is currently Monitoring & Reporting Specialist at UN Women West & Central Africa. He obtained his Ph.D. in 2006 (Demography) at Institut de Démographie de l'Université de Paris 1. He has extensive experience in the field of population studies in Europe (France, Belgium) and Africa (Senegal, Ghana, DRC, Zimbabwe, Kenya).

References

Agadjanian, V. 2002. 'Men"s talk about "women"s matters": gender, communication and contraception in urban Mozambique', *Gender and Society* 162: 194–215.

_____ 2005. 'Fraught with ambivalence: reproductive intentions and contraceptive choices in a sub-Saharan fertility transition'. *Population Research and Policy Review* 21(6): 617–645.

Agence Nationale de la Statistique et de la Démographie ANSD [Sénégal], et ICF International 2012. *Enquête Démographique et de Santé à Indicateurs Multiples au Sénégal EDS-MICS 2010-2011*. Calverton, Maryland, USA: ANSD et ICF International

Andro, A. and V. Hertricht 2002. 'Demand for contraception in Sahelian countries: Are men and women"s expectations converging? Burkina Faso and Mali compared to Ghana'. *Population-E* 57(6): 929–958.

Antoine, P. 2002. 'Les complexités de la nuptialité: de la précocité des unions féminines à la polygamie masculine en Afrique', in G. Caselli, J. Vallin and G. Wunsch (eds), *Démographie: analyse et synthèse. II Les déterminants de la fécondité*. Paris: INED, pp. 75–102.

Antoine, P. and M. Djire 1998. 'Un célibat de crise', in D. Ouedraogo, P. Antoine, and V. Piché (eds), *Trois générations de citadins au sahel: trente ans d'histoire sociale à Dakar et à Bamako*. Paris: L'Harmattan, pp. 117–45.

Antoine, P., and F.-B. Dial. 2005. 'Mariage, divorce et remariage à Dakar et Lomé', in K. Vignikin and P. Vimard (eds), *Familles au Nord, Familles au Sud*. Brussels: Academia Bruylant, pp. 205–32.

Avogo, W., and V. Agadjanian. 2008. 'Men's Social Networks and Contraception in Ghana', *Journal of Biosocial Science* 40: 413–29.

Bankole, A., and S. Singh. 1998. 'Couples' Fertility and Contraceptive Decision-Making in Developing Countries: Hearing the Man's Voice', *International Family Planning Perspectives* 24(1): 15–24.

Bawah, A.A. 2002. 'Spousal Communication and Family Planning Behaviour in Navrongo: A Longitudinal Assessment', *Studies in Family Planning* 33(2): 185–94.

Bawah, A.A., P. Akweongo, R. Simmons and J. Phillips. 1999. 'Women's Fears and Men's Anxieties: The Impact of Family Planning on Gender Relations in Northern Ghana', *Studies in Family Planning* 30(1): 54–66.

Becker, S. 1996. 'Couples and Reproductive Health: A Review of Couple Studies', *Studies in Family Planning* 27(6): 291–306.

Benefo, K., and V. Pillai. 2005. 'The Reproductive Effects of Family Planning Programmes in Rural Ghana: Analysis by Gender', *Journal of Asian and African Studies* 40: 463–77.

Blanc A.K. 2001. 'The Effect of Power in Sexual Relationships on Sexual and Reproductive Health: An Examination of the Evidence', *Studies in Family Planning* 32(2): 189–213.

Casterline J., Z. Sathar and M. ul Huque. 2001. 'Obstacles to Contraceptive Use in Pakistan: A Study in Punjab', *Studies in Family Planning* 32(2): 95–110.

Castle, S. 2003. 'Factors Influencing Young Malians' Reluctance to Use Hormonal Contraceptives', *Studies in Family Planning* 34(3): 186–99.

Castro, R. 2001. '"When a Man is with a Woman it Feels Like Electricity": Subjectivity, Sexuality and Contraception among Men in Central Mexico', *Culture, Health and Sexuality* 32: 149–65.

DeRose, L., and A.C. Ezeh. 2005. 'Men's Influence on the Onset and Progress of Fertility Decline in Ghana, 1988–98', *Population Studies* 59(2): 197–210.

Dial, F.B. 2008. *Mariage et divorce à Dakar. Itinéraires féminins*. Paris: Karthala – CREPOS.

Diop, A-B. 1985. *La famille Wolof: tradition et changement*. Paris: Karthala.

Diop, M.C. 2008. *Le Sénégal des migrations. Mobilités, identités et sociétés*. Paris: Karthala.

Dodoo, F.N.-A., Y. Lup and E. Panayotova. 1997. 'Do Male Reproductive Preferences Really Point to a Need to Refocus Fertility Policy?', *Population Research and Policy Review* 16: 447–55.

Dodoo, F.N.-A. 1998. 'Men Matter: Additive and Interactive Gendered Preferences and Reproductive Behaviour in Kenya', *Demography* 35(2): 229–42.

Ezeh, A.C. 1993. 'The Influence of Spouses over Each Other's Contraceptive Attitudes in Ghana', *Studies in Family Planning* 24(3): 163–74.

Foley, E.E. 2007. 'Overlaps and Disconnects in Reproductive Health Care: Global Policies, National Programs, and the Micro-politics of Reproduction in Northern Senegal', *Medical Anthropology* 26(4): 323–54.

Greene, M.E., and A.E. Biddlecom. 2000. 'Absent and Problematic Men: Demographic Accounts of Male Reproductive Roles', *Population and Development Review* 26(1): 81–116.

Gribaldo, A., M.D. Judd and D. Kertzer. 2009. 'An Imperfect Contraceptive Society: Fertility and Contraception in Italy', *Population and Development Review* 35(3): 551–84.

Hollos, M., and U. Larsen. 2004. 'Which African Men Promote Smaller Families and Why? Marital Relations and Fertility in a Pare Community in Northern Tanzania', *Social Science & Medicine* 58: 1733–49.

Hulton L.A., and J. Falkingham. 1996. 'Male Contraceptive Knowledge and Practice: What Do We Know?' *Reproductive Health Matters* 7: 90–101.

Izugbara, C., and A.C. Ezeh. 2010. 'Women and High Fertility in Northern Nigeria', *Studies in Family Planning* 41(3): 193–204.

Johnson-Hanks, J. 2005. 'When the Future Decides: Uncertainty and Intentional Action in Contemporary Cameroon', *Current Anthropology* 46(3): 363–85.

———. 2006. *Uncertain Honor: Modern Motherhood in an African Crisis*. Chicago: Chicago University Press.

Kaag, M. 2011. *Islam et engagements au Sénégal: résultats d'un programme de recherche demandé par l'Ambassade du Royaume des Pays Bas à Dakar*. Leiden: African Studies Centre.

Kulczycki, A. 2008. 'Husband-Wife Agreement, Power Relations and Contraceptive Use in Turkey', *International Family Planning Perspectives* 34(8): 127–37.

LeGrand T., T. Koppenhaver, N. Mondain and S. Randall. 2003. 'Reassessing the Insurance Effect: A Qualitative Analysis of Fertility Behaviour in Senegal and Zimbabwe', *Population and Development Review* 29(3): 375–403.

Maharaj, P., and J. Cleland. 2005. 'Women on Top: The Relative Influence of Wives and Husbands on Contraceptive Use in KwaZulu Natal', *Women and Health* 41(2): 31–41.

Mason, K.O. 1997. 'Gender and Demographic Change: What Do We Know?', in G.W. Jones, R.M. Douglas, J. Caldwell and R.M. D'Souza (eds), *The Continuing Demographic Transition*. Oxford: Clarendon Press, pp. 158–82.

Miller, K., E.M. Zulu and S.C. Watkins. 2001. 'Husband-Wife Survey Responses in Malawi', *Studies in Family Planning* 32(2): 161–74.

Mondain, N., A. Diagne and S. Randall. 2012a. 'Migrations et responsabilités intergénérationnelles : implications pour la transition à l'âge adulte des jeunes migrants sénégalais', in M. Gomez-Pérez and M-N. Leblanc (eds), *L'Afrique des Générations*. Paris: Karthala, pp. 259–300.

Mondain, N., S. Randall, A. Diagne and A. Elliot. 2012b. 'Les effets de l'émigration masculine sur la situation des femmes au Sénégal : renforcement ou ébranlement des équilibres traditionnels?', *Autrepart* 61: 81–98.

Musallam, B.F. 1983. *Sex and Society in Islam*. Cambridge: Cambridge University Press.

Navarra, C., and E. Salis. 2011. 'L'associationnisme sénégalais en Italie : une revue de la littérature', Document de travail UMR DIAL, DT/2011-02.

Omran, A.R. 1992. *Family Planning in the Legacy of Islam*. London: Routledge.

Osei, I. 2009. 'Exploring the Opportunities and Challenges to the Use of Emergency Contraception in Accra, Ghana', unpublished Ph.D. thesis. London: University of London.

Perry, D.L. 2005. 'Wolof Women, Economic Liberalization and the Crisis of Masculinity in Senegal', *Ethnology* 44(3): 207–36.

Pezeril, C. 2007. 'Réflexivité et dualité sexuelle : Déconstruction d'une enquête anthropologique sur l'islam au Sénégal'. *Journal des Anthropologues* 108–9: 353–80.

Pinelli, A. 2001. 'Genre et démographie', in G. Caselli, J. Vallin and G. Wunsch (eds), *Démographie: analyse et synthèse, VI – Population et société*. Paris: INED, pp. 419–52.

Randall, S., and T. LeGrand. 2003. 'Reproductive Strategies and Decisions in Senegal: The Role of Child Mortality', *Population-E* 58(6): 687–716.

Randall, S., and T. Koppenhaver. 2004. 'Qualitative Data in Demography: The Sound of Silence and Other Problems', *Demographic Research* 11(3): 57–96.

Riccio, B. 2006. '"Transmigrants" mais pas "nomades". Transnationalisme mouride en Italie', *Cahiers d'Etudes Africaines* XLVI(1): 95–114.

Sachedina, Z. 1990. 'Islam, Procreation and the Law', *International Family Planning Perspectives* 16(3): 107–11.

Sargent, C. 2007. 'When the Personal is Political: Contested Reproductive Strategies among West African Migrants in France', in M. Inhorn (ed.), *Reproductive Disruptions: Gender, Technology and Biopolitics in the New Millennium*. Oxford: Berghahn Books, pp. 165–82.

Smith, D.J. 2004. 'Premarital Sex, Procreation and HIV Risk in Nigeria', *Studies in Family Planning* 35(4): 223–35.

Tall, S.M., and A. Tandian. 2010. 'Entre regroupement familial et migrations autonomes des femmes sénégalaises. Quelle analyse de genre des migrations sénégalaises?', CARIM Notes d'analyse et de synthèse 2010/69, Robert Schuman Centre for Advanced Studies.

Takyi, B., and F.N.-A. Dodoo. 2005. 'Gender, Lineage and Fertility-Related Outcomes in Ghana', *Journal of Marriage and the Family* 67: 251–57.

Timaeus, I., and T. Moultrie. 2008. 'On Postponement and Birth Intervals', *Population and Development Review* 34(3): 484–510.

Towriss, C. 2014. 'Birth Intervals and Reproductive Intentions in Eastern Africa: Insights from Urban Fertility Transitions', unpublished Ph.D. thesis. London: University of London.

Vignikin, K. 2007. 'Famille et relations intergénérationnelles. Réflexions sur les évolutions en cours en Afrique', in P. Antoine (ed.), *Les relations intergénérationnelles en Afrique. Approche plurielle*. Paris: CEPED, pp. 19–30.

Wolff, B., A.K. Blanc and J. Ssekamatte-Ssebuliba. 2000. 'The Role of Couple Negotiation in Unmet Need for Contraception and the Decision to Stop Childbearing in Uganda', *Studies in Family Planning* 31(2): 124–37.

Chapter 6

ACCOUNTING FOR REPRODUCTIVE DIFFERENCE

SOCIALITY, TEMPORALITY AND INDIVIDUALITY DURING PREGNANCY IN CAMEROON

Erica van der Sijpt

Introduction

The last few decades have witnessed a booming interest in the minutiae of human reproduction within anthropology. Starting off in the 1970s and 1980s as an 'anthropology of birth' aiming to document the relatively unknown childbirth practices from all over the world (Kay 1982; MacCormack 1982), the anthropological study of reproduction took a radically different turn from the 1990s onwards, when earlier normative and holistic descriptions of 'birthing systems' came under criticism. Influenced by poststructuralism, third-wave feminism, and an emerging global health discourse denouncing differentials in reproductive rights and decision-making power, anthropologists started to pay greater attention to the variations, contestations and politics of reproduction. What resulted was a proliferation of studies 'situating' people's reproductive agency, or the lack thereof, within the conflicting forces and power dynamics of daily life (Ginsburg and Rapp 1991, 1995; van Hollen 1994; Greenhalgh 1995).

This approach has yielded many new insights with regard to reproductive decision-making – an issue that had remained largely unaddressed in ethnographic accounts before the 1990s. Reproduction and its related choices have been shown to be 'stratified' issues: women and men from different backgrounds have different reproductive options at their disposal (Ginsburg and Rapp 1995). These options are intrinsically related to constantly changing social contexts and larger political arenas. Studies focusing on how people in different settings seize the reproductive options at hand have generated the common understanding that reproductive decision-making is less a matter of rational calculation than the outcome of an uncertain process of *navigation* (Vigh 2006) through complex social situations and other contingent circumstances (Lock and Kaufert 1997; Bledsoe 2002; Wardlow 2006; Cornwall 2007; Cole 2010; Van der Sijpt 2010, 2013).

In order to understand the particular dynamics of this navigation, Jennifer Johnson-Hanks (2006) has proposed viewing reproductive moments that require some form of decision-making as 'vital conjunctures'. Defined as 'socially structured zones of possibility that emerge around specific periods of potential transformation in a life' (2006: 22), vital conjunctures capture the structures, constraints and options that people encounter at possible turning points in their lives. The concept proved to be of direct empirical and theoretical relevance in Johnson-Hanks' study on first pregnancies in Cameroon. Analysing the experiences and decisions of her Cameroonian informants as part of a vital conjuncture allowed her to highlight not only the extreme uncertainty that such fertility events brought about, but also the contingent character of the choices that women made at those moments. In the face of the different scenarios for the future – or, in Johnson-Hanks' terms, 'horizons' – that could be imagined during these potential turning points, women constantly adapted their aspirations and their reproductive decisions. Johnson-Hanks' broader argument posits that in the current precarious Cameroonian context in which horizons constantly appear and disappear, people do not direct their life trajectories on the basis of prior strategies or fixed aspirations. Instead, their actions and choices are based upon 'judicious opportunism' – the pragmatic seizure of options that present themselves at certain points in life (Johnson-Hanks 2005).

Such an approach is very valuable for illuminating the ambiguities, complexities and inventiveness of reproductive behaviour. It also offers a useful starting point for exploring how the seemingly improvised individual manoeuvres that Johnson-Hanks captures with the term 'judicious opportunism' are nevertheless related to wider social structures – or stratifications – and to the passage of time. All vital conjunctures are, in the end, socially structured and temporally situated; individual manoeuvres are not endless or completely random, but always circumscribed by larger forces. These forces might play out differently for different (groups of) people and at different times, leading to divergences in reproductive behaviour and outcomes.

In this chapter, I would like to take the idea of vital conjunctures forward by investigating exactly those social and temporal forces[1] that systematically inform the possibilities of and constraints to reproductive action in Cameroon. In other words, I examine how women's reproductive decision-making during such conjunctures is *inherently* connected to their positions within the stratified landscape of fertility, and to their own and others' changing life courses. By linking women's belonging to certain subgroups and their position on the reproductive life trajectory to the options and horizons that appear and are explored during vital conjunctures,[2] I intend to give a substantiated account of *why* Cameroonian women make particular choices at critical moments in their reproductive lives (see also Guyer 2005; Slama 2007). The aim is to develop a more systematic understanding of (patterns in) 'reproductive navigation' – i.e. the ways in which people give direction to their reproductive conjunctures and trajectories – without, of course, overlooking the spontaneity, flexibility and 'judicious opportunism' that pervade everyday reproductive practice.

Such an endeavour is particularly relevant in light of the contemporary discussion among Africanist scholars about the *nature* of (reproductive) decision-making. A dominant argument in this debate states that, in so-called 'sociocentric' African settings, people's actions and experiences should not be situated in the individual body or mind alone; rather, they should be comprehended within the framework of a 'social body' that interconnects and integrates the self with its social relations (Turner 1995; Piot 1999). Reproductive decision-making, in this view, can never be purely individual; it is always intrinsically tied to the social fabric in which persons are embedded. Critics of this claim have argued that even in the most relational realities of African daily life, people *do* have the freedom to pursue personal goals and to be creative (Jackson and Karp 1990; Nyamnjoh 2002).[3] According to them, the empirical question should be how the individual and the social come to be negotiated in any process of achievement. This debate, then, has put the extent to and manner in which certain structural configurations affect people's reproductive navigation explicitly on the research agenda.

It is exactly this issue that I will take up in the remainder of this chapter. After outlining the context in which I did research, and in which Cameroonian women conceive, bear and lose their children, I will present the stories of two of my informants, both of whom conceived a pregnancy against their will or expectation. Their stories will form the starting point for an analysis of sociostructural, temporal and individual forces that influenced the nature and outcomes of these reproductive conjunctures. The resulting account of reproductive navigation will be both 'situated' and systematic: it will be grounded in local contingencies and yet will reveal some patterns that may help us make sense of heterogeneous reproductive practices in Cameroon and in other parts of our stratified world.

Methodology

The empirical data provided in this chapter were obtained over fifteen months of anthropological fieldwork, spread between 2004 and 2009, in a Gbigbil village in eastern Cameroon. The aim of the research project was to disentangle Gbigbil women's experiences with, and decisions around, different forms of interrupted fertility – such as miscarriages, stillbirths, induced abortions, infertility or child death. To gain an insight into women's perceptions and practices during such critical reproductive events, I was in close contact with twenty-five purposefully selected informants who had experienced at least one instance of interrupted fertility in their lives. This group included women from all ages, with different educational histories, economic backgrounds, marital statuses and reproductive experiences.

The longitudinal character of the research project allowed me to follow my informants over time and to observe and discuss the many developments in their reproductive trajectories. I investigated their reproductive experiences both retrospectively and on the spot. The situational dynamics of important past happenings were captured through multiple and extended life history interviews with these women as well as with some key persons in their lives. Through participant observation, I took part in the real-time reproductive events my informants experienced during my stays in the field, as well as in the health-seeking itineraries that ensued. The valuable knowledge thus obtained was complemented with insights gathered through numerous thematic interviews and twelve focus group discussions with other women and men in the village. Group discussions that focused explicitly on reproductive health decisions were often initiated with 'vignettes', or hypothetical case studies, upon which informants were asked to reflect together. On other occasions, I invited groups of women to re-enact certain decision moments; each of the participants would assume a different social role and try to affect the actions of the 'decision-maker' in ways that they thought were most representative for the particular social position they were asked to occupy. As such, I developed an insight into how women themselves 'situated' their reproductive decisions within the social fabric that made up their daily lives.

Because of the highly confidential and often secret information that my informants would share with me in personal conversations, I always asked for their explicit consent when interviewing them and recording our interactions. All names appearing in the case studies are fictive; personal details that could potentially lead to the identification of my informants have been omitted from the descriptions. Before presenting those particular stories, however, I will give an overview of the most important historical and contemporary dynamics in which the reproductive conjunctures under study should be situated.

The Landscape of Fertility: Old Expectations and New Horizons

In the east of Cameroon, motherhood has long been the most important marker of womanhood. Historically, it was through bearing children that women contributed to the successes of men; in the semi-nomadic communities that inhabited this vast rainforest area until the nineteenth century, to become a male adult was to separate oneself from the patriliny, create an autonomous settlement and become the chief of a new family unit. Power and respect depended on the number of followers (such as family members, wives, children, devotees or slaves) a man could subsequently subject to himself – a 'wealth in people' principle that was widespread throughout the region (Laburthe-Tolra 1981; Geschiere 1982; Guyer 1984; Copet-Rougier 1985, 1987; Johnson-Hanks 2006) and that eventually led to the development of large polygynous households after sedentarization in the nineteenth century. Although women could not be 'honourable' themselves, by bearing the children that would expand a man's group of followers, they were essential contributors to the masculine honour upon which societal organization was based.

Yet, as rules of exogamy demanded that potential wives were chosen among those groups with which war was possible – i.e. non-related patrilinies – a married woman's position, and her reproductive capacities in particular, was fraught with ambiguity (de Thé 1970; Geschiere 1982; Copet-Rougier 1985; Houseman 1988). For her husband and his family, she was a (potentially dangerous) outsider on whom they depended for the continuation of their lineage; for her own family, she became an outsider as well, since she would leave her paternal home and bear children that would belong to another patriline. Upon marriage, the latter would therefore demand some compensation for the 'loss' of their daughter and her childbearing capacities to an unrelated group. This compensation – several gifts, social duties and brideprice payments over time – created an enduring reciprocal alliance between the lineages and appeased the inherent ambiguities of the exogamous marriage rule. Fertility, then, was at the crux of societal organization and continuation.

Although the last century has witnessed drastic societal changes, many contemporary expectations with regard to marriage and motherhood are rooted in this historical context. In the Gbigbil village in which I conducted fieldwork, exogamy and virilocality[4] still define with whom and where marital unions are formed; family members reserve the right to be involved in partner choice and the marital lives of their children; and people maintain high hopes with regard to brideprice transactions. Yet, while marriage norms and expectations have probably always diverged to some extent from actual conjugal practices in the region, several recent developments have certainly contributed to a discrepancy between historically rooted marital ideals and reality: First, in the context of a longlasting economic crisis that started in the second half of the 1980s, payment of (parts of) the brideprice is often delayed or completely discarded.[5] As a consequence, definitions of marriage have become more flexible (with brideprice no longer its *sine qua non* condition) and the belonging of children born in the union more contested (with family members of the woman claiming their daughter's children in the absence of any matrimonial compensation).

Second, in the face of multiple urban horizons and alternative forms of honour related to schooling and formal employment, marriage and parenthood have ceased to be the only means to attain respect. Many Gbigbil women alternate their stay in the village with shorter or longer periods in urban realms, where different lifestyles and imagined futures offer attractive alternatives to the rural ethics of production and reproduction that frame 'good womanhood' in terms of agricultural work and conjugal childbearing. This is not to say that marriage and motherhood are not important for those exploring urban horizons; yet, these goals seem to become relevant only later in life (see also Goheen 1993; Calvès 1999; Johnson-Hanks 2006, 2007; van der Sijpt 2011).

Both developments have engendered a proliferation of premarital sexual relationships, which might or might not culminate in what is finally agreed to be a marriage. Both partners take time to explore each other's traits: women want to be ensured of the good character and (financial) responsibilities of a man before settling down in his family, whereas men await a proof of a woman's fertility before engaging more formally. These informal unions, in which brideprice payments are most often lacking, are easily dissolved and replaced when more attractive horizons arise. Municipal or religious unions, which formally restrict this marital freedom, are rare in the village. With polygyny being a widespread phenomenon, men especially seem hesitant to preclude the option of taking another wife in the future – much to the lamentation of women who indicate that relations between co-wives are often characterized by jealousy and conflict.

Within this flexible and competitive marriage setting, bearing children is not always the primary aim of either partner, nor does it necessarily lead to the consolidation of a union. To conceive a pregnancy *can* be an important strategy for women to convince their partners of their worth and of the necessity of initiating negotiations between families. But, at the same time, many youngsters indicate that their partners often miraculously disappear upon the discovery of a pregnancy, while married mothers denounce the complete lack of (financial) commitment of their husbands or in-laws. Furthermore, women themselves may, for several reasons, refuse to get pregnant or to carry their pregnancies to term. Abortions are common events in women's reproductive life trajectories; since an early pregnancy is believed to contain only 'water water' (*medii medii*) and is traditionally shrouded in silence, it can be easily interrupted, without too many moral scruples or interventions from others.

Thus, although motherhood is, just like marriage, an ultimate goal in life that most women will eventually choose to pursue (preferably within a conjugal framework), reproductive events are often contested and their outcomes are contingent. Pregnancies, then, are uncertain conjunctures in which aspirations may come to be reconsidered and previous pathways to be redirected; fertility outcomes are largely unpredictable as a result. The stories of two informants, both of whom experienced an unexpected pregnancy during my fieldwork, will illustrate the complexity of such reproductive navigation. Set against very different personal backgrounds and conjunctural circumstances, their stories allow us not only to disentangle the particularities of their decisions, but also to understand some structural factors that seem to shape the possibilities for those decisions. On the basis of these two cases, as well as many others that I have observed in this east Cameroonian village, I will present some general insights about the social, temporal and individual forces at play in reproductive navigation.

Nadine

Nadine was born as the sixth of ten children in a relatively rich and respected family owning several cocoa and coffee plantations. Her father had been eager to grant all his children an honourable future; he arranged respectable marriages for his first sons and daughters, while he sent his younger children, like Nadine, to school. When his sudden death and the concomitant loss of revenues in the family jeopardized the future education of these children, his sister, who resided in the provincial capital, decided to foster the then thirteen-year-old Nadine and allow her to continue high school in the city. However, Nadine's urban lifestyle ended when she got pregnant; after a failed abortion attempt, she returned to the village where she eventually gave birth to a son whom her mother had decided to raise. After the death of this boy, Nadine entered and left two informal marriages, both of which were arranged by her mother. Two of the four children she had borne in those marriages died; the other two remained with the second ex-husband, the son of the village chief (an old friend of Nadine's father). Nadine's decision to leave the latter for the much younger and poorer Didier had raised eyebrows within her family. Knowing that their father *and* their mother, who had recently died, would surely have opposed this move, Nadine's brothers and older sisters, representing parental authority, strongly disapproved of the union.

The subsequent death of the son who was born in this relationship left Nadine with no children to care for, no stable relationship with Didier, no family support and no clear future perspectives. She therefore gladly left the village when a family member offered her a job as a servant in Douala, Cameroon's economic capital. However, disappointed with the hard working conditions and with the poor and irresponsible lovers she met, she decided to return to her natal village nine months later. Here, another disappointment awaited her as it turned out that Didier had been having relationships with two other women. The anticipated return to her previous 'marriage' was no longer so evident; she had to seek refuge with her brothers.

It is in this situation that Nadine finds out that she is again pregnant – probably from a married lover in Douala. With her current position and marital future being uncertain, the pregnancy opens a reproductive conjuncture in Nadine's life: what to do? After an initial wish for an abortion of what will become a 'bastard child', Nadine decides to keep the pregnancy; this pregnant state might enable her to undergo treatment for the affliction (*iwō*) that she suspects caused her previous children's deaths.[6] At the same time, this pregnancy might help her find a marriage somewhere in the city; now that gossip about her marital instability abounds in the village, Nadine would like to restore her honour by marrying a respectable man elsewhere. This might at the same time prevent her child from becoming the 'bastard child' she initially feared it would be.

The question thus becomes to who to 'give' her pregnancy. Three men at this point enter the stage: next to the biological father from Douala and her socially recognized husband Didier in the village, she recognizes another promising candidate: the driver of the car she travelled with on her way back from Douala. As a man without a wife and with a formal job in the provincial capital, this driver quickly turns into one of Nadine's lovers worthy of imagining a shared future with – more than the two other men at the moment. For, she contemplates, the man in Douala will never acknowledge paternity; a formal engagement with that married man is highly unlikely. Didier, on the other hand, has proven to be promiscuous and is moreover based in the village – a place that she seriously considers leaving now that it is associated with deception, child death, family frictions and gossip. She decides that if the driver shows commitment, she will try to convince him that he is the father-to-be.

Starting her treatment itinerary while still contemplating a possible father, Nadine is then told by an indigenous healer in the village that in order to heal her affliction effectively, she needs the cooperation of the father of the pregnancy – which is assumed to be Didier. Due to his physical proximity and her desire to be treated, Nadine switches focus, telling Didier that the pregnancy she carries is his. Didier agrees to cooperate in the treatment, but her brothers and sisters object to this strategic move. Nadine's older sister discloses the truth about the origin of Nadine's pregnancy to Didier, who immediately breaks off all contact.

With no other men in the direct neighbourhood to run to, and with the burden of shame and family curses caused by her capricious marital behaviour, Nadine decides on an abortion. Supported by some female friends in the village, she attempts to interrupt the pregnancy with a toenail, with some herbal concoctions and with an overdose of antimalarial drugs. After repeated failures, Didier begs her to keep the pregnancy, despite his ambivalence regarding his paternity. A future marriage with him is again envisaged and negotiated: Didier proposes to fully engage once a blood test on the newborn baby confirms his paternity; Nadine demands his future faithfulness and their relocation to the city.

However, when Didier traces several of Nadine's lovers on her mobile phone, his uncertainty about his paternity is exacerbated and he retreats again. This, together with the additional curses she receives from several family members, strengthens Nadine's wish to leave the village forever. When she coincidentally receives a phone call from the taxi driver, she immediately tells him she carries his pregnancy. The man is overwhelmed and asks her for time to reflect. In this undecided period Nadine points at the radical uncertainty of this reproductive conjuncture: 'The ball is still turning. My chance will fall wherever it falls. If it is with Didier, I will return to the village. But he knows my conditions; I have decided I want to live in the city. Even if he doesn't agree, I will leave. And if I succeed at the other side [i.e. with the driver], I will block him [i.e. Didier] for sure.'

Two years later, I find Nadine living with her only surviving twin daughter in the house of a friend in the village. None of her marriage attempts had been successful, but her priority now is to ensure the survival of her baby girl. All the rest is secondary, she asserts. 'What comes next, comes next.'

Yvette

Unlike many Gbigbil women, Yvette grew up among her maternal family members. Left behind by her mother who went back and forth between different marriages, Yvette spent her youth, together with her younger brother, next to her maternal grandmother. The grandmother, who herself also settled down in her own family after several failed marriages, was a hard-working woman whose aim was to provide good care and education for Yvette and all the other grandchildren in her household. However, school ended for Yvette when she conceived a pregnancy with an urban lover at the age of fourteen. Intending to bear many children, whom she would consider as the brothers and sisters she never had, Yvette decided to keep the child, but refused a future with the urban lover. After delivering her son in her maternal grandmother's house, Yvette met Daniel, the son of a chief in the village, who made her pregnant and married her as a second wife.

While the beginning of the marriage was good and harmonious, problems came when – after bearing a daughter and a son – Yvette started losing her children. Three sons in a row died immediately after birth. After a daughter was born who stayed alive, another son did not survive an extremely problematic delivery that almost cost Yvette's life. Left without the baby and with serious physical problems, Yvette was advised by doctors and village *mamas* never to conceive again and to focus instead on raising her four living children. Although the marriage had become fraught with conflict – her husband and in-laws suspected her of having killed her children and those of her co-wife (who also lost three children) through witchcraft – Yvette decided just to cling to her position of married wife and mother, and to reduce her vulnerability by assuming the associated responsibilities.

It is in this situation that Yvette, despite all her intentions and efforts to 'prevent a pregnancy from entering', conceives again. This conception opens a critical conjuncture in her life. Carrying another pregnancy so quickly after her 'near-miss' experience, from which she is still recovering, poses not only serious physical risks but also jeopardizes her social status as a *responsible* wife and mother. Initially, therefore, she tries to get rid of this pregnancy. But her ignorance of effective abortion methods, the unwillingness of other women to share this knowledge with her, and especially her fear of abortion-related death eventually lead her to accept the fact that she is, in the end, 'a married woman and supposed to bear children'.

Yvette's husband and in-laws disagree. Still remembering the financial costs incurred by her last problematic delivery and remaining suspicious about the wave of child deaths in their household, they refuse to support the pregnant Yvette in any way until they see the results of the delivery. Their explicit financial neglect infuriates her to such an extent that she repeatedly throws all her kitchen utensils outside – thus indicating her readiness to leave the marriage. Yet, her strong determination to abscond stands in stark contrast to the weak support networks outside of the conjugal context: with the recent death of her grandmother, there are no maternal family members left who would support her plans or accept her to come home; her paternal relatives, who would normally interfere in conjugal disputes, are rather indifferent to her, as she did not grow up in their midst. Moving to the city is not an attractive option either. Without a school diploma or social contacts there, she feels unequipped for urban life. And, in her view, her physical state would also not allow her to move away from the village. She therefore sees no other option than to 'stay and endure', i.e. carry the pregnancy to term and hope that she and her child will survive; only then will the future that she envisages for herself be safeguarded.

Despite very critical circumstances requiring a long period in hospital both Yvette and her baby boy survive the delivery. Her husband and in-laws seem satisfied with the situation, now that a new son has been added to the family. They agree to her using the contraceptive pill to prevent further fertility-related dramas. The reproductive conjuncture seems over: she can stay in the marriage and focus on raising her children again, without having to fear risky reproduction in the future. But then, after a few weeks, the baby dies. This death triggers much upheaval and contestations about Yvette's position as a wife and a mother; it reopens the conjuncture. Daniel and his relatives decide that since so much money and so many descendants were lost and since no children are to be expected from Yvette in the future, no brideprice payments should ever be transferred to her family.

Furious about this neglect of conjugal obligations, Yvette considers leaving the marriage, but finds herself, once again, obliged to stay:

> Since I don't even have any family to support me . . . If I had such a person, I would not even be here anymore. But now, if I left, where would I stay? My grandmother is dead. Others don't care. And to still find another marriage with these children behind me, that would not be easy either. Going into a new marriage is anyway dangerous for me. It will always be the same thing: the man will first want to have intercourse in order to give me a pregnancy. And that's not possible anymore. No, I am in this marriage and I will stay – brideprice or not. What can I do? It's the village. You have to be married.

It is only when Yvette's brother dies a few months later and when Daniel refuses to fulfil his financial duties that her paternal relatives openly denounce Daniel's financial irresponsibility. Among different sanctions, they set an ultimatum for a first brideprice transaction: if nothing is paid within a few months, they will come to take Yvette home. And so it happens. After more than fifteen years of marriage, Yvette leaves her husband and children behind and settles in the village of her paternal uncles. The reproductive conjuncture that surrounded her last pregnancy has come to a close; thanks to the ones from whom she expected it least, she has embarked upon a new pathway into the future.

Situating Reproductive Navigation: Social Stakes and Subgroups

These two cases tell the stories of two women from different backgrounds who found themselves in completely different circumstances when they encountered a similar reproductive event – an unexpected pregnancy. The sequence of conjunctures in which they and those around them came to terms with that event present particular convergences of past reproductive pathways, existing options, constraints and future aspirations. To recount all the options and horizons that Gbigbil women can possibly encounter and explore during such conjunctures – conjunctures that are multiple and situated in wider, ever-changing historical, political and economic conditions – would be an endless enterprise. The two stories illustrate this variation.

However, all reproductive conjunctures in this eastern Cameroonian region eventually touch upon similar (locally grounded and shared) dilemmas. Broadly, what is at stake is (embracing or rejecting) motherhood and/or wifehood, and (continuing or abandoning) one's pathway towards rural or urban respectability. The question is why certain women favour one horizon while others cling to another, and which structural configurations make women more or less liable to prefer certain horizons from the outset. My analysis of the stories of Nadine, Yvette and many others suggests that there are several forms of sociality that affect this navigation.[7] Women's reproductive pathways and possibilities are informed by their positions in a number of social subgroups.

First, one's position among siblings matters. It makes a difference whether a woman is her mother's first or last daughter and whether she has few or many siblings. First or only daughters are often highly valued for the brideprice they are expected to bring to the family, and are therefore most likely to be put on a pathway leading to marriage and childbearing (in order to encourage in-laws to fulfil their financial obligations). This happened, for instance, to the first daughters of Nadine's father. Later daughters, such as Nadine, can benefit from the marital careers of their older sisters and are likely to have more freedom in pursuing alternative respectable futures (at least temporarily).

Second, one's position within a wider body of kin relations matters. It makes a difference whether a woman was born within or outside a conjugal framework, and whether she grew up in her own patrilineage or among her maternal uncles. Women who grow up among paternal kin are more likely to be encouraged to achieve motherhood (within or outside of marriage) as their children can be claimed and added to the patriline in case of unacknowledged paternity or marital disruptions. The ease with which Nadine's mother decided to take care of Nadine's first child shows the point. Women like Yvette who were born outside of a marital union and grew up among their maternal uncles experience less pressure in this respect, as the matriline generally does not profit from brideprice payments and the offspring of daughters. At the same time, such women also receive less support if they encounter problems on their marital or reproductive pathways, as we saw in Yvette's case. They may therefore have fewer possibilities to change those pathways when confronted with a critical reproductive conjuncture.

Third, the position of a woman's kin group within wider networks matters. In the current atmosphere of political and economic nepotism, daughters from families in which important persons have informal political power, formal employment or large urban networks are better positioned to profit from such established financial and social capital. Women like Nadine, whose father was quite influential, are thus more likely to embark upon pathways towards urban respectability from a young age – through schooling or well-off foster parents in the city, for instance. During unexpected reproductive conjunctures, these women may be less inclined to cling to motherhood and wifehood, and may be supported by their family members and other villagers in this deviation from rural respectability (based on the ethics of production and reproduction). That this is less the case for women whose relatives occupy a vulnerable or isolated position in the wider community becomes clear if we look at Yvette's story. Backed up only by her maternal grandmother and (to a lesser extent) her mother, both of whom had precarious positions in the compound of their maternal uncles, Yvette did not have the freedom to drastically change her plans and pathways when she was confronted with critical reproductive events. Alternative horizons were simply few and far between.

Fourth, one's position in the marriage market matters. It makes a difference whether a woman has many or few boyfriends, and whether her partner(s) is (or are) ready to become engaged or not. A woman who has multiple partners in both rural and urban zones, like Nadine, may feel less inclined to accept or pursue marriage and motherhood with one particular partner than women like Yvette who, due to social or physical circumstances, occupy a less solid position in the wider marriage market. Multiple partners may offer multiple horizons and thereby create more room for changing pathways, aspirations and decisions in case of critical reproductive events. Further, the eagerness of one's partner(s) to become engaged influences one's navigation of reproductive conjunctures. Especially when paternity is acknowledged and financial commitment is shown, motherhood and marriage can become immediate priorities informing reproductive decisions. However, in the absence of signs of commitment, alternative pathways and partners may be preferred instead. Faced with the disengagement of multiple partners, for instance, Nadine considered the interruption of her pregnancy to be the only way out of her unexpected reproductive conjuncture.

Fifth, if already married, one's position within the marriage matters. It makes a difference whether a woman is the first, second or third wife of her husband and whether she has a good or bad relationship with her in-laws and co-wives (if present). The pressure to be a good wife and mother is often greatest for first wives, as a husband and in-laws are generally most eager to see their patriline expand at the beginning of a marriage. Subsequent wives are often granted a bit more freedom – as seen in Daniel's approval of Yvette's use of contraceptives. At the same time, later wives occupy a more competitive and contested position; their fertility events are usually surrounded by more conjugal complications and explicit reconsideration of their pathways and aspirations. Fights with in-laws and co-wives, often inspired by fertility-related matters, are common reasons to abandon one's marital pathway. The ease with which this is done depends on whether (parts of) the brideprice has been paid. Although instances of divorce after brideprice exchange are certainly not rare, the transfer of sums of money from one's in-laws to one's own family members (who often immediately consume it and would not be able to pay it back in the event of divorce) complicates one's decision to abandon a marriage during critical reproductive events.

Together, these five configurations circumscribe, to a greater or lesser extent, the availability of options in reproductive conjunctures, and thereby form possibilities and/or constraints to women's decision-making. Reproductive navigation is thus always a socially contingent affair, inherently dependent on one's social positioning in relation to relevant others. Yet, both this position and the social subgroups themselves are constantly in flux, as time passes by and people move forward in their life trajectories. Such changes influence the processes and outcomes of reproductive navigation. The next section therefore explores the implications of temporality for the decisions women can (or cannot) make during particular conjunctures.

Reproductive Navigation in Flux: Locating Conjunctures in Time

The very notion of a conjuncture indicates a critical *duration* – a longer or shorter period of uncertainty and potential transformation provoked by the convergence of certain circumstances. Restricting our focus to one such conjuncture – such as an unexpected pregnancy – allows us to unravel the minutiae of that duration, as well as the contingencies of its onset, unfolding and outcomes. Yet, when we look beyond its boundaries and follow people longitudinally, taking their broader life courses into account, we discover that a reproductive trajectory is, in fact, a long string of conjunctures. The dynamics in these different conjunctures are not fully independent of one another; outcomes of previous reproductive conjunctures inform the possibilities at later critical moments. Thus, when systematically analysing the appearance of such possibilities, and women's navigation at particular reproductive conjunctures – as is my aim in this chapter – we should locate the conjuncture not only within concurrent structural contexts but also within the wider flux of the life trajectory. For Gbigbil women, past reproductive happenings and choices inform their reproductive navigation in several ways.

An important factor in decision-making during any reproductive conjuncture is whether a woman has already borne children before or not.[8] How the presence (or absence) of children influences the outcome of the conjuncture at hand depends, in turn, on how much that woman has advanced on her life trajectory. For young Gbigbil women, the absence of children and of a 'mother' status may provide an opportunity to focus on ambitions unrelated to maternity, such as education, employment, small-scale trade or relations with affluent sexual partners. When confronted with an unexpected pregnancy at this point in life, such youngsters often choose to have an abortion.[9] Others may keep the pregnancy, but as pregnancies do not necessarily imply social motherhood or marriage in this area, they can still remain focused on alternative projects for the future. The presence of children does not necessarily preclude options. Nadine and Yvette, for instance, both left their first babies with female family members and moved on.

However, such decision-making patterns are only tenable up to a certain point. The more a woman moves forward on her life trajectory, the greater the social pressure to start bearing children or, if babies have been borne already, to find a suitable husband and to take care of her children. Thus, over time, marriage and motherhood are likely to increase their saliency as aspirations and proposed pathways directing women's reproductive navigation. Nadine's desperate attempts to find a respectable husband after she discovered her pregnancy, as well as her siblings' admonitions when she appeared unsuccessful, are a case in point.

Options and horizons may change again when a history of successful and respectful childbearing has been established. The presence of (live) children confirms one's worth as a woman and a real (or potential) wife and mother, and can thereby open up new horizons that are less related to maternity. In contrast, a long history of unsuccessful fertility can foreclose marital options and diminish maternal ambitions. Women with such experiences turn their focus more easily to urban horizons or virtues unrelated to wifehood and/or motherhood. This was seen in Yvette's clear wish to not conceive anymore and, eventually, to leave marriage in a village context altogether.

A young woman's position on her reproductive trajectory is not the only temporal dimension that is subject to change. The positions of relevant others – members of the various subgroups outlined above – on their respective trajectories are also changing. As a consequence, the influence that siblings, parents, partners, in-laws, co-wives and other villagers have on a particular woman's decisions depends in turn on *their* life contingencies, *their* previous pathways and *their* stakes at that moment. Seen in this dynamic and diachronic light, reproductive navigation is not only socially *contingent* but also *inter*contingent (Becker 1994). In other words, life stories intersect; a woman's navigation never happens independently from the dynamic navigations of those around her. The outcomes of reproductive conjunctures are informed by women's position in relation to the social networks around them, and by the ways in which their position and networks adjust to each other at a particular point in time. Reproductive navigation is thus both socially structured and temporally constrained.

And yet, despite such intersections of social and temporal forces in any reproductive conjuncture, Gbigbil women seem to have plenty of room for manoeuvre. The next section will explore the relevance of notions and expressions of individuality – the presence of creativity, tactics and inventiveness – in daily Gbigbil life and in reproductive navigation more particularly.

Room for Individual Manoeuvre: The Power of Personal 'Politiques'

The stories of Nadine and Yvette have shown that these women – irrespective of their personal background, social network or position on the reproductive trajectory – *did* find room to manoeuvre through complex circumstances when striving after their own goals. Both of them had clear ideas about the stakes and the desired outcomes of their reproductive conjunctures, even if these ran against what others had in mind. Nadine, for instance, expressed a very strong wish to enter an urban, respectable union and used her pregnancy to try to realize this personal aspiration. Yvette's priority was to stay healthy and to avoid future fertility events; it was therefore in her interests to remain in a rural marriage and enforce the use of modern contraception – a remarkable achievement in a rural setting where an enduring marriage is inextricably connected to childbearing. Given the inherent sociality of reproductive experiences and decisions as discussed above, the question is how we should understand and situate such individual moves.

First of all, it should be pointed out that notions of individuality are not unheard of in this village. In fact, they have a long history in this region, where social relations prior to colonization were organized according to principles of separation and resettlement: once individual men attained a certain age and independence, they would leave their kin group to found an autonomous village elsewhere in the rainforest. On the basis of personal talent and characteristics, men attempted to enlarge their group of followers and gain wider respect and power (Laburthe-Tolra 1981). Social organization was based upon what Guyer (1996: 7) has described as a 'self-valuation/realization process whereby the singular pathways of personal expertise were competitively/performatively valued and validated'. Individuality *mattered* for the attainment of social status and power.

While this self-realization could historically be only achieved by adult men, nowadays it is something that women can and do aspire to as well. Individual achievements, inventions and improvisations are even considered constitutive of good and successful womanhood; my Gbigbil informants proudly called their individual manoeuvres 'politiques' without which they would not be able to succeed in life. Self-realization – and the concomitant preoccupation with one's own pathways in life – thus comprises a historically rooted 'social asset' (Guyer 1996: 6) that is highly valued in the contemporary social fabric of this east Cameroonian village.

As for the relationship between such particular pathways and social structures, Guyer (1996: 23) claims that 'to the degree that the creation of a life trajectory is a prominent principle in the social organization of assets, to the same degree will agency and improvisation have structural salience'. Indeed, Gbigbil women's celebration of their personal projects and 'politiques' can be related to some structural configurations that make up their daily lives. First, it is a result of their ambiguous positions as women and wives in society. Due to longstanding virilocal and patrilineal norms, and the reality of most brideprice obligations not being respected, women are not only considered 'outsiders' in their partners' households, but are also often moving between multiple, fragile partnerships and their own families. This situation both demands constant improvisation from women and offers them space for manipulation.

Second, beyond the marital framework, women and men face structural circumstances that require constant individual creativity. In the present era, when the economic crisis seems never-ending, (urban) opportunities are rare and unpredictable, the practice of witchcraft is believed to be omnipresent (Geschiere 1997, 2003) and longstanding norms of social interaction are often breached, 'horizons' may vanish as quickly as they appear. The mechanism underlying women's navigation of their reproductive conjunctures is indeed therefore one of 'judicious opportunism' (Johnson-Hanks 2005) – a matter of pragmatic improvisation rather than following a pre-established, rationalized itinerary. Instead of having clear trajectories in mind, my informants take promising chances.

Perhaps paradoxically, then, women's decision-making in the inherently *social* domain of reproduction is often an *individual* affair, with women exploring and evaluating promising horizons individually, inventively and often also secretly. Indeed, although nothing is more *social* than reproduction – enabling the continuation of the social order and imbuing parents with social status – nothing is more *individual* either. This is especially the case in a cultural context in which women are considered individual outsiders to the patrilineage into which their children are officially born, and where the first few months of pregnancy are shrouded in silence and denial. Both norms can leave the management of fertility largely in the hands of individual women: individuality and privacy offer pregnant women a secret space for decision-making.[10] Even if these decisions are never 'free choices', but are informed by social and temporal configurations, they may run counter to social norms. Due to this potential tension between individual experience and influence over fertility on the one hand and social interests and expectations on the other, reproduction – and even more its interruption – is often an extremely ambiguous affair.[11]

Conclusion

In this chapter, I have attempted to make sense of the 'messiness', heterogeneity and contingency of reproductive practice. While acknowledging that individual lives are unique and unpredictable, I have argued that a systematic investigation of the 'reproductive conjunctures' experienced by different Gbigbil women allows us to identify some structural issues that seem to be at play in all of them. Specifying the social subgroups, temporal dimensions and possibilities for individual manoeuvre that circumscribe action has revealed some mechanisms of reproductive navigation. Insight into such mechanisms is relevant for at least two reasons.

First, it offers a more nuanced understanding of the nature of decision-making. The ambiguous interplay between sociality and individuality that this chapter has highlighted sheds new light on a debate that has long divided those who focus on the social dependency and interconnectedness of reproductive decision-makers, and those who stress the potential for individual autonomy in fertility matters. I argue that, at least in the Gbigbil case, one does not exclude the other. Women can be intrinsically tied to social others – in different ways over time – and at the same time enact forms of individuality that are rooted in (and even encouraged by) that same social order.

Conceptually, such dynamics would be best captured through a combination of 'vital conjunctures' as proposed by Johnson-Hanks and 'social bodies' as proposed by Africanists such as Piot and Turner, as each of these terms makes up for shortcomings in the other. The concept of the vital conjuncture allows us to lay bare the minutiae of individual decision-making *within* social contingencies, but tends to overlook the *inter*contingencies and *inherent* sociality of agents as well as of the horizons that guide their navigation; the concept of the social body stresses exactly this state of interconnectedness, but often ignores its impact on individual decision-making. Taken together, they allow for a more comprehensive view of reproductive navigation – one that offers new avenues for theorizing the interrelationship between individual agency and the surrounding structural contexts.

Second, an in-depth understanding of the mechanisms of reproductive navigation is crucial for unravelling the nature of reproductive differences and stratifications. Identifying *which* specific subgroups and *which* developments in the life course are relevant to reproductive practice allows us to trace some regularities in the midst of heterogeneity – or, in Guyer's terms, to discover 'new aspects of "ordering" out of apparent randomness' (2005: 379). It is a first step towards accounting for the creation and reproduction of differentials in reproductive behaviour. Further, the identification of such structuring (and stratifying) forces in one particular setting might enable us to start comparing case studies in the same or different societies. For, even if locally grounded and continually in flux, the salient features of reproductive conjunctures in one setting may resonate with those in another. An exploration along these lines could shed new light on the wider implications of certain social and temporal dynamics for the local and global stratifications in the domain of reproductive health.

Erica van der Sijpt is a medical anthropologist at the University of Amsterdam who works on reproductive health issues. She has published several articles, chapters and a book on decision-making around pregnancy loss in Cameroon. Currently, she is conducting a postdoctoral research project on the challenges of motherhood in postcommunist Romania.

Notes

1. As I have argued elsewhere (Van der Sijpt 2013), aside from social structure and time, the *material body* can be considered another force informing the options and limitations that women encounter during critical fertility events. However, a discussion of such physical dynamics falls outside the scope of this chapter.
2. In the remainder of this chapter, I will speak of 'reproductive conjunctures' rather than 'vital conjunctures', since the prefix 'vital' renders the concept too broad and general for my purposes. After all, life is full of vital conjunctures of many different sorts – not only those related to fertility. I thus limit the scope of this chapter to critical moments around *reproductive* events and do not wish to claim that the described dynamics and proposed conclusions apply to other vital conjunctures in people's lives.
3. These critics are part of a wider group of scholars questioning the dichotomy between a Western ego-centric 'individual' and a non-Western sociocentric 'dividual' (see also Spiro 1993; Li Puma 1998; Sökefeld 1999; Carsten 2000, 2004; Halliburton 2002). Instead of interpreting the distinction between dividualistic and sociocentric notions of bodies and personhood in terms of Western and non-Western, they argue that both aspects are present in persons all over the world, but become variously dominant in different cultures or contexts.
4. Virilocality refers to the social system in which a married woman lives in the compound of her husband and his kin.
5. The quantity, quality and actual initiation of brideprice payments always seem to have been subject to change and negotiation (Guyer 1986). Studies among the neighbouring Beti show how men often preferred to postpone brideprice payments until they had seen proof of the fertility of their wives, and how women exerted considerable influence on marriage negotiations and on premarital or extramarital sexuality (de Thé 1970; Laburthe-Tolra 1981; Houseman 1988; Ombolo 1991).
6. *Iwō* is the Gbigbil word for a condition in which a woman's children repeatedly die. Several indigenous treatments of *iwō* exist, which are all to be initiated during pregnancy.
7. It is exactly because of their divergences that I have selected the cases of Yvette and Nadine to illustrate this argument. In case study research, such a strategy for choosing cases is called a 'diverse case method' (Gerring 2007: 97). The underlying idea is that by capturing as much variation as possible along relevant dimensions – here, women's belonging to social subgroups – common patterns and mechanisms can be revealed.
8. As Bledsoe (2002) has also argued, a woman's exact age (i.e. her position on a linear, temporal trajectory) seems to matter less than her contingent reproductive history.

9. Often, such a situation is preferred over the prevention of pregnancies through contraception. Given the importance attached to a large number of offspring in this village, young Gbigbil women like to have proof of their fecundity and be reassured that children can be borne in the future – even if they do not wish to bear them now.
10. Although a discussion of the perspectives and practices of Gbigbil men falls outside the scope of this chapter, it must be noted here that men are often aware of the existence of such secret 'politiques'. Acknowledging that the fate of any pregnancy is, eventually, largely in women's own hands, many of my male informants claimed to feel powerless in reproductive matters and to experience feelings of distrust towards their sexual partners – despite their attempts to control women's behaviour (van der Sijpt 2011).
11. This ambiguity finds a clear expression in the witchcraft accusations that easily erupt around reproductive conjunctures, as seen in Yvette's case. To accuse someone of being a witch is to insinuate that this person's actions are led by an occult and individual appetite for blood, flesh and wealth that is detrimental to social stability. The ubiquity of such suspicions reflects a local and historically embedded preoccupation with forms of individuality that have long been *recognized* but also *feared* – in society in general and in reproductive matters in particular (see also Geschiere 1997).

References

Becker, H.S. 1994. '"Foi por Acaso": Conceptualizing Coincidence', *Sociological Quarterly* 35(2): 183–94.

Bledsoe, C. 2002. *Contingent Lives: Fertility, Time, and Aging in West Africa*. Chicago: University of Chicago Press.

Calvès, A.E. 1999. 'Marginalization of African Single Mothers in the Marriage Market: Evidence from Cameroon', *Population Studies* 53(3): 291–301.

Carsten, J. 2000. *Cultures of Relatedness: New Approaches to the Study of Kinship*. Cambridge: Cambridge University Press.

———. 2004. *After Kinship*. Cambridge: Cambridge University Press.

Cole, J. 2010. *Sex and Salvation. Imagining the Future in Madagascar.* Chicago: University of Chicago Press.

Copet-Rougier, E. 1985. 'Controle Masculin, Exclusivité Féminine dans une Société Patrilinéaire', in J.C. Barbier (ed.), *Femmes du Cameroun. Mères Pacifiques, Femmes Rebelles*. Paris: Karthala, pp. 153–80.

———. 1987. 'Du Clan à la Chefferie dans l'Est du Cameroun', *Africa* 57: 345–63.

Cornwall, A. 2007. 'Taking Chances, Making Choices: The Tactical Dimensions of "Reproductive Strategies" in Southwestern Nigeria', *Medical Anthropology* 26(3): 229–54.

De Thé, M.P. 1970. *Des Sociétés Secrètes aux Associations Modernes. La Femme dans la Dynamique de la Société Beti, 1887–1966*. Paris: École Pratique des Hautes Études.

Gerring, J. 2007. *Case Study Research: Principles and Practice.* Cambridge: Cambridge University Press.

Geschiere, P. 1982. *Village Communities and the State: Changing Relations among the Maka of South-Eastern Cameroon since the Colonial Conquest.* London: Kegan Paul International.

———. 1997. *The Modernity of Witchcraft: Politics and the Occult in Postcolonial Africa*. Charlottesville: University of Virginia Press.

———. 2003. 'Witchcraft as the Dark Side of Kinship: Dilemmas of Social Security in New Contexts', *Etnofoor* 16: 43–61.

Ginsburg, F.D., and R. Rapp. 1991. 'The Politics of Reproduction', *Annual Review of Anthropology* 20: 311–43.

———. 1995. *Conceiving the New World Order: The Global Politics of Reproduction.* Berkeley: University of California Press.

Goheen, M. 1993. 'Les Champs Appartiennent aux Hommes, Les Récoltes aux Femmes: Accumulation dans la Region de Nso', in P. Geschiere and P. Konings (eds), *Itinéraires d'Accumulation au Cameroun*. Paris: Karthala, pp. 241–72.

Greenhalgh, S. 1995. *Situating Fertility: Anthropology and Demographic Inquiry.* Cambridge: Cambridge University Press.

Guyer, J.I. 1984. *Family and Farm in Southern Cameroon,* vol. 15. Boston: Boston University, African Studies Center.

———. 1986. 'Indigenous Currencies and the History of Marriage Payments: A Case Study from Cameroon', *Cahiers d'Études Africaines* 26(104): 577–610.

———. 1996. 'Traditions of Invention in Equatorial Africa', *African Studies Review* 39(3): 1–28.

———. 2005. 'Comment on "When the Future Decides: Uncertainty and Intentional Action in Contemporary Cameroon" by Jennifer Johnson-Hanks', *Current Anthropology* 46(3): 379.

Halliburton, M. 2002. 'Rethinking Anthropological Studies of the Body: *Manas* and *Bodham* in Kerala', *American Anthropologist* 104(4): 1123–34.

Houseman, M. 1988. 'Social Structure is Where the Hearth is: A "Woman's Place" in Beti Society', *Africa* 58(1): 51–69.

Jackson, M., and I. Karp. 1990. *Personhood and Agency: The Experience of Self and Other in African Cultures*. Uppsala: Acta Universitatis Upsaliensis.

Johnson-Hanks, J. 2005. 'When the Future Decides: Uncertainty and Intentional Action in Contemporary Cameroon', *Current Anthropology* 46(3): 363–86.

———. 2006. *Uncertain Honor: Modern Motherhood in an African Crisis.* Chicago: University of Chicago Press.

———. 2007. 'Women on the Market: Marriage, Consumption, and the Internet in Urban Cameroon', *American Ethnologist* 34(4): 642–58.

Kay, M.A. 1982. *Anthropology of Human Birth.* Philadelphia: F.A. Davis.
Laburthe-Tolra, P. 1981. *Mínlaaba. Les Seigneurs de la Fôret.* Paris: Karthala.
Li Puma, E. 1998. 'Modernity and Forms of Personhood in Melanesia', in M. Lambek and A. Strathern (eds), *Bodies and Persons: Comparative Perspectives from Africa and Melanesia.* Cambridge: Cambridge University Press, pp. 53–79.
Lock, M., and P.A. Kaufert. 1997. *Pragmatic Women and Body Politics.* New York: Cambridge University Pres.
MacCormack, C.P. (ed.). 1982. *Ethnography of Fertility and Birth.* New York: Academic Press.
Nyamnjoh, F.B. 2002. '"A Child is One Person's Only in the Womb". Domestication, Agency and Subjectivity in the Cameroonian Grassfields', in R. Werbner (ed.), *Postcolonial Subjectivities in Africa.* London: Zed Books, pp. 111–38.
Ombolo, J.P. 1991. *Sexe et Société en Afrique Noire: l'Anthropologie Sexuelle Beti. Essai Analytique, Critique et Comparatif.* Paris: L'Harmattan.
Piot, C.D. 1999. *Remotely Global: Village Modernity in West Africa.* Chicago: University of Chicago Press.
Slama, M. 2007. 'Review of Uncertain Honor: Modern Motherhood in an African Crisis', *European Association of Social Anthropologists* 393–94.
Sökefeld, M. 1999. 'Debating Self, Identity, and Culture in Anthropology ', *Current Anthropology* 40(4): 417–48.
Spiro, M.E. 1993. 'Is the Western Conception of the Self "Peculiar" within the Context of the World Cultures?', *Ethos* 21(2): 107–53.
Turner, T. 1995. 'Social Body and Embodied Subject: Bodiliness, Subjectivity, and Sociality among the Kayapo', *Cultural Anthropology* 10(2): 143–70.
Van der Sijpt, E. 2010. 'Marginal Matters: Pregnancy-Loss as a Social Event', *Social Science & Medicine* 71(10): 1773–79.
———. 2011. '"The Vagina Does Not Talk": Conception Concealed or Deliberately Disclosed in Cameroon', *Culture, Health, and Sexuality* 14(1): S81–S94.
———. 2013. 'Complexities and Contingencies Conceptualized: Towards a Model of Reproductive Navigation', *Sociology of Health & Illness* 36(2): 278–90.
Van Hollen, C.C. 1994. 'Perspectives on the Anthropology of Birth', *Culture, Medicine and Psychiatry* 18(4): 501–12.
Vigh, H. 2006. *Navigating Terrains of War. Youth and Soldiering in Guinea-Bissau.* New York: Berghahn Books.
Wardlow, H. 2006. *Wayward Women: Sexuality and Agency in a New Guinea Society.* Berkeley: University of California Press.

Chapter 7

Understanding Childlessness in Botswana

Reproduction and Tswana-nization of Middle-Class Identities in the Twenty-First Century

Astrid Bochow

Introduction

Sandra, aged thirty-two, is one of many working women I met in the course of my research on urban professionals in Botswana and their uses of reproductive medicine. Her husband is member of the Botswana Defence Force (BDF) and she works in a local administration. With her high school degree and her job in lower-level management, she may count as belonging to a group of rising urban professionals, though she has not quite reached the economic standard of many in the economic and political elite. Sandra married two years ago and has a child aged fifteen. Her husband has no children, and the couple now wishes to have a child together. They have been 'trying' for about a year and are now seeking medical assistance in one of the private hospitals in Gaborone (interview, 11 November 2010).[1]

Sandra's story fits well into the findings of Botswana's national statistics, which show a rapid decline of fertility since the 1990s. These statistics indicate that the total fertility rate has fallen from 6.6 in 1985 to 2.9 in 2006 (Botswana Central Statistics Office 2009: 4). This development is astonishing in view of the ever-growing fertility rates across the continent in the 1970s, which have proven modernization's theory of demographic transition to be wrong (Caldwell 1977). Drawing upon experience of what is called the fertility transition in European countries, the theory assumed that increased standards of living and levels of industrialization, as well as growing response to formal education, would impact on family sizes (Goode 1963; Caldwell 1982). In fact, Sandra's life course seems to feature some of modernization theory's assumptions on the causes of fertility decline, such as the correlation between level of education and a drop in family size. As our understanding of demographic transition has advanced, it has been realized that one of the important indicators of fertility decline, next to ceasing or postponing births, is child spacing. In the 1970s, when family planning methods were introduced into Botswana and other African countries, the hope was that contraceptives would enable women to postpone and or space their births, and that this would reduce overall fertility rates (Namboodiri 1964; Wray 1971; Page and Lesthaeghe 1981; Westoff and Charles 2000). Counter to this hypothesis, anthropological demographers, such as Caroline Bledsoe (Bledsoe 2002), have shown that child spacing might indeed serve to *enhance* fertility in some African communities, such as those she studied among the Kpelle in Cameroon.

In this chapter I will show that Sandra's child spacing may be viewed as a specific form of fertility reduction that comes with the popularization of elite lifestyles among upwardly mobile urban professionals and that has also been induced by the spread of HIV/AIDS. Sandra and her husband are representative of this group. However, the exceptional life courses of educated professionals who have experienced fertility problems in twenty-first-century Botswana also need to be placed against the backdrop of historical patterns of childbearing; in this way we see how reproductive changes have been integral to changing Tswana ethnic and national identities.

Contested Modernization: Notes on a Paradigm of Fertility and People's Identities

With its steadily dropping overall fertility rates, Botswana seems to counter a long-observed trend of population growth in many African countries since the 1970s. The latter trend has alarmed demographers and policy-makers in the global North and contributed to the conviction that fertility is a constant and unchanging cultural value in African societies (Caldwell and Caldwell 1987; Caldwell 2002).

This conviction is still prevalent in recent writings, even though the problem of infertility has long been widespread in some African countries – referred to as the so-called 'infertility belt' – due to the high precedence of venereal infections causing medical problems in large sections of the population and poor environmental conditions further reducing fertility (van Balen and Inhorn 2002: 23; Kreager 2004: 23–27). The perception of Africa as the pronatalist continent has led to a bias in which researchers begin from the premise that the main economic, demographic and social issue is the question of how best to reduce fertility. Yet in many African societies, successful reproduction – perceived as imperilled in view of the many couples who experience difficulties – is necessary to making a person a full member of society. Personal and ethnic identities are heavily invested in reproduction (Feldman-Savelsberg 1999a).

Infertility as a source of medical and social suffering, although remarked upon some time ago in major studies (e.g. Frank 1983; Larsen 1994), has long remained secondary in African demographic research and population programmes. This is evident in reviews of research on childlessness (Hunt 2005). Childlessness can be seen as an extreme form of suffering from infertility, as pathological sterility more often strikes after a woman has already had some children. People who have remained entirely childless may thus appear to be a minority in Botswana, as elsewhere in Africa, even though they are a significant subpopulation. This observation runs counter to a long tradition of anthropological research stressing the importance of fertility in African populations, for instance, as undertaken by Isaac Schapera in the 1930s in Bechuanaland. In Tswana-speaking ethnic groups, fertility came to represent both personal and ethnic identities. Schapera reports the great anxieties over fertility among Tswana speakers and found that one in every ten women remained childless (Schapera 1993).[2] Despite this and later evidence, countries like Botswana have not seen major government health initiatives addressing the issue of infertility. Apparently, infertility/ childlessness continues to be viewed as exceptional in the African context, and suffering from it is regarded a personal problem rather than a social one.

The problem of infertility/childlessness illustrates some of the shortcomings of conventional postwar demographic inquiries, which have often seen little interest in accounting for what are – from a statistical point of view – insignificant cases. Infertility/ childlessness may, however, be a key indicator of previous or changing fertility problems that differentiate subpopulations. Conventional demographic approaches, from this point of view, have not provided sufficient analytical space to examine variations in fertility and how they arise and may continue in important groups. This blind spot is closely related to a characteristic methodological problem. In calculating correlations between, on the one hand, levels of education, economic status or other so-called 'independent variables' and, on the other, what then become 'dependent variables' (e.g. age of marriage or fertility), demography creates the idea that entirely external factors are what chiefly direct people's reproductive behaviour. In consequence, it appears, for instance, that being educated and female, and coming from Germany and being Protestant, determine why a person has children at a certain age and limits childbearing in a characteristic manner. These theories correspond well with the sociological theory of standardization of individual lifetimes, as outlined, for example, by the German sociologist Martin Kohli.[3] Kohli finds that life courses became standardized in the nineteenth century in the age of industrialization as new labour market requirements fostered a formalization of education and imposed a new time regime on individual life courses (Kohli and Meyer 1986; Kohli 2007). The individual life course appears as sequenced in several stages, with reproduction having a fixed place in them. With this theory of standardization, Kohli points out that social stratification is identifiable not only vertically across social strata but also horizontally across people's lifetimes. Accordingly, with regard to reproduction, demographic studies have shown that age of marriage impacts on a couple's fertility in Northern Europe (e.g. in the United Kingdom) as it postpones birth and pregnancy (Szreter and Garrett 2000). An associated factor impacting on the timing and numbers of births is the formal education of men and women. Reproduction thus has a fixed place in the life course sequence of modern European individuals. Plausible analogies exist in other parts of the world. In many African societies, for instance, it is often not the age of first marriage that impacts on the timing of first childbirth – because children are often born before people's first marriage – but rather puberty rites (Sommer 2009) or schooling (Johnson-Hanks 2006).

However, speaking to individuals about their reproductive histories and decisions readily introduces other critical factors for which standardizing approaches leave no room. One finds, for example, the contingencies that make up an ordinary person's biography – such as the question of partner choice or unfixed educational and professional preferences. Demography, in other words, provides us with a limited and usually preconceived set of ideas about how factors that influence childbirth translate into individuals' decisions, and even then what is at issue may not be, as demographers have commonly assumed, a choice about numerical family size, but about when, how and with whom to have children. Person-centred approaches, put forward by anthropologists like Andrea Cornwall (2007), Jane Guyer (1994) and Liv Haram (2004), have focused on these contingencies. They develop a more refined analysis of the situationality and contextuality of reproductive decisions. These researchers show how individuals use their reproductive capacities to achieve other social goals, and how these decisions are embedded into wider processes of producing meaning and moral contestations of family planning practices. They demonstrate that reproductive decisions and outcomes may be subject to complex negotiations, and that people's tactics may change from one moment in the life course to another. A good example is given by one of the authors in this volume: in Chapter 6, Erica van der Sjipt describes how Nadine negotiates the fatherhood of her pregnancy and how, with each suitor, she develops new visions of a bright and hopeful future. This approach often succeeds in giving insights into the complexity of individual fertility decisions, thus showing the importance of taking full account of the influence of a person's social and cultural environment. The social complex in which reproduction takes place entails specific hierarchical kin relations, ideals of marriage, love, motherhood and fatherhood, cosmologies and ideas of the body – all of which will be influenced by social and cultural institutions such as marriage or schools (Lesthaeghe 1989). A question remains, of course, as to how frequent or typical the particular situations of a given individual are.

In addressing these issues, anthropologists working on infertility have coined the term 'reproductive disruption' to refer recurring events that are indicators at the subpopulation level of variations that have potentially much wider implications for women's and men's reproductive experience (Hörbst and Schuster 2006; Sundby and Larsen 2006; Inhorn 2007). Scholars working on childlessness have pointed out that infertility is likely to appear in women's life courses if unexpected events interrupt the – often standardized – life courses in which pregnancy and birth have an expected place. Infertility often results from unusual circumstances in a person's life, circumstances that are due to social dynamics beyond individual control. Poor healthcare for women who have had an abortion is one example, often related to the illegal status of abortion (Hörbst and Schuster 2006). Other examples include changing gender roles, professionalization or position in a kinship system. Thus, it has long been known that in eighteenth-century Europe, educated but not extremely wealthy women who were the youngest in a set of female siblings found it impossible to marry, as their older sisters had to be married first. In the case of Botswana, educated professional women search for suitable husbands, i.e. those who are both educated and rich enough for them to marry, and tolerant enough to accept educated women's altered self-perceptions. Therefore, the seeming exceptionality of disrupted life courses leading to recurring issues of infertility and fertility may point to underlying breaks and ruptures in cultural norms and expectations governing kinship, family life, marriage and shifting material realities.

An important approach to understanding disruptions as both contingent on, and regulated by, social dynamics is provided by Jennifer Johnson-Hanks' concept of 'vital conjunctures' (Johnson-Hanks 2002). This suggests an analytical perspective on individual reproductive lives that allows both for understanding how individual life courses are shaped by cultural and social institutions, and how gendered norms and expectations that shape a person's reproduction and materialities of life are negotiated. While there are prefigured paths through life-generating normative expectations about the point in time when a person should enter reproductive life, the actual event (and when or whether it happens) is accompanied by many contingencies. Vital conjunctures are those moments in a person's life that open up a new future and require decisions. A typical example is teenage pregnancy. A woman who is pregnant may marry and be forced to leave school, or may leave the child in the care of her mother or other female relatives and continue schooling (cf. Johnson-Hanks 2002: 876; Ringstedt 2008). Analysing these vital conjunctures opens up perspectives both on people's reproductive agency and on the cultural and social structural conditions of their decision.

With reference to Johnson-Hanks, I shall argue that disruptions in some people's life courses encountered during my fieldwork in Botswana follow recurring patterns that indicate changing reproductive dynamics of a wider scope; these patterns speak to new gender roles, new approaches to the body, new spiritualities and alternative ways of how to bear and beget children. Looking at an individual's biographical circumstances, I propose, allows us to understand several of the factors that have shaped gender relations, reproductive moralities and reproductive decisions.[4] As we shall see, they also have an important bearing on wider ethnic and national identities.

Fertility in Tswana-Speaking Communities since the Beginning of the Twentieth Century: Relevant Datasets

There are three main datasets I wish to discuss here. The main corpus of my research consists of reproductive histories of eighty female and fifteen male educated professionals over three generations. For interviews, I met women (as well as men) mostly in public spaces, cafés or restaurants. The interviews, lasting between forty-five minutes and two hours, resemble the intimate chats that urban women are used to. My interactions with men outside the context of my research were limited, so that I do not know how men usually speak about these issues outside the interview situation. Chatting with me gave women the opportunity to share some of their troubling conditions, such as HIV infection or infertility. Narrating their lives involved interpreting events and relationships; looking at how people construct meanings in this way enables us to see interviews as reflecting people's reproductive ethics and how moral issues shape subjectivity. During the conversations, I took notes[5] and later finalized a protocol based on these notes and my memory. Twenty-five of the women sought medical assistance in order to conceive; only nine had not given birth to any child so far. Their ages, and therefore also their chances of conceiving, varied considerably, from twenty-eight to fifty-five. During the interviews, respondents were very open about highly sensitive and taboo subjects such as infertility and their HIV status. However, they would rarely agree to a follow-up interview.[6] Therefore, my data, while of high quality concerning sensitive information, could not in many cases be verified by triangulation or by repeating a conversation.

The data are complemented by participant observation, media analysis and official reports. I used national statistics to complement material from my interviews, mainly the Population and Housing Census (PHC) (Botswana Central Statistics Office 2001), and the Botswana Family Health Survey (BFHS) (Botswana Central Statistics Office 2009) conducted in 2007. Botswana's first population census was conducted in 1904, and thereafter censuses were performed after independence in 1971, 1981, 1991, 2001 and 2011. Botswana's population is estimated at about two million over the past three decades. Results of the latest census have not yet been disseminated and we need to keep in mind that methodological shortcomings may have given rise to undercounting; one consequence is that projections and survey samples based on the census series may therefore include significant biases. This is particularly important, for example, for estimates of HIV prevalence. Estimating HIV prevalence in a population is a very difficult undertaking, not only on account of incomplete data, but because of the nature of the spread of the virus itself, notably its long incubation period. As it takes about ten years for a patient to develop AIDS and there are often delays when this information is finally reported to a hospital, infections commonly go undetected for a long time. As such prevalence only becomes 'countable' statistically at a very late point in time, estimations about prevalence need to be adjusted repeatedly (Chin 2007). The many insecurities in HIV prevalence estimates have led to vast discrepancies between estimates made by UNAIDS and by national statistics. The former estimates prevalence in the adult population at 40 per cent, while the figure in national statistics is 30 per cent.

Survey compilation and analysis have in consequence developed long experience in handling HIV prevalence data. Pretests and pilot studies are conducted in selected areas, in which case questions can be adapted to local population structures and dynamics. A particular challenge is that Botswana is a sparsely populated country with a low population density. As rural areas were not fully mapped heretofore, unregistered settlements and single compounds have had to be mapped with the help of GPS. One of the questions that was crucial for gaining accurate data was the question of how to define a 'household', i.e. who should be counted as members in order to avoid underenumeration or overenumeration. The census followed a de facto approach in which each household was asked to count those members resident in the past six months. Thereby interviewers avoided children being counted twice. (Children are usually regarded as members of a household even if they have moved away, commonly resulting in their being counted both in the households of parents and in their own households in the city.) This issue is of considerable importance due to the high mobility of the population, particularly internal migration. In fact, due to the high mobility of men in the age group of 35–49, they were likely to be undercounted in the 1981 census (Bulatao 2003: 59). In consequence, projections show a deficit of at least five thousand males in each five-year group from thirty to thirty-nine in 1991 and from thirty-five to forty-nine in 2001. Given the relatively low population size of a country, this number represents a considerable proportion. As noted, the deficit is likely to be explained by the high volume of net migration not captured by the census.

In sum, over the past few decades, Botswana's Central Statistical Office has tried to develop questionnaires that respond to sociocultural dynamics within populations and to avoid one of the important fallacies of questionnaire-based research, namely producing misrepresentations owing to standard classifications that do not fit local categories. Nevertheless, questionnaires still do not respond to research requirements for dealing with sensitive personal questions, notably the number of 'I don't know' answers that have remained high in data on household economy and fertility (Buthali 2003: 44).

The Botswana Family and Health Survey of 2007 is the fourth in a series since independence. The first was conducted in 1984 and was followed by a second two years later in 1988, and a third in 1996. The BFHS 2007 was conducted in close cooperation and with the support of UNICEF. It covers data about standards of sanitation in households, fertility and access to healthcare. Selected households were interviewed in all districts, in total 7,800. Sampling was done on the basis of the 2001 census. The overall response rate was quite high, at almost 90 per cent (89.5); the percentage of women interviewed was slightly higher at 94.7 per cent than of men at 90.9 per cent. In sum, statistical data in national surveys and censuses have been quite well developed and monitored over the past thirty years, and thus represent a valuable resource in conjunction with ethnography.

It is further remarkable that there is a lot of reflection and discussion of rural poverty, especially with regard to female-headed households (Lesetedi 1989, 2003; Mookodi 2003). However, in view of the fact that Botswana counts as one of the few middle-income countries in Africa, it is astonishing that there is comparatively little differentiation of the wealth of households. Rich households are taken to have an income of 8,000 BWP, or about £600, and are mostly found in big cities such as Gaborone, Francistown, Lobatse and Selibe Phikwe. This information is provided in one unofficial UN document, which states that educated professionals (i.e. the group I write about) mainly work in the Civil Service. Civil servants constitute 40 per cent of the nation's total workforce and claim over 54 per cent of total wages, enjoying 40 per cent higher wages than the rest of the private and parastate sectors (Partow 2010: vii, 15). Among these professionals, education is coupled with wealth and (most often) political influence. In view of the fact that 30 per cent of the country still lives below the poverty line (Partow 2010: 82), mostly in rural areas, I refer to these privileged, educated groups as 'elites'. Otherwise, there is comparatively little differentiation that would enable a clear socioeconomic stratification of better-off and other households in Botswana. Qualitative data on educated professionals' life histories are therefore an important addition to national household survey and allow micro-analysis of processes of social differentiation in a historical perspective that is otherwise missing in Botswana.

A third set of data needs to be remarked upon, at least briefly. This is the first survey of fertility and marriage undertaken by the anthropologist Isaac Schapera in 1932 in a compound near Mochudi in southeastern Bechuanaland. Even though conducted on a small scale, his survey is likely to be highly reliable as he had built up long-standing relations with people in Mochudi over a research period of about two years (Schapera 1993).

Out-of-Wedlock Children: Shifting Reproductive Dynamics among Tswana in the First Half of the Twentieth Century

When Schapera conducted his research in southeastern Tswana, he could already observe a shift in the organization of reproductive relationships and dynamics in Tswana-speaking societies. This shift had been motivated by economic diversification and its impact on the political economy of reproductive relationships, as well as by Christianity. Schapera was confronted by a society with a strong emphasis on fertility. High regard for fertility was expressed, notably, in anxieties about infertility (Schapera 1966, 1993). 'To have children is the destiny of every woman' (Schapera 1993: 166). Fertility was seen as a central feature of female personhood and the most important function of a marriage. If a marriage remained childless, the husband was allowed to divorce and remarry. If the husband was suspected of being infertile, special arrangements between his wife and his brother were made so that the wife would conceive by the brother. Having many children was associated with spiritual blessing and wealth. In other words, having many children was seen as an index of a successful, wealthy way of life. This view still applies today to rural women, as demonstrated by my conversations with women aged 60–100[7] in Molepolole in 2009. An eighty-eight-year old women emphasized the importance of having many children in order to have sufficient support in old age. She had ten children, of whom seven had died. The other three were now taking care of her. 'If I had only three, imagine!' she exclaimed. Having many children guaranteed social and economic survival (interview, 10 April 2010).

In the 1930s, men who had spent long periods of time outside the home, either because they were at the cattle post or because they had migrated to the mines in South Africa, often had a second wife and children at the place they worked. As long as these relationships did not jeopardize reciprocal relationships with kin and wives, such affairs were tolerated (Schapera 1966: 182–85). Women's extramarital sexual affairs were less accepted than those of men. However, the children born of extramarital relationships during the husband's absence were welcomed, as it was understood that a woman should have as many children as possible (Schapera 1966: 186–87). The institution of marriage was important in order to determine lineage rights over children, but reproduction did not need to take place within marriage.

In 1973 Roberts repeated one of Schapera's surveys in a small ward in Mochudi, Rampedi. Together with Comaroff, he argued that during the 1930s, there was a shift in the legal handling of cases of childbirth outside marriage (Comaroff and Roberts 1977). Before, fathers were seen to be responsible for claiming compensation in the case of pregnancy before marriage. Now these cases were brought to the attention of the *kgotla*, the chief and court of the community. Furthermore, women themselves (and not their guardians – i.e. the woman's father or another older male relative from her patrilineage (Schapera 1993)) could now claim compensation for a child from a man who had made a promise of marriage he did not fulfil. This development went hand in hand with increasing marriage payments, *lobola*, which the husband was supposed to pay to the women's father. In consequence, the paying of *lobola* was often postponed to sometime after the woman had given birth. Women could bring their claims in front of the *kgotla* without necessarily being accompanied by their affinal relatives.[8] This shift in the handling of legal cases demonstrates that claims on *lobola* as well as claims on the right to children born out of wedlock were moving out of the sphere of kinship and became subject to communal politics; they were seen as being of wider public concern.

Comaroff and Roberts (1977: 102) interpret this change as an indicator of the fact that women gained property rights over their own body. These rights were attributed to the fact that women could increasingly choose to stay in their own households, also due to the fact that they migrated from their homestead to find paid labour elsewhere. Women's contribution to a common income (such as running a shop) played a role in successful claims to compensation (Comaroff and Roberts 1977: 101). Therefore, women's rights for compensation in cases of betrayed marriage promises can be seen as being strongly attached to women's increasing economic position in their societies in the course of the monetarization of labour in the first half the twentieth century. As we shall see, this forms part of a pattern in which reproductive events and relationships that had previously been family and kin matters became indicators of wider shifts in personal and group identities.

The detachment of reproduction and marriage was a product of historical circumstances that Schapera came to witness. By the end of the 19th century, the fathers of extramarital children were heavily fined by the guardian of the woman. The claim to fines was made on the argument that the woman's prospects for marriage, and therefore the prospect to a high bride price (*lobola*), was spoilt (Comaroff and Roberts 1977). These claims were handled in the private sphere and were not brought in front of the *kgotla*. Nevertheless, the number of children born out of wedlock was considerable. Schapera's 1930 survey of Mochudi, a village with a population of one hundred, shows that two-thirds of children were born out of wedlock (1993: 99). In the course of the second half of the century, cases of children born out of wedlock increased: by 1961, when Comaroff and Roberts repeated Schapera's survey, 65 of the 162 children (40 per cent) living in the ward had been born to women who were regarded as unmarried, whereas in 1934 it had been only 12 per cent (Comaroff and Roberts 1977: 101). Cohabitation also became more common, and Comaroff and Roberts see a connection between this development and the practical abolition of polygyny due to Christian influence. During the course of the twentieth century, cohabitation was established as a quasi-institutionalized form of relationship, and became identified with ethnic membership. This is indicated by the fact that 'living together' appears as a category in national statistics next to the category of 'married', 'divorced' and 'single' (Mookodi and Fuh 2004).

This trend persisted throughout the twentieth century and brought forward matrifocal household structures, i.e. households headed by women living alone with their children. Ethnographers attest to the great economic independence of women who chose to have children without the obligations of marriage (Helle-Valle 1999). Others point out the economic precariousness of such living arrangements, mostly in the rural area (Gaisie 2000).[9] What is important for this chapter is the fact that these new residential patterns became popular across the region and came to be considered as cultural markers embodying ethnic identities (Adesina 2010). The matrifocal model favours childbirth before marriage and the birth of a high number of children who are supposed to provide for their mothers in old age. In the second half of the twentieth century, out-of-wedlock children and cohabitation have been incorporated into national statistics and thus associated not only with ethnic but also national identities. Werbner (2004: 63–85) has described how Tswana-ness advanced to become a source of national identity in the course of postcolonial state formation; cohabitation, as a pattern specific to the Tswana, exemplifies this development as providing a template for national statistics.

Controlling Birth: Emerging National Identities of Educated Professionals

Next to this development, a second trend emerged among educated professional women. In the 1930s professional women tended to postpone their age at first childbirth. Influenced by Christian doctrine, they married before they had children. Take, for instance, MmaMusi. Her parents were already educated and living in a small town in Botswana. Like many of these first-generation educated professionals, they demonstrated modesty vis-à-vis other people in their community and did not display wealth. MmaMusi was one of two sisters among seven siblings who pursued schooling. She stood out from her peers and siblings, who went to South Africa to work as maids or in the mines (in the case of her brother, for instance), and also by managing to avoid early pregnancy, which would have caused her to stop schooling. Instead, she finished school and afterwards went to Lesotho to receive training as a nurse. She married her husband at the age of twenty-three; they met during her practical training in Botswana. She had her first child when she was twenty-five after she took up her first post as a nurse. After three years she had another child, and upon her return to professional nursing was given the opportunity to go for special training in Scotland. When she came back to Botswana, she was offered a job as head nurse in the National Hospital and had her third child soon after (interview, 20 September 2011). There are no statistical data available on how widespread this trend might have been among educated professionals of her generation. Of my own sample, all seven women in her age group narrated a similar life history. MmaMusi's biography demonstrates that many educated women of this first generation postponed first childbirth and practised birth control. The demands of their education and later of their jobs motivated them to reduce childbearing to a level below the national fertility rate.

This generation also witnessed a radical restructuring of Botswana's national politics and economy. In the 1930s and 1940s, when people like MmaMusi were educated, Botswana was under the British Protectorate and was seen as one of the poorest countries in the world, with an underdeveloped infrastructure. Its wealth lay in its vast pastures. Cattle was the main source of wealth (migrant labourers invested mainly in cattle), an occupation that did not result in a high GDP. However, in the mid 1970s, new diamond fields were discovered, and from the 1980s the Botswana government invited South African companies to invest in mining. After 1975, the country experienced rapid economic growth that accelerated especially in the years 1985–91. Its GDP growth was one of the highest in the world and the number in employment doubled. President Quett Masire led the process of forming a government that developed institutions and a welfare system covering the education and healthcare of its citizens. The first educated African professionals in the colonial period were teachers and health workers (mostly nurses), and there were only a handful of university graduates by the end of the colonial period. The lack of trained personnel was a challenge to the government (Werbner 2004). Over the past thirty years, the growing apparatus of government institutions as well as the diamond industry have created a need for specialist personnel, and this has enabled rapid social mobility for some. Women and men of MmaMusi's generation, as well as their children, were in great demand as Botswana's economy expanded. Their experience shows that education has been, and is still, key to elite formation. In particular, this process has fostered the formation of cosmopolitan elites, mostly of Christian orientation. The new ruling class was recruited of educate professionals often coming from the north and mostly represented by members of the ethic group of the Kalanga or wealthy people from the south, mostly represented by Tswana-speaking people (Werbner 2004: 48). Many members have studied in South Africa, the United Kingdom or the United States, frequently travelling to these places. Most importantly, child birthing was an important conjugal strategy of these groups. Unlike the situation in Lesotho, where birth spacing was a conjugal strategy of working women as described by Kroeker (this volume), in Botswana the restriction of fertility was mostly practised by the educated classes.

Individuals of this generation often spoke about their jobs as 'service to the nation'. Women felt they had to contribute to the project of nation-building by advancing their qualifications, and hence they needed to reconcile their private life with their work. In order to combine work with motherhood, they spaced their births and actively engaged in family planning. Trained women, like MmaMusi, were familiar with the biological components of reproduction. In the first years of their marriage they used the calendar method to prevent pregnancies. Later, in the 1960s, when the birth control pill became available, they switched to using this. Botswana was one of the few African countries to agree to take part in the population control programme of the UN in 1971; by 1973, fifty family planning centres had been built around the country. Compared to other African countries, the pill achieved a remarkable acceptance of 11.7 per cent in 1981 (Lucas 1992: 150).

In the 1930s Schapera witnessed the elite pioneering of techniques of birth control, noting that some educated men used condoms they had bought in town or from local traders. Due to the lack of general access to contraception, Tswana-speaking people's emphasis on birth control was practised most often using *coitus interruptus*. The Tswana practised birth spacing in order to allow newborn babies to grow before they had to share love and breast milk with siblings. Educated professionals, however, controlled reproduction and reduced childbearing under the added incentive of dedication to their jobs, and thus began to live with an alternative set of values concerning their fertility. At the same time, they benefited from the country's economic development since the late 1970s, many of them reaching a high occupational level and gaining considerable income and wealth. In that sense, these early educated professionals were pioneers simultaneously of the project of nation-building and of biomedical contraception. Their reproductive practice soon came to embody a new national identity that stood in contrast to more specific regional and ethnic reproductive practices and identities.

In the generation who were in their late twenties to early forties when I conducted my research, elite women were used to controlling their fertility. They nonetheless felt it was difficult to combine their demanding jobs with their tasks as mothers. One or two children, many of them stated, would be enough, or even more than they could handle. Most of them took care of at least one or two other children from their kin group.[10] In addition to time-consuming jobs and the increased need to fulfil the emotional demands of motherhood, educated professionals also stated that raising costs of childcare, especially school fees, contributed to their wish not to have more children. Although historical examples existed of this pattern (often unnoticed by those to whom I spoke), these mothers' childbearing strategies drew comments and questions from relatives and friends. Notably, they had designed their lives according to an alternative model of parenthood in which stress was placed on emotional ties between parents and children, and mothers and their children in particular. The pattern is similar to the gender roles that emerged in the rising middle classes of nineteenth-century Europe: women perceived motherhood in a framework that included emotional demands related to their employment. In other words, parenthood came to belong to a framework entailing emotional and economic commitments rather than social recognition of the value of fertility as an indicator of family or ethnic group status. In Botswana, emotions had thus entered the political economy of parenting before the start of the twenty-first century.

Young educated professionals' attitudes to birth control went along with a heightened awareness of the biology of reproduction, similar to their mother's generation. In addition, they went for regular gynaecological checkups and cancer screening. These technologies were unknown and unavailable to their mother's generation. These consultations are offered only by private gynaecological clinics and are not covered by health insurance. Nor does public healthcare provide for regular fertility checkups.[11] Taking all of these costs together, including consultation fees, x-rays, laboratory tests, and the primary and secondary costs of ordinary gynaecological examinations (for instance, for women who suffer heavy bleeding), the total can range between £125 and £300. This sum far exceeds the average costs of healthcare in households in the city, which is estimated at an average 63.5 BWP, or about £5 (Botswana Central Statistics Office 2004: 23). These figures suggest that only those households classified as wealthy – i.e. that have an income of 8,000 BWP or about £600 – are able to afford this expense. Most likely, these educated middle-class and elite groups are the only beneficiaries of Botswana's private health sector. Only they are able to pay for advanced reproductive healthcare.

Reducing fertility through birth spacing therefore now appears as normal behaviour in the context of the lives of urban educated professionals. The Botswana Family Health Survey confirms this trend: fertility rates are lower in urban than in rural areas across the country (Botswana Central Statistics Office 2009: 31). The economic argument that motivated older rural generations to have many children has turned around in this group. At the age of thirty, educated professionals do not worry about their upkeep in old age, but rather about the costs of childcare. In addition to the time constraints they face due to their demanding jobs, they construe motherhood as a fundamentally personal, emotional enterprise. All of this fits classical modernization theory's assumption that fertility reduction requires modernizing societies. But, as noted, there is another dimension to this change: childbearing and reproductive levels remain central markers of individual and group identity, while different levels and contraceptive methods, and a different construal of the nature of childbearing have become keys to this identity. However, the life courses behind these apparently modern adjustments reveal a sequence of vital conjunctures that do not conform to the smooth transition to modernity that postwar demography and development theory presupposed. It is to these conjunctures that we now turn.

New Attitudes towards Fertility among Urban Professionals: Late Fertility Care and Early Lifetime Childbearing

After postponing birth or after having a first child when they were unmarried and still in school, most women have come to desire having a further a child in their thirties. National statistics support my interview data. With an average of 5.8 pregnancies in the age group of the 30–34-year-old women, most pregnancies fall within this period in life, albeit not significantly (Botswana Central Statistics Office 2009: 30).[12] Among educated professionals, these 'late' children are usually born within marriage to prove the couple's fertility. Even though in rural Tswana communities reproduction may well take place outside marriage, a marriage without children is still regarded as a failure. This valuation applied to my educated professional interview partners, who experienced the scorn and ill-wishes of their families, relatives and colleagues. Sandra and her husband were well aware of the social pressure on their marriage. Moreover, the intended second child was the fulfilment of Sandra's personal goals and for her would signify that she had made it in life. Sandra had several bad relationships with boyfriends who had cheated on her before she met her husband. They became friends, both complaining about their former partners, and soon became a couple. To Sandra, this relationship gave life a positive turn. She felt secure and her husband respected her – although she felt that the foundation of their relationship was friendship rather than passion. She wished to experience the joy of motherhood within marriage. Now, within this marriage, she would have the child that she and her husband had wished for, and this child would establish their relationship: she would really be the wife. Her mother and her mother-in-law would then care for her and spoil her, the young mother. And people would come and admire her and her child (interview, 12 September 2010). Sandra's history exemplifies that childbearing becomes important in the prestige economy of educated urban professionals. A child within a marriage completes the union. In her vision of personal fulfilment and the completion of social success through a child, Sandra harks back to old established institutions of fertility care, the *botsetsi*, i.e. the confinement of mother and child after childbirth. During that time, the woman's mother takes care of the infant and the young mother. Albeit accompanied by several taboos, this period is seen as a celebration of life and fertility. Its closure, when the newly born is brought out of the house and presented to neighbours and friends, signifies the success of the marriage and intergenerational cooperation on the health of the child (Schapera 1966). Sandra's case demonstrates that these old established notions of infant care continue to serve as a powerful imagery of successful womanhood, in which fertility has not lost its cultural value. A similar attitude towards fertility is shown by the use of reproductive services in the wider age group of urban professionals to which Sandra belongs. Educated professionals in their thirties, who are married and established in their jobs, will now use often costly advanced fertility services in order to conceive.[13]

Some research has considered the trend of teenage pregnancies, first observed in the 1930s by Schapera, to be a widespread phenomenon in the region. The anthropologist David Suggs, for instance, comments on this trend in the 1980s, explaining it in terms of peer pressure and ideals of female maturity that Tswana girls adhere to and that drive them into early pregnancies (Suggs 1987). National statistics allow for a slightly altered view on this trend: the percentage of women being pregnant at the age of fifteen to nineteen decreases from 1988 to 2007 from 5.5 to 1.7 (Figure 7.1). Somewhat counterintuitively, the trend of teenage pregnancies is slightly higher among educated women than among noneducated women. The highest peak in fertility rates is found among 20–24 year olds in rural as well as in urban areas (Table 7.1), while fertility rates tend to be lower in urban areas than in rural areas. At that age,

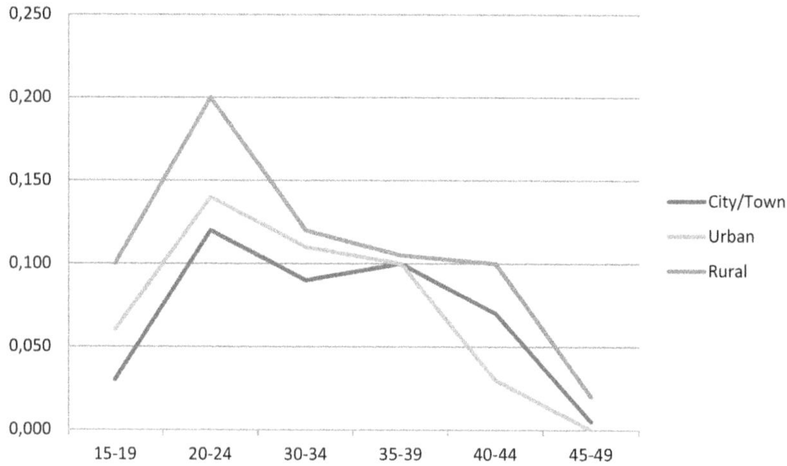

FIGURE 7.1 Prevalence of Women Aged 15–49 Who Were Pregnant during BFHS II, BFHS III and BFHS IV in 2007 (Botswana Central Statistics Office 2009: 42)

TABLE 7.1 Number of Pregnancies, by Age of Mothers (Botswana Central Statistics Office 2009: 42)

Age	BFHS II (1988)	BFHS (1996)	BFHS IV (2007)
15–19	5.5	3.3	1.7
20–24	0.8	7.4	5.5
25–29	10.2	4.8	5.3
30–34	8.0	3.5	5.8
35–39	6.6	0.6	4.0
40–44	3.9	3.6	2.5
45–49	1.4	0.0	0.0
Total (average number of pregnancies per women)	**7.1**	**4.6**	**3.7**

women are most often not yet married, with the average age of first marriage being 26.4 for women (and 30.9 for men) (United Nations 2013). These figures indicate that the trend of having children early in life and before marriage continues. In that sense, Sandra's story reflects a common, albeit regressive, trend. Some of these women, especially if they were students at the time they conceived, stated that their child was a product of their love. Their statement reflects both an adaptation of global ideas of romantic love[14] and of Tswana ideals of romance, previously described by Schapera ([1940] 1971).

They had loved the father of their child, often a student like themselves, who had promised to marry them. Some women indicated that their partners had insisted on having a child. However, during their pregnancies, or soon after, the relationship broke down and they were left alone to care for the child.

Other women reported these first pregnancies as resulting from a 'mistake'. In several cases, women indicated that the pregnancies were a result of 'broken condoms',[15] thus demonstrating that their pregnancies were unplanned. This was the case in Sandra's story. Her son was the result of such a mistake during a party. At that time she had not yet settled in life and liked to go out with her friends to drink. Often they were invited by older men for drinks. Sometimes these contacts ended up with the man sleeping with them. After her first pregnancy, she tried an IUD, which, however, led to an infection. For some time the infection went undetected and she only discovered it when it was already well advanced. The infection may be related to her subsequent HIV status, given the greater susceptibility to HIV following other venereal infections. Such sequences are often the cause of infertility. However, few women suffering from infertility in my sample had medical histories that suggested that this was the case. Rather, first pregnancy and an HIV infection are both attributes of a partying lifestyle that young people entertain in cities and towns across the country. Going out with friends and drinking alcohol promises to be an adventure. As in many African societies, alcohol represents a drink of luxury and power, and drinking means partaking in adult privileges as well as in affluent modernity (Akyeampong 1996).

Sandra's story sheds new light on the fertility-seeking strategies of educated professionals in their thirties. In her case, child spacing was not merely a strategy related to her education or job development, but rather resulted out of the circumstances of her HIV infection. Epidemiological studies show that HIV prevalence correlates with lower fertility on a national level (Lewis et al. 2004). In addition, a wave of death has affected a whole generation of reproductive age, over one-third of the 30–34 and 35–39 age cohorts having contracted AIDS (Velkoff and Kowai 2006: 54). HIV is a further and major factor leading to the drastic reduction of overall fertility rates at the national level. It is therefore likely that Botswana's remarkably low fertility level is in part epidemiologically induced. Sandra's story allows insights into the more specific reproductive dynamics that underpin this low fertility. Some of these women became pregnant at young ages when they were partying with friends. Many also appear to have been infected with HIV during these contacts. Whether HIV has been an impediment to finding a suitable husband or whether it is bound up with other venereal infections leading to infertility, stories like Sandra's indicate the emergence of a new and general understanding of childbearing that reflects Botswana's current historical, demographic and epidemiological conjuncture. Education, demanding jobs, the necessity of creating emotional space for children, and the personal and medical complications of HIV all combine to favour low fertility.

This point leads to my last consideration regarding new approaches to fertility among urban professionals in twenty-first-century Botswana, and to how they link up with ideas of modernity and elite ways of life. On top of her own anxieties about conception, Sandra also experiences the impatience of her relatives, especially of her mother-in-law, who earnestly desires a grandchild. In order to protect Sandra from her relatives' criticism, she and her husband told their relatives that they wanted to 'wait' a little before they started having children. They pointed to their financial 'projects' – a term commonly used in Botswana – by way of explanation. 'Projects' involve, for example, building houses and buying cars. Some newlywed couples also want to get rid of debts incurred by their extremely expensive wedding celebrations – occasions of conspicuous consumption in which couples demonstrate their belonging to the newly emerging economic elite. However, often couples take on large amounts of debt[16] and it is common to postpone childbearing in the first year of marriage in order to deal with it. Having fewer children, and sometimes having children later in life, enables these women and men to get around the cultural emphasis on high fertility. At the same time, they continue to emphasize the high value of reproduction by using advanced fertility services after having postponed childbearing, for example, after a long period of child spacing. Among these women and men, the economic rationale for having children has turned from children as a means of security in old age to children as a major expense of private households, representing a new urban lifestyle. The story of Sandra demonstrates that this new urban lifestyle has gained recognition among rising sections of society at the turn of the twenty-first century, and may now legitimize postponing childbearing within marriage. The economic argument enhances the plausibility of postponing children or, as in Sandra's case, child spacing. Sandra's case demonstrates that this rationale gains new weight in a situation in which the total fertility of the population has decreased for epidemiological reasons. Young couples may draw upon these examples to legitimize child spacing and to help launch the ideals of a modern and wealthy family.

In sum, these women's lives may be understood as a sequence of three main vital conjunctures: (1) early birth related to youthful lifestyle, whether 'mistakes' or not; (2) middle childbearing, with spacing and delaying, arising from various causes, including uncertain partnerships, contraceptive problems and HIV; and (3) later childbearing, which can be understood as reaffirming many traditional values, albeit at lower overall TFRs, and complicated by choices made at previous conjunctures. Altogether the picture we get is of the costs as well as the benefits of Botswana's modernization, not an untroubled path to blissful modernity.

Conclusion

Jennifer Johnson-Hanks' concept of vital conjuncture as a perspective on individual life courses has allowed us to understand disrupted reproductive biographies as, in effect, windows that open up the way to shifts in reproductive dynamics. This chapter has shown a series of such shifts in the fertility strategies of educated professionals in the context of HIV/AIDS in twenty-first-century Botswana. Using Sandra's history as an extensive case study, I have argued that while new practices of child spacing have emerged among educated professionals, these practices continue to follow historically established patterns of reproduction, namely, early childbearing by unmarried women. These women's subsequent entry into the elite then justifies a period of birth postponement and a reduction of childbearing altogether. The case of Sandra shows that child spacing among rising educated groups may also be epidemically induced, as a first pregnancy may come with an HIV infection prior, or after, the pregnancy. Jennifer Johnson-Hanks has pointed to vital conjunctures as moments in which alternative futures and life course possibilities are opened up for young people. In the case of Sandra and of many other women, a first pregnancy accompanied by an HIV infection can also close options and futures; after an HIV infection, future navigations of life require continued social and medical efforts by women (and their men) if they are to get pregnant again. Interpreting their fertility-seeking strategy in the framework of elite lifestyles, upcoming educated professionals like Sandra and her husband attribute new meaning to reproductive practices that originated in specific regional ethnic identities. Thus reinterpreted, reproductive practices also come to serve as a source for constructing new national identities among young urban professionals.

Acknowledgements

This contribution is inspired by a seminar lecture series that was conducted under the auspices of the Fertility Reproduction Studies Group at the University of Oxford in collaboration with the Max Planck Institute for Social Anthropology, during Michaelmas term 2012. I thank Günther Schlee, who has supervised my project, for his support, and Philip Kreager for the cordial welcome and fruitful collaboration. The chapter has been finalized during my stay at the Centre for Advanced Studies, Constance. I thank the Centre for its generous scholarship. This research was made possible by the support of the Fritz-Thyssen Foundation and the Max Planck Institute for Social Anthropology, Halle, and was conducted with the permission of the Botswana Ministry of Labour and Home Affairs, the Ministry of Health, the Gaborone Private Hospital (Dr Music and Dr Eaton) and Bokamoso Private Hospital (Dr Abebe). I thank all institutions and the people involved who have supported my research financially and intellectually. My special thanks go to Abigail Morgan (a women's health nurse at Bokamoso) and Pastor Seithamo, who actively helped me make contacts with patients and church members. Pearl Sechele, and Abigile and John Hamathi also assisted me greatly during my research. I especially thank John Hamathi for his inspiring words and his help in establishing connections with the right people; I also thank Sethunya Mosime, Godisan Mookodi and Treasa Galvin from the Department of Social Science, and Musa Dube and Francis Nkomasana from the Department of Theology and Religious Studies at the University of Botswana. Last, but not least, I would like to thank Rijk van Dijk from the ASC, Leiden, who introduced me to these colleagues.

Astrid Bochow is Lecturer in Social Anthropology at Georg August Universität Göttingen, an associate of the Fertility and Reproductive Studies Group at the Institute of Social and Cultural Anthropology, University of Oxford, and a member of the Steering Committee of the Research Network: Religion, HIV/AIDS and

Social Transformation. She has conducted extensive field research in Botswana and Ghana.

Notes

1. All names of participants have been changed and some aspects of their social identity have been disguised to guarantee their anonymity. If not stated otherwise, interviews took place in Gaborone.
2. Other widely read ethnographers document high anxieties over infertility/childlessness among African populations. Take, for instance, the seminal studies of Victor Turner (1969: 1–34) or Edwin Ardener (1962). Even international organizations appeared to be aware about these anxieties in the 1950s, for instance, Frank Lorimer (1954).
3. Simon Szreter (1993) has also pointed out that the inspiration for sorting of variables derived largely from Talcott Parsons' modernization theory that postwar demography had taken on. It seems that the idea that fertility could be understood according to standardized variables appeared when Europe was busy with repairing the damages of the Second World War and was finding a new modus operandi, politically as well as socially.
4. Cf. also Leonard (2002).
5. Most respondents did not feel comfortable having interviews tape recorded.
6. My explanation for their attitude is that informants did not want to integrate me into their social environment after having delivered such sensitive information on their lives, in order to avoid subsequent embarrassment. My presence and my knowledge would have endangered their position. My colleague who accompanied me during this research agreed to this interpretation.
7. In fact, the oldest women indicated she was 102 years old. Her excellent English indicated that she had enjoyed some formal education. It is therefore quite possible that she had an informed idea about her exact date of birth.
8. However, women came unaccompanied only in four out of thirty-five cases brought in front of the *kgotla* in the years 1955–70. The number of thirty-five also suggests that very few cases were brought to court.
9. While the tendency of matrifocality has been noted for Namibia as well as for Lesotho (cf. Pauli and Kroeker, this volume), there is a fundamental difference between the situation in Lesotho and Botswana: urbanization has been noted only since the 1980s for Botswana and it was not predominately a female problem.
10. Some of these children's parents had died, while others were living in poor and underprivileged conditions. The extent to which educated

professionals took care of their relatives' children varied: some children came to live in their households, while others were supported by having their school fees paid.

11. Fertility treatments are offered only by Princess Marina Hospital, the National Hospital in Gaborone, and during some hours at the hospital in Molepolole.
12. This is compared to an average of 5.3 in the 25–30-year-old group and 5.5 among 20–24-year-old women. In 1988 the highest number of average pregnancies was recorded among women aged 25–30 (10.0), followed by those aged 30–34 (8.0) (Botswana Central Statistics Office 2009: 30). This indicates a shift in fertility trends with fewer babies born to women at a later age.
13. Here, Botswana's private healthcare sector offers only limited possibilities. Therapies most often offer hormone therapies or an operation to remove fibroids, which are commonly held to be the cause of infertility. Other services such as IVF or ISCI are only offered in South Africa.
14. Cf. Cole and Thomas (2009).
15. The frequency with which I received reports about broken condoms made me doubt whether condoms had indeed been used. These self-reports are perhaps best read as indications that condoms had advanced to be the preferred method of contraception by the beginning of the 2000s. This fact can be seen as a success story for HIV prevention policies, which launched condom use in Botswana.
16. Botswana is one of the few countries in Africa in which banks readily give out loans to individuals. One of the advantages of being employed in the public service sector, like Sandra and her husband, is that they are given private loans and mortgages to buy houses and cars.

References

Adesina, J.O. 2010. 'Re-appropriating Matrifocality: Engdogeneity and African Gender Scholarship', *African Sociological Review* 14(1): 2–19.

Akyeampong, E. 1996. 'What's in a Drink? Class Struggle, Popular Culture and the Politics of *akepeteshie* (Local Gin) in Ghana 1930–67', *Journal of African History* 37: 215–38.

Ardener, E. 1962. *Divorce and Fertility: An African Study*. London: Nigerian Institute of Social and Economic Research and Oxford University Press.

Bledsoe, C. 2002. *Contigent Lives: Fertility, Time and Aging in West Africa*. Chicago: University of Chicago Press.

Botswana Central Statistics Office. 2001. *Population and Housing Census (PHC)*. Gaborone: Botswana, Central Statistics Office.

———. 2004. *Household Income and Expenditure Survey 2002/03*. Gaborone: Botswana, Central Statistics Office.

———. 2009. *2007 Botswana Family Health Survey (BFHS) IV Report*. Gaborone: Botswana Central Statistics Office.

Bulatao, R. 2003. 'Population Projections', in Botswana Central Statistics Office, *2001 Population and Housing Census Dissemination Seminar*. Gaborone: Botswana Central Statistics Office, pp. 57–81.

Buthali, D. 2003. 'Methodological Aspects of Census, Quality Control Measures and Outcome', in Botswana Central Statistical Office, *2001 Population and Housing Census Dissemination Seminar*. Gaborone: Botswana Central Statistics Office, pp. 40–56.

Caldwell, J.C. 1977. *Population Growth and Family Change in Africa: The New Urban Elite*. London: C. Hurst & Co.

———. 1982. *Theory of Decline*. London: Academic Press.

Caldwell, J.C., and P. Caldwell 1987. 'The Cultural Context of High Fertility in Sub-Saharan Africa', *Population and Development Review* 13(3): 409–37.

———. 2002. 'Africa: The New Family Planning Frontier', *Studies in Family Planning* 33(1): 76–86.

Chin, J. 2007. 'How Credible are HIV/AIDS Estimates?', in J. Chin, *The AIDS Pandemic: The Collision with Political Correctness*. Oxford: Radcliffe Publishing, pp. 120–39.

Cole, J., and L.M. Thomas (eds). 2009. *Love in Africa*. Chicago: University of Chicago Press.

Comaroff, J.L., and S. Roberts. 1977. 'Marriage and Extra-marital Sexuality: The Dialectics of Legal Change among the Kgatla', *Journal of African Law* 21: 97–123.

Cornwall, A. 2007. 'Taking Chances, Making Choices: The Tactical Dimensions of "Reproductive Strategies" in Southwestern Nigeria', *Medical Anthropology* 26: 229–54.

Feldman-Savelsberg, P. 1999. *Plundered Kitchens, Empty Wombs: Threatened Reproduction and Identity in the Cameroon Grassfields*. Ann Arbor: University of Michigan Press.

Frank, O. 1983. 'Infertility in Sub-Saharan Africa; Estimates and Implications', *Population and Development Review* 9(1): 137–44.

Gaisie, S.K. 2000. 'Family Structure, Gender and Fertility in Botswana', *Pula: Botswana Journal African Studies* 14(2): 130–47.

Goode, W.J. 1963. *World Revolution and Family Patterns*. New York: Free Press.

Guyer, J. 1994. 'Lineal Identities and Lateral Networks: The Logic of Polyandrous Motherhood', in C. Bledsoe and G. Pison (eds), *Nuptiality in Sub-Saharan Africa. Contemporary Anthropological and Demographic Perspectives*. Oxford: Clarendon Press, pp. 231–55.

Haram, L. 2004. '"Prostitutes" or Modern Women? Negotiating Respectability in Northern Tanzania', in S. Arnfred (ed.), *Re-thinking Sexualities in Africa*. Uppsala: Almquist & Wiksell Tryckerei, pp. 211–32.

Helle-Valle, J. 1999. 'Sexual Mores, Promiscuity and 'Prostitution in Botswana', *Ethnos* 64(3–4): 372–96.

Hörbst, V., and S. Schuster 2006. 'Introduction', *Curare (Special Issues: Reproductive Disruptions? Perspectives on African Contexts)* 29(1): 5–16.

Hunt, N.R. 2005. 'Fertility Fires and Empty Wombs in Recent Africanist Writing', *Africa* 75(3): 421–35.

Inhorn, M. (ed.). 2007. *Reproductive Disruptions: Gender, Technology and Biopolitics in the New Millennium*. Oxford: Berghahn Books.

Johnson-Hanks, J. 2002. 'On the Limits of Life Stages in Ethnography: Towards a Theory of Vital Conjunctures', *American Anthropologist* 104(3): 865–891.

———. 2006. *Uncertain Honour: Modern Motherhood in an African Crisis*. Chicago: University of Chicago Press.

Kohli, M. 2007. 'The Institutionalization of the Life Course: Looking Back to Look Ahead', *Research in Human Development* 4(3–4): 253–71.

Kohli, M., and J.W. Meyer 1986. 'Social Structure and Social Construction of Life Stages', *Human Development* 29(3): 145–49.

Kreager, P. 2004. 'Where are the Children?', in P. Kreager and E. Schröder-Butterfill (eds), *Ageing without Children: European and Asian Perspectives*. Oxford: Berghahn Books, pp. 1–76.

Larsen, U. 1994. 'Sterility in Sub-Saharan Africa', *Population Studies* 48(3): 459–74.

Leonard, L. 2002. '"Looking for Children": The Search for Fertility among the Sara of Southern Chad', *Medical Anthropology* 21(1): 79–112.

Lesetedi, G.N. 2003. 'Household Perspectives of Women and Men in Botswana', in Botswana, Central Statistical Office, *2001 Population and Housing Census Dissemination Seminar*. Gaborone: Botswana, Central Statistics Office, pp. 408–22.

Lesetedi, L.T. 1989. *Botswana Family Health Survey II, 1988*. Gaborone: Botswana, Central Statistics Office.

Lesthaeghe, R.J. 1989. 'Introduction', in *Reproduction and Social Organisation in Sub-Saharan Africa*. Berkeley, California: University of California Press, pp. 1–12.

Lewis, J.J., C. Ronsmans, A. Ezeh and S. Gregson. 2004. 'The Population Impact of HIV on Fertility in Sub-Saharan Africa', *AIDS* 18(2): 35–43.

Lorimer, F. 1954. *Culture and Human Fertility*. Paris: UNESCO.

Lucas, D. 1992. 'Fertility and Family Planning in Southern and Central Africa', *Studies in Family Planning* 23(3): 145–58.

Maruatona, T. 2003. 'Cartographic Methodological Aspects and Quality Control Measures for the Census Cartographic Preparatory Work', in Botswana, Central Statistical Office, *2001 Population and Housing Census Dissemination Seminar*. Gaborone: Botswana, Central Statistics Office, pp. 32–39.

Mookodi, G. 2003. 'Household Perspectives of Women and Men in Botswana', in Botswana, Central Statistical Office, *2001 Population and Housing Census Dissemination Seminar*. Gaborone: Botswana, Central Statistics Office, pp. 337–46.

Mookodi, G., and D. Fuh. 2004. 'Finding the "Missing" Male in Gender Discourses in Botswana', *Pula: Botswana Journal of African Studies* 18(1): 31–42.

Namboodiri, N.K. 1964. 'The Wife's Work Experience and Child Spacing', *Milbank Memorial Fund Quarterly* 42(3): 65–77.

Page, H.J., and R.J. Lesthaeghe 1981. *Child-Spacing in Tropical Africa: Traditions and Change*. New York: Academic Press.

Partow, Z. 2010. 'Botswana Public Expenditure Review'. Gaborone: World Bank (unofficial report).

Rafalitnanana, H. and C. F. Westoff 2000. 'Potential Effects on Fertility and Child Health and Survival of Birth-Spacing Preferences in Sub-Saharan Africa', *Studies in Family Planning* 31(2): 99–110.

Ringstedt, M. 2008. 'Collision in Life-Courses: Teenage Motherhood and Generational Relations in North-East Tanzania', in E. Alber, D. van der Geest and S. Reynold-Whytes (eds), *Generations in Africa. Contrasts and Connections*. Hamburg: LIT: 357–380.

Schapera, I. [1940] 1971. *Married Life in an African Tribe*. Harmondsworth: Penguin.

———. 1966. *Married Life in an African Tribe*. Evanston: Northwestern University Press.

———. 1993. 'Some Kgatla Theories of Procreation', in D. Suggs and A.E. Miracle (eds), *Culture and Human Sexuality: A Reader*. Boston: Brooks/Cole: 165–82.

Sommer, M. 2009. 'Ideologies of Sexuality, Menstruation and Risk: Girls' Experiences of Puberty and Schooling in Northern Tanzania', *Culture, Health & Sexuality* 11(4): 383–98.

Suggs, D.N. 1987. 'Female Status and Role: Transition in the Tswana Life Cycle', *Ethnology* 26(2): 107–20.

Sundby, J., and U. Larsen. 2006. 'Health Care Service for Infertility in Sub-Saharan Africa: The Case of Moshi in Northern Tanzania', *Curare (Special Issues: Reproductive Disruptions? Perspectives on African Contexts)* 29(1): 47–57.

Szreter, S. 1993. 'The Idea of Demographic Transition and the Study of Fertility Change: a Critical Intellectual History', *Population and Development Review* 19(4): 659–702.

Szreter, S., and E. Garrett. 2000. 'Reproduction, Compositional Demography, and Economic Growth: Family Planning in England Long before the Fertility Decline', *Population and Development Review* 26(1): 45–80.

Turner, V. 1969. *The Ritual Process: Structure and Anti-structure*. Chicago: Aldine.

United Nations. 2013. 'UNData. Age of First Marriage', June 2013. Retrieved 1 February 2017 from http://data.un.org/Data.aspx?d=GenderStat&f=inID%3A20.

Van Balen, F., and M.C. Inhorn. 2002. 'Introduction. Interpreting Fertility: A View from the Social Sciences', in M.C. Inhorn and F. van Balen (eds), *Infertility around the Globe: New Thinking on Childlessness, Gender, and Reproductive Technologies*. Berkeley: University of California Press, pp. 3–32.

Velkoff, V.A., and P.R. Kowai. *Population Aging in Sub-Saharan Africa: Demographic Dimensions 2006.*Washington DC: United States Bureau of the Census.

Werbner, R. 2004. *Reasonable Radicals and Citizenship in Botswana: The Public Anthropology of Kalanga Elites.* Bloomington: Indiana University Press.

Wray, J.D. 1971. 'Population Pressure on Families: Family Size and Child Spacing', *Reports on Population/Family Planning* 9: 404–61.

Chapter 8

Low Fertility and Secret Family Planning in Lesotho

Lena L. Kroeker

Today, Basotho women are having fewer children on average than in many other African countries (Lucas 1992; DSD and HRSC 2003; MoHSW 2010: xix) and the total fertility rate still continues to decline. While the 1976 census recorded 5.4 children born per Basotho woman, by 2009 the number had decreased to 3.3 (MoHSW 2010: 47). Since the late 1960s, the Ministry of Health and Social Welfare (MoHSW) has followed a fertility reduction plan and currently aims at achieving a total fertility rate of 2.8 by 2025 (UNFPA 2012; cf. Tuoane et al. 2004). Even in a regional comparison of Southern African countries, Lesotho seems outstanding. This chapter therefore addresses the question of what has impacted on fertility in Lesotho in recent decades, highlighting from a historical and anthropological perspective some of the key factors of an ongoing process of social and economic change.

The Kingdom of Lesotho, with a population of 2.1 million in 2012, is inhabited predominantly by the Basotho people. It is a constitutional monarchy landlocked within the Republic of South Africa. The population is often described as ethnically homogeneous, even though composed of various tribes united under King Moshoeshoe in the course of the nineteenth century. Today, the Basotho define themselves as one ethnic group, even though some cultural differences still show, for instance, in clan-related practices during rites of passage. While other ethnic groups were incorporated into the

Republic of South Africa, Lesotho opposed the Cape Colony under white rule and apartheid, and remained independent. During apartheid, Lesotho's government not only opposed South Africa's apartheid regime by supporting the African National Congress (ANC) (Gill 1993: 203; Rosenberg et al. 2004: 23, 27), but allowed numerous Western organizations to operate against apartheid from Lesotho's territory. Welcoming Western organizations as well as Christian (mostly Catholic) missionaries resulted in further advancement in the fields of education and healthcare (Gill 1993: 190). Economically, however, the small country is dependent on its only neighbour, the Republic of South Africa, due to scarce resources in Lesotho that result in high levels of labour migration. Diamonds were found in Kimberley in 1870 and gold mines opened at Witwatersrand in 1885, and Basotho men left their agricultural production to work in them. Of course, the absence of a large share of the male population for several months a year had an impact on family planning and fertility rates; however, this does not necessarily distinguish Basotho from other groups of labour migrants in the homelands or Botswana. Of course, South Africa is the economic heavyweight of the region and underwent historic developments such as the apartheid system that distinguish it from other Southern African countries. The multiethnic dimension in South Africa, in addition to ethnic segregation during apartheid (1948–94), impacted on many people's views of gender, fertility, partnership and family support. By 1996, just after the end of apartheid, fertility rates in South Africa averaged 2.9 children per woman (SADHS 1998: 18). However, this figure disguises large differences in relation to 'race'. The highest rates were recorded for African women and the lowest rates for whites.[1]

In contrast, Lesotho, with an ethnically homogeneous population of African origin and without a politically driven fertility policy, had an even higher fertility rate of 4.1 children born per women, as the 1996 census indicates. Yet in the longer term, Lesotho's fertility rate was in constant decline from the 1970s (see Figure 8.1).[2]

In this chapter I shall argue that various factors need to be taken into consideration to explain Lesotho's trend. I support Caldwell (1982), who has argued in his theory of fertility decline that social change entails economic changes that then impact on fertility and its control. However, I would like to add that in Lesotho, political and economic changes have affected women more than men, and that health issues, as well as the complex gender relations in times of social change, need to be taken into the equation too. My thesis is trifold.

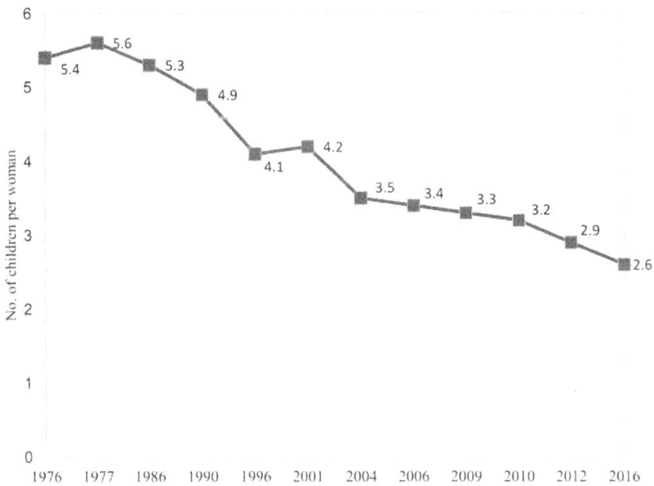

FIGURE 8.1 Decline of the Total Fertility Rate in Lesotho, 1976–2016. Sources: MoHSW, ICPD, Indexmundi.

TABLE 8.1 Low Fertility and Secret Family Planning in Lesotho

Year	**1976**	**1977**	**1986**	**1990**	**1996**	**2001**	**2004**	**2006**	**2009**	**2010**	**2012**	**2016**
TFR	5.4	5.6	5.3	4.9	4.1	4.2	3.5	3.4	3.3	3.2	2.9	2.6
Source	Census	Lesotho Fertility Survey	Census	ICPD 2012	Census	MoHSW 2005	MoHSW 2005	Census	MoHSW 2010	ICPD 2012	Index mundi	Index mundi

First, giving an historical overview of male and female labour migration, I shall illustrate its impacts on family planning during the second half of the twentieth century. Second, in addition to historical changes in the economy, biological factors affected the decline of fertility in Lesotho. High HIV rates and early death due to AIDS-related diseases limited the number of reproductive years and, hence, the number of children born. HIV/AIDS reached Lesotho in the mid 1980s and the high HIV-prevalence stands currently at 23 per cent of the population aged 15–49 (UNAIDS 2013). This represents the third-highest rate worldwide after Swaziland and Botswana. The third section deals with gender relations, delineating why many women prefer hormonal contraceptives that can be used without their partners' knowledge. I argue that, while sexuality and procreation may be dissociated, sexuality remains a male-dominated sphere. These complex gender issues and women's control over their fertility make hormonal contraceptives (like the pill or Depo-Provera) preferred methods of fertility control. In summary, my thesis is that Basotho women not only took over family responsibility as breadwinners and heads of household, but silently took responsibility for the right timing of children, family obligations and partnership arrangements.

Economic Changes and their Effects on the Household

Lesotho was founded during the first half of the nineteenth century in a period of constant conflict in the Southern African region. During the Lifaqane troubles, several agripastoralist clans, deprived of fertile portions of land, united under King Moshoeshoe. They managed to defend a mountainous and scarce part of the Drakensberge and Malouti mountains, and grew together as one nation of Basotho people. However, the land hardly allowed sufficient agricultural production and Basotho became predominately dependent on trade and labour migration during the first half of the twentieth century. At that time, men of reproductive age (15–49) easily found work in South Africa's mining centres and towns, and increasing numbers of Basotho labourers began to migrate to South Africa to supplement the arduous agricultural production at home. By the 1960s and 1970s, almost half of Lesotho's adult male labour force worked for months at a time in South Africa's gold and diamond mines. Male migrant labourers would spend only ten weeks or so in a year at home (Gay 1980: 74) and, in the remaining time, women would serve as provisional heads of households. These changes in the economy over the course of a century did not alter patrilineal and patrilocal descent or access to land. Basotho men continued to perceive rights of property and status patrilineally, and women were, even in absence of their father or husband, regarded as minors. Gay, on the basis of research in Lesotho in the late 1970s, has argued that women received recognition only through marriage, unless they had the opportunity to join the urban working class by their own means:

> Since most rural Basotho women have no hope of joining the employed urban elite, early marriage is regarded as essential to provide cash and productive resources and the rights to utilize such resources. It is only through legal marriage that a girl can break from childhood dependence, be respected as a woman, and obtain lifelong

> rights to a homestead and a house of her own, to the labour and cash support of a man, to fields and livestock, and be assured the legitimate right to the labour and earnings of her children. (Gay 1980: 45)

The number of male migrants, usually from low-educated and rural backgrounds, peaked in the early 1990s at 112,000 workers (Mapetla and Moultrie 2011). Birth records give proof of oscillating migration, since many children were born nine months after the Christmas holidays of mine workers. Around that time, the fertility rate stood at 5.4 according to the population census (1976), or 5.6 following the Lesotho Fertility Survey (1977).

Only a few years later, the economy had to adjust again to new conditions that affected household income generation and thereby fertility rates and family planning. Technological developments in the mines, declining global prices for gold and diamonds, and shifts in South African labour policy following the end of apartheid aggravated the situation of male migrant labourers from Lesotho in the 1980s and 1990s. Many labourers were dismissed and returned home as the opportunities for men in South African mines reduced. Meanwhile, the opening of Chinese textile factories in Lesotho offered new opportunities for seamstresses. Lesotho gained approximately 60,000 jobs in the ready-made garments industry and the jobs were filled almost exclusively by female employees (Rosenberg et al. 2004: 384). Employment enabled women to supplement or compensate for the loss of family income. Many women additionally combined formal and informal[3] occupations to generate income and serve as breadwinners, since male breadwinners were no longer able to provide sufficiently for their families (Gay 1980: 295; Kimane and Ntimo-Makara 1998: 119). These economic developments had major effects on demography, and changes in the fertility rate can be read in correlation with rising female participation in Lesotho's economy. By 2009, around 72 per cent of the formal labour force in Lesotho were women (Hausmann et al. 2010: 193) and the fertility rate stood at 3.2 (MoHSW 2010: 47). Hence, employment rates of women went along with a change from natural fertility to controlled fertility.

The Easterlin hypothesis proposes that with couples' increased income, the number of children born decreases due to costs and benefits of children (Easterlin and Crimmins 1985). The economist Easterlin argued that fertility can be directly linked to relative income and a 'fertility revolution' will come along with social and economic shifts following the modernization of states. He argues:

'The principal changes in reproductive behaviour associated with modernization relate to fertility and fertility control. The change in fertility is from an average of six or more births per woman over the reproductive career to around two' (Easterlin and Crimmins 1985: 4). This fertility revolution will start from Western, modernized states and will spread to 'pre-industrialized' countries in Asia, the Pacific and Africa, where 'a network of sociological and biological factors' have determined or controlled fertility so far (1985: 5). Easterlin explains that contraceptive usage in developing countries is limited by factors such as the accessibility of family planning services as well as a lack of motivation to limit family size – neither of which can fully explain fertility decline in Lesotho.

In his theory of fertility transition, Caldwell (1982: 72) argued that economic and social change alters the flow of wealth between generations, making children more expensive, and thus fertility declines. In his quantitative and qualitative study of household economy and fertility decline in Nigeria, he states that the benefits of having many children will be superseded by the costs of upbringing, education and the like. Employed parents in urban centres are therefore more likely to reduce the number of offspring and invest instead in more intensive care and financing for their fewer children. Moreover, contraceptive use correlates with employment and education of women, with their age and with place of residence (a positive impact if living in an urbanized area) (Caldwell 1982: 18). The number of children is reduced on average by one child with the higher level of education of the mother and/or father. In summary, higher education and employment lead, according to Caldwell's study, to a nucleation of household investments.

Formal schooling, which Caldwell (1982: 74) mentions as the most powerful influence on social change, had been introduced in Lesotho in 1848 on a small scale, and by the beginning of the twentieth century it was widely established (Rosenberg et al. 2004: 90). Over the twentieth century, enrolment rates were higher at all levels among girls than boys, since school attendance was more easily combined with girls' work chores in the household.[4] Due to more education and their household management in the absence of men, women were better prepared for the challenges of the second half of the twentieth century. Women were substantially involved in building the country following Lesotho's independence in 1964. Female workers dominated many areas of local infrastructural development such as construction, water supply and in the tertiary sector (cf. Matete-Lieb 1995: 64–76). Alongside changes in

Lesotho's household economy in the 1980s, fertility rates changed as women took over responsibility for generating income.

More and more women found work in the lowland belt starting from the 1980s, when jobs were increasingly offered to women. Employment enabled them to supplement or compensate for the loss of family income, and to gain recognition at the same time. Before women achieved high involvement as family breadwinners, their negotiating position was marginal, despite having primary responsibility for the household, and often without a male custodian. Around 70 per cent of the rural households had been managed by women, but major decisions were often made by men on their short visits home from South Africa. Yet male migrants in their brief visits often did not manage to reassert their authority or continue to generate sufficient family income. Marital breakdowns, excessive drinking and domestic violence became common (Gay 1980: 135; Gill 1993: 195; Rosenberg et al. 2004: 399). Caldwell recognizes in his study on Nigeria that predominately young, unmarried and childless women left the villages for Nigeria's urban centres to seek employment. In Lesotho, however, in addition to numerous unmarried women in their early twenties and thirties, married mothers and wives also migrated as a means of escaping from abusive relationships or abandonment by migrant husbands. They sought both more independence and access to consumer goods (Rosenberg et al. 2004: 400). As separated women and widows moved to Lesotho's economic centres in the lowlands in search of employment, the rate of urbanization exceeded 6 per cent (Corno and de Walque 2007: 9), with more women than men staying in the towns. There, the new households were managed de facto and de jure by women and no longer dependent on male custodianship. Social and financial ties nonetheless continued to link female employees in urban areas to the households of their extended family; this structure differs from the rural female-headed households, which still depended on male migrants' remittances.

The developments of the last three decades gave women an inevitable position as economic agents in the economy with effects on livelihood, family relations, household decision-making and labour force participation. Employment increased their autonomy over housing arrangements, in day-to-day decision-making, maintenance of social relations, ownership, formal and informal partnerships and enhanced self-esteem. In the absence of familial control and male custodianship over partnership arrangements, Basotho women started to initiate relationships and even marriages, and, interestingly, fertility rates decreased while attendance of family planning services in the highly industrialized lowlands increased drastically.

As outlined, theories of fertility decline cannot explain falling fertility in Lesotho by employing a merely functionalist economic approach. Geographical and social particularities need to be taken into account, particularly gender relations and social norms that limit fertility. Therefore I will now turn, first, to the industrialized lowland belt with characteristics of higher usage of contraceptives, good access to family planning services and involvement of women in the household economy. Later sections will then take up the impact of AIDS and changing gender relations.

Family Breadwinners and Contraceptive Use

It does not come as a surprise that the history of family planning is closely connected to women's increasing participation in formal employment (cf. Mapetla and Moultrie 2011). During the past thirty years, more women became family breadwinners and thereby responsible for financial decision-making for themselves and their dependants. Over the same period, Lesotho's government advertised family planning in order to reduce population growth, and employed women in particular accepted contraceptives. Especially in the industrialized lowland belt, where the apparel industry relies on an almost exclusively female workforce (counting some 60,000 employees in 2003), contraceptive use increased (Rosenberg et al. 2004: 383). As Lucas (1992: 151) remarks: 'The 1989 population estimates of the Ministry of Health show that in the lowland areas there exists a belt running from Butha Buthe to Mohale's Hoek with attendance ratios [i.e. at family planning services] from 21 to 69 visits per 1,000 population. The remainder of the country, comprising foothill and mountainous areas to the west, has ratios from 3 to 19 client visits per 1,000 population, implying much lower usage.'

Contraceptive prevalence rose from around 7 per cent in the mid 1970s to 47 per cent in 2009 in the whole of Lesotho (Tuoane et al. 2004).

The figures and sources for contraceptive prevalence are shown in Table 8.2.

In the lowlands, 56 per cent of married women used modern contraceptives such as injectables and the pill. Among unmarried women in the whole of Lesotho, contraceptive use stood at 58 per cent (MoHSW 2010: 34, 56).[5] Usage was highest among women aged

TABLE 8.2 Figures and Sources for Contraceptive Prevalence in Lesotho

Year	Contraceptive prevalence in % (Source)
mid 1970s	5.6% (Tuoane et al. 2004)
mid 1970s	5.6% (Tuoane et al. 2004)
mid 1970s	5.6% (Tuoane et al. 2004)
1977	7% (Tuoane et al. 2004)
1995	29% (ICDP 2012)
2001	41% (Tuoane et al. 2004)
2009	41% (Tuoane et al. 2004)
2011	70–75% (Tuoane et al. 2004)

Note: The MoHSW aimed at a contraceptive prevalence of 70-75% by 2011 and replacement-level fertility of 2.2 children per woman (Tuoane et al. 2004: 77).

30–34 and among those with three to four children. These women had apparently reached their desired number of offspring before reaching the end of their reproductive life. In many other African settings a usual statement on how many children are desired would be 'as many as possible' or 'as many as God gives me' (Bledsoe 2002: 9). Among Basotho women I never came across these statements; in fact, everybody desired to have at least one child. This leads to the conclusion that contraceptive use was already very common, widely available and well accepted.

The Lesotho Planned Parenthood Association (LPPA), a member of the International Planned Parenthood Federation (IPPF), has been operating in Lesotho since 1968 and is one of the earliest family planning programmes on the African continent. Contraceptive use rose as more and more women entered the labour market. The government introduced primary healthcare in 1970, of which family planning was part and parcel, and in the 1980s other private practitioners and non-governmental organizations (NGOs), such as the Red Cross, or faith-based clinics[6] offered contraceptives too. The LPPA, being the largest and most widely known institution offering family planning, receives direct and indirect financial support from the Ministry of Health and Social Welfare and from external donors (Tuoane et al. 2004). Since the 1970s, fertility trends have been monitored by the government, and in 1976 and 1977 two representative studies were conducted on the total fertility rate[7] under the auspices of the World Fertility Survey programme. Both Surveys showed 'moderate levels of fertility by Sub-Saharan African standards, around five children per woman, accompanied by very low levels of contraceptive use. These moderate fertility levels have been attributed mainly to long periods of postpartum abstinence and long term breastfeeding as well as lengthy absence of adult males working in South Africa' (Tuoane et al. 2003).

Beginning in the early 1980s, the National Population Policy foresaw the need to promote family planning services at mother and child units of hospitals and health centres, as part of their public health approach. Pregnant women were in this way introduced to family planning services and contraception by the time they were postpartum. In the following years, public health nurses who were based at each of the ten district hospitals made efforts in their outreach programmes to increase the number of expectant women attending antenatal checkups. Pregnant women were considered highly receptive to information on family planning and reproductive health (Field notes Kroeker: Public Health Nurse June 2008). Moreover, all twenty-two textile factories in Lesotho except for one also employed a nurse who took care of the employees' reproductive health and family planning needs. Counselling and care for HIV-positive women were offered right in the workplace. With this sexual and reproductive health initiative, employers – supported by the government and NGOs – aimed at a reduction of absenteeism due to sickness and maternity, and thereby to facilitate productivity. Women for their part appreciated children as being a gift, but also that having many children may be too expensive (Field notes Kroeker: 27 November 2008). Financial pressure from their families discouraged them from taking leave for childcare. MaThloni, for instance, did not consider having a second child due to financial constraints:

> MaThloni, aged 28, came to town to work as a maid and became pregnant in 2005 by her employer. She quit her employment and took up a job in the textile factory not only to support herself in town, but also her aunt (who minded the baby in the village), and her unemployed sisters. MaThloni's experience of being the breadwinner, as well as financial hardship, have both played a role in MaThloni's delaying or refusing marriage and having a second child until now. (Field notes Kroeker: 11 June 2008 – 2012)

Many female breadwinners were actually not only responsible for their own offspring but also supported larger family networks (Mapetla 2005). Thus, employed women mentioned that they did not expect to get pregnant in view of their unfavourable financial situation, such as the case of my informant[8] Leshome:

> Leshome, aged 36, started to migrate between village and town in 2001 when she found employment in Mafeteng's textile sector. Leshome, being the firstborn, committed herself to the family hardships and

> generated income to sponsor her younger siblings' education. Now that the last-born was about to graduate, she and her long-term boyfriend started planning their own family. (Field notes Kroeker: 7 November 2008–21 May 2009)

For both women, their own desire for children or marriage came second to supporting family members. Both supported relatives in the rural area who were not generating income, but had to look after children. Moreover, MaThloni and Leshome postponed their plans and intended to wait for a more financially and socially stable situation, including a supportive partner and eventually marriage.

For married women, contraceptives were of even greater importance in town. Since many women rented small one-roomed houses near their workplace, their husband, if there was one, had to stay behind. At the same time, contraceptives allowed women to engage in sexual relationships in the absence of their partner and of familial control, without fear of illegitimate offspring. Hence, contraception allowed sexual intercourse to be dissociated from producing offspring, at the same time guaranteeing uninterrupted income generation and thus the financial support of family members.

HIV/AIDS: A Threat to Reproductive Health

Campaigns addressing sexual and reproductive health in Southern Africa gained momentum in the 1990s with the rapid spread of HIV/AIDS. The first case was detected in Lesotho in 1986 and a national commission was founded the following year to coordinate activities for preventing and controlling the spread of the virus. The Kingdom of Lesotho showed high rates of new HIV infections in the 1990s and 2000s, which currently seem to stagnate at 23 per cent of the population aged 15–49 years (UNAIDS 2013). While other governments in the region were still dithering, Lesotho's government recognized early on a potential loss of the economically most productive segment of society, and governmental and non-governmental structures to contain the further spread of the virus were established. In the mid 1990s, the Lesotho government already recognized HIV and AIDS as not only a threat to public health but also as a general scourge of development in all sectors (GoL 2007: 13). HIV prevalence nevertheless increased, leaving women widowed, families without breadwinners, and children becoming household heads. In the following years, a further decline in the number of children born continued for two reasons. The first was that life expectancy and fecundity dropped as a consequence of the deterioration of people's health condition resulting from the HIV/AIDS crisis. Hence, HIV/AIDS can be named as one of the biological factors that decreased fertility (Dhont 2010; Bochow 2012).[9]

Life expectancy fell to below fifty years of age and only started slowly to rise again after antiretroviral medication became available and kept people living with HIV in better physical condition. Nevertheless, earlier deaths due to AIDS before individuals reached the end of their reproductive age limited the number of offspring (Du Plessis 2003: 78, 83). Moreover, du Plessis lists 'lower coital frequency due to illness', 'less sperm production' and 'foetal loss' among other reasons for lower numbers of offspring to HIV-positive couples. A foetus may miscarry early due to the mother's deteriorated health, particularly if an expectant mother finds herself in an advanced stage of AIDS. However, the introduction of medication that prolongs the life of HIV-positive people could result in rising numbers of offspring, although this has not been the case.

A second factor behind declining fertility was that Lesotho had already adopted a recommendation of the 1994 United Nations International Conference on Population and Development in Cairo: to link family planning and reproductive health services. In the aftermath of the conference, Lesotho's government implemented a National Population Policy and defined targets aiming at the provision of adequate family planning services: contraceptive use of about 70–75 per cent in married couples, and achieving replacement-fertility level by 2011 (Tuoane et al. 2004). Its purpose was also to reduce the adverse effects of high fertility in Lesotho, such as high rates of male unemployment, the limited availability of women to the labour market due to maternal responsibilities, and high demand for social welfare due to sickness and absenteeism. Consequently, campaigns to contain further HIV transmission by promoting condoms were seen by health practitioners as an entry point to teach about family planning in general.

By 2000, the Lesotho government had declared HIV/AIDS a national disaster (GoL 2007: 1), at a time when leading South African politicians were still in denial regarding the crisis in their own country (cf. van Rijn 2006). The MoHSW implemented an ambitious plan of prevention, treatment, testing and care. National strategic plans to combat the spread of HIV thereafter made it a key topic in reproductive health. Family planning was promoted for economic reasons as a valuable strategy to prevent HIV/AIDS in children (USAID 2006).[10] Preventing conception was considered a cheaper and more fruitful alternative to preventing HIV transmission from mother to child during pregnancy, delivery and breastfeeding. Hence, in the following years family planning services were rolled out and many clinics and rural health centres were able to provide contraceptives for free or at little cost (from 10 cents for male condoms to 15 Rand for implants; cf. Tuoane et al. 2004).[11]

Advisers of Lesotho's MoHSW argued that 'efforts to decrease the level of [HIV transmission from mother to child] can also focus on reducing fertility among HIV-positive women', and strategies need to be identified to target the unmet need for contraception (Adair 2007: 1). Hence, family planning should be introduced into medical services provided to HIV-positive women in particular (cf. Singh et al. 2009: 30). However, Warren et al. (2008: ii) point out that there was no consequent follow-up of HIV-positive mothers after delivery, and Adair (2007: 2) claimed a consequent follow-up to be an undervalued and little-used strategy. In 2009 family planning was made a cornerstone of the new HIV/AIDS strategy, published by the MoHSW in collaboration with the Lesotho National AIDS Commission (GoL 2009: 73). Antenatal clinics were identified as valuable entry points (Adair 2007: 2).

Basically, the government intended to reduce fertility, particularly among HIV-positive mothers. Yet in practice not much difference was made between HIV-positive and HIV-negative women. In my observation, HIV-negative mothers were simply considered as potentially at risk of contracting HIV, whether sooner or later. In addition, we might expect numbers of children to show a difference between HIV-positive women who received counselling and HIV-negative women who did not. However, this difference is not confirmed by quantitative studies. Rather, the Demographic and Health Surveys for Lesotho 2004 and 2009 indicate that the desire for children correlated with the number of live children (MoHSW 2005: 99; MoHSW 2010: 83; cf. Moultrie et al. 2012) and was therefore independent of the mother's HIV status. Preventing offspring in HIV-positive women has thus not shown significant effects as yet.

However, it is noteworthy that the rollout of contraceptives starting from the mid 1990s targeted predominately women, not their male counterpart(s) (cf. Silberschmidt 2004: 245–46). Condoms are, of course, the main tool in the fight against HIV transmission, but require the active involvement of men during intercourse. Yet campaigns used female agency in family planning first and foremost as the vehicle to put their messages across, rather than targeting male-dominated sexuality as an entry point. Consequently, while entry via the female sphere was well accepted, it did not result in a public or domestic debate between spouses on sexuality and fertility control. To understand this absence, we need to look into gender relations and how they were affected by women's rise in the household economy and their reproductive health decision-making.

Changing Conjugality and Family Planning

As we have seen, Basotho women entered the labour market, headed their own households and orchestrated sexual relationships. With the new housing situation based on one-roomed dwellings near industrial quarters rented to female labour migrants, family life came to be dissociated from reproductive life. Female sexuality was no longer necessarily tied to conjugal life, and one naturally wonders how this affected gender relations.

Anthropologists like Haram (2004) and Silberschmidt and Rasch (2001), who have studied female employee's reproductive life in East Africa's urban centres, show how conjugal life can be affected. Silberschmidt (2004) highlights that men in Kenya and Tanzania lost their 'biologically given' status of being heads of household since they ceased to be able to provide bridewealth and daily needs for their family. However, with respect to sexuality being key to masculinity, men have tried to maintain traditional role models, even by force. In Silberschmidt's analysis, as men became more and more disempowered by socioeconomic change, there was not only a breakdown of masculine roles, reduced male self-esteem and a general lack of social value associated with men; men attempted to compensate for this loss by dominating sexual relationships, domestic violence and 'escalating gender antagonism'. In the face of poverty, unemployment and a lack of access to education, masculinity has turned to a show of irresponsive, promiscuous and aggressive sexual behaviour towards women and a challenging of HIV awareness campaigns (Silberschmidt 2004: 234, 242).

Moreover, Haram (2004) shows that East African women use their fertility strategically, either as a means to generate income or to establish partnership(s). On the one hand, having a child can bond partners if a liaison looks promising to the woman; limiting the number of children offers better chances to generate future relationships that will result in joint offspring. On the other hand, a steady partnership that comes with male dominance and control may limit economic chances and autonomy (Haram 2004: 226). Being an economically independent town woman who is free to accept sex for its sexual and financial gratification offers opportunities for negotiating relationships and new identities as a 'modern' and 'free' women (Haram 2004: 211).

For Lesotho, Boehm (2006) describes the relation of industrial labour and changing family life from the perspective of young women. He argues that labour migration has replaced marriage as point of transition from adolescence to adulthood. Many moved to the towns being single mums, and only one-fifth of young women aged between eighteen and thirty in the village he studied – a labour reserve for labour migrants – were married. While the picture Boehm describes appears similar to developments in gender relations in Tanzania and Kenya, I disagree with Boehm's analysis in the case of Lesotho. Women indeed entered labour migration and plural informal sexual relations, just as men do whenever normative familial controls weaken. However, marriage never lost its value in Lesotho, in contrast to other African societies, and remains part of a woman's normal biography, as does having at least one child. As women are now usually more educated and better equipped to support themselves financially, good 'husband material' is not so easily found. That said, in the privacy of a female-headed, single-roomed dwelling, relationships of shorter or longer duration, and with or without financial benefits, have become easier to establish for town women. One way, then, of indicating that the right partner has been found is to stop the use of contraceptives and become pregnant. This, as we shall discuss later in this chapter, can be considered a female way of proposing marriage. While women may take their chances in choosing a partner and 'trapping him' by pregnancy, gender relations still do not allow them to ask for their hand in marriage. Women have not (yet) acquired the right to ask: like sexuality, proposing marriage is a male domain.

Silberschmidt (2004) concludes that while women were empowered by socioeconomic changes, the role of men remains neglected. A similar observation was made some time ago by Comaroff (1985), who recognized that gender relations did not change fundamentally among the Barolong, a South African ethnic group closely related to the Basotho. She argues, from a religious and political point of view, that despite women's increased participation in social change, elders and men in authoritative positions could prevent radical shifts. Certain spheres of social life were strongly defended by those in control of the central religious, political and economic media needed to initiate sustainable social change. Women did not have access to this sphere (Comaroff 1985: 48, 60, 80–81; Boehm 2006). In practice, this meant that when a 'traditional' family stayed together, 'traditional' contracts of gender also remained more or less intact on a daily basis.

Lesotho's gerontocratic and patriachal structure demands respect from young women, which is evident in communication between men and women as well as between elders and the young. During interaction between these parties, certain norms apply that, in addition to discourse, include body language, nonverbal communication and avoidance of certain sensitive topics. As outlined elsewhere (Kroeker 2011), patterns of interaction and communication are merely transformed for everyone's comfort. Urban women, despite geographical distance from their family members, have no intention of overturning the social hierarchy, but can make room for themselves by installing separate households in urban spaces (Mapetla 2005) and thereby avoid uncomfortable situations. Whenever the parties meet, normative power relations are reasserted. Consequently, gender roles are not contested. Taboos on speaking about sexuality with persons of the opposite sex, or to those of a different generation, also remain in place (cf. Mturi 2003). Usually same-sex friends deliberately use vulgar terms to talk about private parts and sexual activity in the local language. Sesotho often employs euphemisms, synonyms or comparisons – apparently unrelated metaphors like 'he was hungry', 'swinging the curtains' or 'sharing blankets' – to describe the sexual act. A lack of words and courage often prevents conversation between sexual partners. Women noted that men take the lead in bed or even that women are 'like sex toys' for their partners (Field notes Kroeker: Tsasaniana July 2008). A woman's speech would be considered impolite and vulgar, a sign of disrespect. In addition, women were not interested in getting into conflicts with their parents or partner(s) over topics of sexual pleasure and contraceptives. In consequence, topics of sexuality were silenced between sexual partners and spouses, and women often decided alone on the use of contraceptives without informing their partner(s) (cf. Hall and Malahleha 1989: 10).

The contexts of contraceptive use and arguments surrounding it were, in sum, often based on people's attempts to find a more comfortable social and physical situation. Women often manipulated contexts to further this and to lie about their marital situation. Thus, married women who intended to enter a temporary sexual relationship lied about their marital status, while unmarried women in antenatal care units claimed to be married in order to avoid stigma. Others argued that they would be getting married to the father of the child soon, even if marriage negotiations were not even under way. A fair number of expectant girls were actually waiting for the outcome of marriage negotiations, or at least for the child's father to acknowledge and hopefully accept paternity. In such cases, the parents of a pregnant girl could then approach the boy's parents and discuss marriage arrangements rather than simply accepting a child being born out of wedlock (Kroeker Field notes September 2008–May 2009).

Attitudes towards Premarital Pregnancy

In the precolonial era, as well as in some current Southern African settings, marriage and childbirth guaranteed important networks of social security (Radcliffe-Brown and Forde 1950; Fortes and Evans-Pritchard 1964). Structural-functionalists argued that having many wives – and in consequence many children – would secure support of an ever-larger number of family members. Moreover, a higher number of children would make it more likely that some of them would arrive at an age to produce and reproduce for the sake of the family. In precolonial times, Swazi, Zulu, Sotho and Tswana, like most other Southern African tribes, practised polygyny. In contrast to Basotho and Tswana, no proof of virginity was expected for marriage arrangements among the Swazi; rather, a prenuptial pregnancy or child would guarantee the fertility of a woman and thus make it easier for a man to agree to marry her. A child, even if not biologically the man's own, would be accepted as his offspring once marriage with the mother was agreed (Kuper 1950: 88). Thus, offspring would assure family wellbeing and enhance prestige, while having many children increased the chance of an heir and caretaker in the parents' old age.

Today, Botswana records high rates of pregnancy of about 20 per cent for women up to twenty years of age, and 70 per cent for women aged 20–25 years. Even in a regional comparison, this seems a rather young age to have children, and we also find high numbers of unmarried mothers. However, in Lesotho, many women in my ethnographic study stated that marriage is still important to them, which contrasts with the case of contemporary Botswana.

The Basotho have generally discouraged premarital sexual relationships and encouraged abstinence until marriage. Nevertheless, secret premarital relationships must have been considered the norm rather than the exception, just as today, when premarital meetings between boys and girls are still expected to be modest. Early initiation in nonpenetrative sexual contact simply has to be considered a fact in today's Lesotho, and in many cases parents appear to turn a blind eye provided there are no consequences. As a means of preventing premarital pregnancies in precolonial times, Basotho girls were usually married off at an early age (Maqutu 2005: 36). Moreover, food taboos were placed upon adolescent girls to limit their sexual appetite. While there were no such restrictions for boys, girls from the onset of puberty until marriage were not allowed to eat animal intestines and eggs. Such foods were believed to stimulate maidens to mature more quickly, as their consumption encourages the growth of secondary sexual characteristics and consequently raises their interest in sexuality and the likelihood of illegitimate children (Sechefo 1900: 19; Field notes Kroeker 21: 5 December 2008; Field notes Kroeker: Theko 28 July 2009). Eggs in particular resemble the amniotic sac and their consumption may result in a miscarriage or 'burn the girl from inside' (Field notes Kroeker: MaThloni 10 January 2011). Cooked sheep's tripe, following Sechefo's account (1900: 19), would also harm young girls as its consumption would cause heavy menstruation. A limited intake of proteins has therefore been associated with the prevention of teenage pregnancies (Romero-Daza and Himmelgreen 2004: 962).

In earlier times, traditional initiation for girls taught these principles upon the onset of puberty. Today few girls attend initiation and food restrictions no longer apply. Nevertheless, a stigma for unmarried teenage girls remains in place and many schools expect girls who become pregnant to leave. Even worse, Sesotho culture is still strict when it comes to unmarried young women with children. While the situation of reproductive health awareness and family planning has changed, the stigma of being pregnant and unwed continues, and girls with children may be called derogative names; in Mturi and Moerane's (2001) account, premarital pregnancy results in 'social ostracism and was locally referred to as *o senyehile*, meaning that she is spoiled or destroyed'. Even today I found children with given names that were meant to stigmatise their mother as morally weak or loose:

> The baby is given a bad name when it is born out of wedlock. I say that this is actually unfair, because everybody will know by the first meeting. Everybody will know that something is wrong with the mother of this child. (Field notes Kroeker: Maletsie 15 March 2009)

Having many children can no longer be associated with social security as it did in rural farming families, yet some children do provide social security. For instance, in the Cape Flats, a low-income and high-crime-rate area of Cape Town, single motherhood is well known among coloured and black inhabitants. Families are based on two-generational maternal solidarity, and income depends predominately on government welfare. In total, over twelve million South Africans receive cash grants and child support of monthly 250 Rand in the largest programme, which not only alleviates child-poverty, but provides for 8.5 million poor households (Orderson 2011). In such cases, having offspring secures a family's sole income, while the value of marriage as the foundation of familial alliances and solidarity has waned.

In the absence of government child benefits, social security in Lesotho relies predominantly on the family as a fallback system and on income from wage labour. As larger networks due to marriage are recognized to guarantee a better social standing, perhaps the link between marriage and fertility has not eroded despite increasing female education and wage labour in recent decades. First pregnancy for Basotho women occurs in their early twenties, and teenage pregnancies were recorded less often than in Botswana.[12] In fact, the age for having a first child rose in recent years in Lesotho and marriage was likewise delayed. The average age for marriage is now at twenty-one for women and twenty-six for men (MoHSW 2010: 72). First pregnancy is also delayed to approximately twenty-two for first mothers in urban areas and twenty in rural areas. The correlation of marriage and childbirth is already implied by the mother's average age for these events. A first child is born on average one year into the marriage and the number of desired children stands at 1.7 in this region (MoHSW 2010: 92). Age at marriage and first childbirth rises with education, urban residency and higher wealth quintile (MoHSW 2010: 50), just as Caldwell argued in his demographic study of Nigeria. Caldwell compared rural farming households with urban families relying on formal sector incomes, concluding:

> The kind of prestige and power (very much interlinked in the traditional community) that the illiterate farmer derives from having a considerable number of grown-up children in the village has no counterpart among the white-collar workers of the town; they derive their prestige from their education and job, the size of their house, and from throwing parties and other conspicuous expenditures. (Caldwell 1982: 57)

In an urban workforce that does not rely on high numbers of children and where education and jobs replace large family networks as security systems, women who have completed their school education may delay or refrain from getting married as a guarantee of home and familial security. Instead, they rely on their own labour, in contrast to the above-mentioned case from the Cape Flats.

While in all generations, informal polygamy of both sexes and premarital sexual contacts cannot be denied, childbirth is nonetheless postponed to a later point in life with the help of contraception. In Lesotho, presumably due to male and female labour migration, sexuality turned some time ago into a personal matter and became detached from reproduction. In the absence of husbands, wives had to control their fertility. Today, fertility control remains equally important since childbirth reduces economic chances and lessens marriageability. Meanwhile, being married remains a crucial part of family wellbeing and the legitimacy of offspring. Postponed childbearing is crucial for Basotho women until their social situation allows for it.

Limiting, Spacing and Postponing Children

Having outlined what factors limit the number of children, I will now turn to the question of which factors contribute to having them. This aspect is hardly discussed in Western-based demographic theory. In the West, the familiar argument is that contraceptives are used predominately to limit the number of children. In contrast, feminist and anthropological studies have shown that modern contraceptives are used in Africa in a different way. As Bledsoe and others (Bledsoe et al. 1998: 45, 50; Bledsoe 2002; Timaeus and Moultrie 2008; Moultrie et al. 2012) have argued, African women accept contraceptives to space children rather than to limit them:

> For several decades now, motivations for contraceptive use in less developed countries have been assumed to fall into one of two exclusive categories: stopping and spacing. We have argued that, in order to explain birth intervals as long as those observed in South Africa, this two-way typology must be expanded to include 'postponement' as a third motivation for contraceptive use. (Moultrie et al. 2012: 241)

Bledsoe shows that for this purpose, hormonal contraceptives are preferred by Gambian women in order to take their time and recover from their last pregnancy. A child should be weaned, able to walk or able to speak before the mother becomes pregnant again (Bledsoe 2002: 113–18). Especially if a pregnancy ends in a miscarriage or stillbirth, women limit their fertility 'to regain strength' (Bledsoe 2002: 4). In contrast to the reasoning of Western-based research, there are no children to space – rather, there is a spacing of affirmative situations for the mother until she is ready to conceive again. In fact, in the Gambia, mothers waited until the time was ripe from their perspective to have a healthy baby again, and therefore to have in the end more rather than fewer children (Bledsoe 2002: 100). In summary, women did not limit the number of children by accepting modern contraceptives, but increased their chances of having healthy offspring by means of managing the right time. This compares to the perspective of Lesotho women's views, notably their desire for well-timed children and or adjusting their contraceptive needs accordingly. However, their criteria were different: an affirmative economic and marital situation rather than biological readiness for conception. Nonetheless, in both cases, women tried to manipulate their conditions by the secret use of contraceptives, as I will highlight now.

The Female Power: Secret Use of Contraception

Unmarried as well as married female labour migrants in Lesotho engage in casual relationships. Due to the use of contraceptives, the majority of these relationships do not result in offspring. Given the difficulty of speaking about contraception openly with a partner, hormonal means of contraception were favoured by far due to their potential for secret use (Hall and Malahleha 1989: 2; Tuoane et al. 2003; Field notes Kroeker 10 February 2009). Hence, the most commonly given methods of family planning are Depo-Provera injections for three-month periods, followed by the pill (MoHSW 2010: 56). Even schoolgirls preferred injections since they would be unrecognized by their parents (Tuoane et al. 2003). Before 1994, the pill was requested more than injectable contraceptives, apparently also for the reason of secret usage (Lucas 1992; Tuoane et al. 2004).

Griffiths (1990), Kaufman (2000) and Boehm (2006) assume that the link between marriage and reproduction slowly but steadily erodes. My interviewees argued decidedly the opposite. Basotho women are well aware that marriage and reproduction should ideally be considered as one (Field notes Kroeker 02 February 2009; 21 May 2009). Boehm's (2006) examples likewise indicate that an interest in marriage is high, only that relationships do not last. Despite the reality of single mothers and couples living at a distance from home communities and kin, the ideal family described by my interviewees consisted of a married couple living together with their children. Generally, Basotho women associated childbearing with marriage, and marriage with childbearing. Socially, the couple would maintain close bonds to extended family members for support and care. Young women nevertheless dreamt of eventually getting married to a husband who would care for their social and financial wellbeing entirely, as well as being the father of their children. However, they described such suitable matches as hard to find and much sought-after (Field notes Kroeker: 02 February 2009; 01 March 2009; 19 July 2010). The temporal and informal nature of some relationships and male dominance in gender relations made it difficult for young women to build relationships and to arrange for marriage once Mr Right was found.

Young women nonetheless found another way to propose marriage, albeit indirectly. In quite a number of cases, young women stopped using contraception without their partner's knowledge. Despite the widespread availability of free condoms as male contraception, safe protection against pregnancies seems to be a female responsibility, and this opens up the way for girls to use fertility for the purpose of marriage when they consider the circumstances to be just right (Field notes Kroeker MaMong: 15 April 2009; Field notes Kroeker Theko 15 April 2009; Field notes Kroeker LeSupa; Field notes Kroeker MaMeli; Field notes Kroeker MaTharo). MaMeli provides a case in point:

> MaMeli planned her pregnancy despite her unmarried status. She moreover calls the father of the child her husband, although no marriage ceremony took place, and explains that the couple intended to speed up the process of negotiations due to their parents' reluctance. MaMeli's parents disapproved of her liaison with a much older miner from their neighbourhood. Yet, a planned pregnancy hastened the process of marital negotiations due to the moral stigma of an unmarried girl with child (Field notes Kroeker MaMeli: 25 November 2008).

For many girls in Lesotho, as well as in South Africa, becoming pregnant is in effect a nonverbal marriage proposal. Discussions with young men in Lesotho showed that while they thought a girl proposing to them was an odd idea, they admitted that a pregnancy would force a boy into commitments (Field notes Kroeker Theko: 15 April 2009; 21: 16 April 2009; 3/2010). Haram (2004: 224), in her study of Northern Tanzania, puts it in a comparable way: 'a common child often cements the relationship between partners'. Despite the several sources of women's agency described in the preceding sections of this chapter, Basotho norms continue to make a girl asking a boy out or proposing marriage verbally inappropriate.

Perhaps more directly, any young women in antenatal care would claim to be in a stable relationship, referring to their lover as a husband as soon as the relationship becomes public. They then wait for his reaction (Field notes Kroeker MaMeli: 25 November 2008; Field notes Kroeker MaTharo: 28 January 2009). In MaMeli's case the pregnancy resulted in marriage, although in many cases the strategy does not guarantee success (Field notes Kroeker MaMong: 16 April 2009; Field notes Kroeker LeSupa; Field notes Kroeker: 09 June 2008). If a boy still denies his involvement with the girl, negotiations will be delayed until after the baby is born, at which point the physical appearance of the child may suggest affiliation (Field notes Kroeker: March 2010).

As a second option, young women consider abortions, even though this practice is prohibited in Lesotho. Mturi summarizes:

> Premarital childbearing is more restricted and children who are born to unmarried women are regarded as illegitimate. For these reasons some adolescents resort to induced abortion, which is illegal in Lesotho unless performed to save the life of the mother, as a means of avoiding unwanted children. (Mturi 2003: 26)

Abortions are thus one option to avoid stigma whenever marriage arrangements fail. Although unwanted and mistimed pregnancies do exist, fertility rates, which only count live offspring, remain low. Despite the fact that abortion officially does not exist in Lesotho, Nzioka (2003) has compiled a report on it for Maseru, the capital of Lesotho. Typical reasons for abortion include unwanted and mistimed pregnancy due to failure to use contraception or contraceptive failure. Often challenging circumstances, like abandonment by the partner or unexpected financial difficulty, turn an initially desired pregnancy into an unwanted one. Young women particularly feared having a child out of wedlock and the disinterest of their partner (Nzioka 2003: 5, 15), which supports the view that strong stigma still exists around premarital motherhood (Mturi and Moerane 2001). In fact, several women I interviewed knew where to have an abortion, either with Chinese doctors or traditional healers (Field notes Kroeker 27 June 2008), and many were able to tell stories about acquaintances who had one. The demand for abortions is, however, unreported or undetected by health statisticians. Since abortions are available in the Republic of South Africa, they are mostly reported as spontaneous rather than as induced abortions in the medical files of Lesotho's health centres. Women with incomplete abortions nevertheless present themselves in Lesotho's hospitals, but the numbers remain in the dark. Here, the dead foetus will be removed and recorded as a perinatal death. If the mother passes away as a result of the abortion, her death is recorded as a maternal death. In conclusion, abortion may contribute significantly to low fertility rates among young women in Lesotho. Despite illegality, abortions count in effect as an additional means of family planning (cf. Shostak 1982: 142, 152; Bledsoe 2002: 80–81; Ampofo 2004: 127).

Conclusion

In the last thirty years, socioeconomic changes, high female employment and a change in marital careers have altered Lesotho's societal structure and, in consequence, fertility control. Three issues seem fundamental when looking at low fertility rates in this context: who carries primary responsibilities as household head and family bread winner? Is there good access to family planning services? And are there social norms that advocate childbearing within wedlock?

The enhancement of women's status and labour force participation in Lesotho is attested by the Global Gender Gap Report. This Report, which is published annually by the World Economic Forum (Hausmann et al. 2010), rates women's participation in politics, the economy, access to health and access to education in Lesotho as comparable to most European countries. In opposition to authors who have considered education the key to a decrease in fertility rates (Caldwell 1982; Caldwell and McDonald 1982; Lucas 1992; Tuoane et al. 2003), I have shown that female participation in economic life is a more valuable parameter than education (cf. also Mapetla and Moultrie 2011). I agree, however, with Caldwell in his basic argument that social change alters economic principles, which in the end impact on fertility control. In Lesotho, household headship seems pivotal. Female household heads were not part of patriarchal gender arrangements. They have become prominent, while the value of marriage and of having at least one child remains untouched in Basotho culture and society. Moreover, my case study indicates that employed women in Lesotho have taken care of generating income for larger family networks and remitted money to next of kin, even though their incomes were never an obligatory part of household bread baskets (cf. Mapetla 2005). This observation contrasts with Caldwell's hypothesis that a reduction of offspring is due to increased investments for a few children rather than larger family networks. In my examples, women instead postponed their own desire for offspring and assisted family members (i.e. younger siblings) financially.

Tuoane et al. (2003: 105) state that the 'use of contraceptive methods allows women to postpone pregnancy, alter the timing between pregnancies, or avoid pregnancy completely'. Biological factors such as high HIV/AIDS rates have in recent decades limited the number of children born due to short life expectancy, which is now often lower than the end of reproductive life. However, since medication to prolong the lives of people with HIV has become available, the low number of children born has remained unchanged. The combination of rising awareness of communicable diseases with family planning has apparently reached the key target group of reproductive control, namely, women of reproductive age. However, their reproductive decisions were already founded on affirmative and viable social conditions. Further, we have seen that while contraceptive use is now common in the urban and industrialized lowland belt, its spread cannot be taken simply as confirmation of functionalist theses about the diffusion of Western economic and familial rationality. Stopping contraceptive use has, in the same period, gained value too. Young women choose to become pregnant, thus initiating marriage negotiations by their own individual agency. Such strategies are conscious attempts to improve their social and material conditions. For the same reason, women who find themselves carrying an unwanted or mistimed pregnancy now terminate these pregnancies to avoid stigma. Figures on abortions remain in the dark due to their illegality in Lesotho.

Men's attitudes were affected to a lesser extent by changes in the social and economic realm, as well as their involvement in reproductive health. Gender relations continue to be followed rather conservatively by men, who have on the whole kept their authority over sexuality as a male domain. Women have allowed men to play out their masculinity when it comes to sexuality, but have taken decisions over family planning and household composition into their own hands. Despite open debates on reproductive health with reference to HIV prevention, in both educational and medical institutions, sexuality remains to date a taboo subject of discussion between men and women, and across generations. Ethnography reveals that the secret use of contraceptives by women is widespread, as this pragmatically avoids awkward discussions that would be needed to initiate fundamental social change in sexual relations. Women have openly contested neither gender relations nor conventional speech etiquette regarding sexuality, but have accepted present norms and social hierarchies. Hence, women drive decisions on family planning, but not on reproductive health as they rarely demand condom use or abstinence. However, the hormonal methods of contraception on which they rely cannot prevent sexually transmitted diseases, like HIV/AIDS. Here, women are not (yet) drivers of change, even if they have silently taken over responsibility for the right timing of children, for economic and social family obligations, and for engineering partnerships. However, in the basic sense of the phrase, 'gender relations' entails the engagement of both sexes with each other. Nonetheless, in many cases, it is mistaken as 'women's issues'. As a matter of fact, many health programmes focus predominantly on women. In particular, family planning units address women as gatekeepers to reproductive health. However, this reading does not grasp the core of the concept. Reducing 'gender issues' to 'women's issues' ignores the much-needed contribution of men. Further engagement of men is needed in the realm of reproductive health to facilitate substantial change.

Lena L. Kroeker is a postdoctoral fellow at the Bayreuth Academy of Advanced African Studies. She holds a Ph.D. in Social Anthropology from the Bayreuth International Graduate School of African Studies (BIGSAS), Bayreuth University. In 2015 her monograph on the obstetric choices of HIV+ mothers in Lesotho was published.

Notes

1. South Africa's population was classified according to four categories during apartheid that guaranteed and limited access to rights and duties. The population policy aimed at increasing birth rates among whites and lowering them among African women (Anderson 2003: 27). The increasing number of black people, together with the decreasing number of whites, was feared to threaten political stability of the apartheid regime. Hence, black women who showed much higher fertility rates than white and coloured women were coerced to agree to Depo-Provera injections; meanwhile, white women were encouraged to have larger families (Hartman 1987: 193). The motives behind this

policy were related to assuring white dominance (Chimere-Dan 1993). It will suffice merely to mention these political aims here, since they are not key to my main argument.

2. The sources for these rates are given in Table 8.1; cf. MoHSW 2010: 47; ICPD 2012; Indexmundi 2012.
3. Formal employment in Lesotho entails skilled manual labour in offices as well as unskilled labour, as in textile factories and shops. Informal occupations include jobs as domestic helpers, selling door-to-door, vegetable and pastry vendors, telephone kiosks, etc. Petty income was also generated by raising and selling small livestock, such as chickens and pigs, and from brewing beer for sale.
4. This has been quite common in many African countries in the first half of the twentieth century (see Lindsay and Miescher 2003). With the changing of family life under Christianity (with men becoming breadwinners) and with education offering reliable opportunities for social mobility, the ratio between girls and boys often changed (though not in all African countries). In addition, from the turn of the century onwards, female education appeared to be a 'problem' often addressed through concerns over school drop-outs due to early teenage pregnancies (Bledsoe and Barney 1993). These concerns might not only express development policy makers' concerns over the status of women in African societies but also local suspicions against schooling women (Cole 2007). For a debate on the gender gap in Lesotho, see also Kroeker (2011).
5. This figure captures the whole of Lesotho, not the lowlands. It must be much higher in that area; however, regional figures were not available.
6. A total of 40 percent of the clinics under the Christian Health Association are Catholic and reject artificial contraceptives (Tuoane et al. 2004). In my experience, many Catholic health practitioners refer clients to neighbouring health centres that offer family planning services, if the client so wishes.
7. GoL 1976; WFS 1977.
8. The author conducted a longitudinal ethnographic study in the Mafeteng District in the Southern Lowlands of Lesotho between 2007 and 2011, which involved thirty HIV-positive mothers, their families, lay counsellors and health professionals. On an institutional and financial level, the study was supported by the Bayreuth International Graduate School of African Studies (BIGSAS) at Bayreuth University, Germany.
9. See also literature on the so-called 'infertility belt', which refers to low fertility rates in some African countries caused by venereal disease, including HIV/AIDS (van Balen and Inhorn 2002: 23). Another biological factor that limits fertility is malnutrition, especially in the mountainous regions of Lesotho where there is little arable land. For a discussion of HIV/AIDS and food insecurity in Sub-Sahara Africa see

Mazzeo et al. (2011), which includes Kroeker and Beckwith (2011) on Lesotho.

10. The MoHSW initiative was taken over subsequently by the Lesotho National AIDS Commission (GoL 2009: 72).
11. During the period of my research, available methods of family planning were the following: male and female condoms, hormonal implants that last for five years, Depo-Provera injections, diaphragm and intrauterine devices, and contraceptive pills (progestin-only and combined type). Hospitals offered sterilisation via tubal ligation and vasectomy. Tuoane et al. (2004) also mention spermicides. These were not provided when I did research in Lesotho between 2007 and 2011. Instead, hormonal emergency contraception was available, and injectables and implants seemed more popular than in 2004. Abortions are illegal in Lesotho, but occur nevertheless to terminate mistimed and unwanted pregnancies (cf. Shostak 1982: 142, 152; Bledsoe 2002: 80–81; and Ampofo 2004: 127 for other African contexts).
12. Teenage pregnancies (15–19 years): Botswana 21 per cent, Namibia 14 per cent, South Africa 13 per cent, Zimbabwe 4 per cent and Lesotho 3 per cent (Mturi and Moerane 2001).

References

Adair, T. 2007. *Desire for Children and Unmet Need for Contraception among HIV-Positive Women in Lesotho*. Calverton: Macro International Inc. Retrieved 1 February 2017 from http://dhsprogram.com/pubs/pdf/WP32/WP32.pdf.

Ampofo, A.A. 2004. 'Whose "Unmet Need"? Disagreement about Childbearing among Ghanaian Couples', in S. Arnfred (ed.), *Re-thinking Sexualities in Africa*. Uppsala: Nordiska Afrikainstitutet, pp. 115–34.

Anderson, B.A. 2003. 'Fertility, Poverty and Gender', in Department of Social Development (ed.), *Fertility*. Cape Town: HSRC Publishers, pp. 27–56.

Bledsoe, C.H. 2002. *Contingent Lives*. Chicago: University of Chicago Press.

Bledsoe, C.H., F. Banja and A.G. Hill. 1998. 'Reproductive Mishaps and Western Contraception: An African Challenge to Fertility Theory', *Population and Development Review*. 24(1): 15–57.

Bledsoe, C.H., and C. Barney (eds) 1993. *Social Dynamics of Adolescent Fertility in Sub-Saharan Africa*. Washington DC: National Academy Press.

Bochow, A. 2012. 'Quest for Conception in Times of HIV/AIDS: (In)fertility Care in Botswana', *ObsGyn* 81–86.

Boehm, C. 2006. 'Industrial Labour, Marital Strategy and Changing Livelihood Trajectories among Young Women in Lesotho', in C. Christiansen, H.E. Vigh and M. Utas (eds), *Navigating Youth, Generating Adulthood*. Uppsala: Nordic Africa Institute: 153–182.

Caldwell, J.C. 1982. *Theory of Fertility Decline*. New York: Academic Press.

Caldwell, J.C., and P. McDonald.1982. 'Influence of Maternal Education on Infant and Child Mortality. Levels and Causes', *Health Policy and Education* 2: 251–67.

Chimere-Dan, O. 1993. 'Population Policy in South Africa', *Studies in Family Planning* 24(1): 31–39.

Cole, C.M. 2007. '"Give Her a Slap to Warm Her up": Post-gender Theory and Ghana's Popular Culture', in C.M. Cole, T. Manuh and S. F. Miescher, *Africa after Gender?* Bloomington: Indiana University Press, pp. 270–85.

Comaroff, J. 1985. *Body of Power, Spirit of Resistance.* Chicago: University of Chicago Press.

Corno, L., and D. de Walque. 2007. *The Determinants of HIV Infection and Related Sexual Behaviors: Evidence from Lesotho.* Policy Research Working Paper 4421. Washington DC: World Bank.

Department of Social Development and Child, Youth and Family (DSD) and Human Science Research Council (HRSC). 2003. *Fertility: Current South African Issues of Poverty.* HIV/AIDS and Youth, Department of Social Development and Child, Youth and Family. Cape Town: Development Research Programme of the Human Science Research Council.

Dhont, N. 2010. 'Clinical, Epidemiological and Socio-cultural Aspects of Infertility in Resource-Poor Settings. Evidence from Rwanda', Doctoral thesis, Ghent University.

Du Plessis, G. 2003. 'HIV/AIDS and Fertility, in DSD and HRSC (eds), *Fertility. Current South African Issues of Poverty.* HIV/AIDS and Youth, Department of Social Development and Child, Youth and Family. Cape Town: Development Research Programme of the Human Science Research Council, pp. 77–116.

Easterlin, R.A., and E.M. Crimmins. 1985. *The Fertility Revolution.* Chicago: University of Chicago Press.

Fortes, M., and E.E. Evans-Pritchard 1964. *African Political Systems.* Oxford: Oxford University Press.

Gay, J.S. 1980. 'Basotho Women's Options. A Study of Marital Careers in Rural Lesotho', Ph.D. dissertation. Cambridge: University of Cambridge.

Gill, S.J. 1993. *A Short History of Lesotho.* Morija: Morija Museum and Archives.

Government of Lesotho (GoL), Bureau of Statistics. 1976. *Population Census 1976.* Maseru.

——. 2007. *Coordination Framework for the National Response to HIV and AIDS.* Maseru.

——. 2009. *Lesotho HIV Prevention Response and Modes of Transmission Analysis.* Lesotho National AIDS Commission/USAID/World Bank Global HIV/AIDS Program, Maseru. Retrieved 1 February 2017 from http://siteresources.worldbank.org/INTHIVAIDS/Resources/375798-1103037153392/LesothoMOT13April.pdf.

Griffiths, A. 1990. *Negotiating Pregnancy: Women's Strategies Concerning Marriage and Compensation among the Kwena in Botswana.* Edinburgh: Centre of African Studies.

Hall, D., and G. Malahleha 1989. *Health and Family Planning Services in Lesotho.* Morija: Morija Printing Works.

Haram, L. 2004. '"Prostitutes" or Modern Women? Negotiating Respectability in Northern Tanzania', in S. Arnfred (ed.), *Re-thinking Sexualities in Africa.* Uppsala: Nordiska Afrikainstitutet, pp. 211–29.

Hartmann, B. 1987. *Reproductive Rights and Wrongs.* New York: Harper & Row.

Hausmann, R., L.D. Tyson and S. Zahidi. 2010. *The Global Gender Gap Report 2010.* Geneva: World Economic Forum. Retrieved 1 February 2017 from http://www.weforum.org/reports/global-gender-gap-report-2010.

Indexmundi. 2012. Lesotho. Demographics, from http://www.indexmundi.com/lesotho

International Conference on Population and Development (ICPD). 2012. *Lesotho Country Implementation Profile.* Retrieved 1 February 2017 from http://icpdbeyond2014.org.

Kaufman, C.E. 2000. *Adolescent Pregnancy and Parenthood in South Africa.* New York: Population Council.

Kimane, I., and M. Ntimo-Makara. 1998. 'The Gender Dimension of Urban Migration in Lesotho', in A. Larsson, M. Mapetla and A. Schlyter (eds), *Changing Gender Relations in Southern Africa.* Rome: Institute of Southern African Studies: 101–128.

Kroeker, L. 2011. 'Lesotho's Performance in the Global Gender Gap Index 2010. Conflicts over Resources and Roles of the Female Breadwinner'. In Daniel, A., K. Fink, L. Kroeker, and J. Schütze (eds), *Women's Life Worlds 'In-Between'.* Bayreuth: BIGSASworks!, pp. 80–100.

Kroeker, L., and A. Beckwith. 2011. 'Safe Infant Feeding in Lesotho in the Era of HIV/AIDS', in J. Mazzeo et al. (eds), *HIV/AIDS and Food Insecurity in Sub-Saharan Africa: Challenges and Solutions.* Hoboken, NJ: Wiley-Blackwell, pp. 50–66.

Kuper, H. 1950. 'Kinship among the Swazi', in A.R. Radcliffe-Brown and C.D. Forde (eds), *African Systems of Kinship and Marriage.* New York: Oxford University Press, pp. 87–110.

Lindsay, L.A., and S.F. Miescher. 2003. 'Introduction: Men and Masculinities in African History', in L.A. Lindsay and S.F. Miescher (eds), *Men and Masculinities in Modern Africa.* Portsmouth, NH, Heinemann: 1–34.

Lucas, D. 1992.' Fertility and Family Planning in Southern and Central Africa', *Studies in Family Planning* 23(3): 145–58.

Mapetla, M.M.T. 2005. 'Perspectives on Living Conditions of Women Factory Workers in Ha Tetsane, Lesotho', in F. Kalabamu (ed.), *Gender, Generation and Urban Living Conditions in Southern Africa.* Lesotho: Institute of Southern African Studies National University of Lesotho, pp. 131–52.

Mapetla, N., and T.A. Moultrie. 2011. 'Fertility and Women's Labour Force Participation in Lesotho'. *6th African Population Conference: African Population: Past, Present, and Future, Ouagadougou, 5–9 December 2011.* Retrieved 1 February 2017 from http://uaps2011.princeton.edu/papers/110714.

Maqutu, W.C.M. 2005. *Contemporary Family Law: The Lesotho Position.* Lesotho: National University of Lesotho Publishing House.
Matete-Lieb, T. 1995. 'Basotho Women's Role in Urban Housing: The Case of Maseru', in S. Sithole Fundirc, A. Zhou and A. Larsson (eds), *Gender Research on Urbanization, Planning, Housing and Everyday Life.* Harare: Zimbabwe Women's Resource Centre and Network.
Mazzeo, J., A. Rödbach and B.P. Brenton (eds). 2011. *HIV/AIDS and Food Insecurity in Sub-Saharan Africa. Challenges and Solutions.* Hoboken, NJ: Wiley-Blackwell.
Ministry of Health and Social Welfare (MoHSW). 2005. *Lesotho Demographic and Health Survey 2004.* Maseru: MoHSW.
Ministry of Health and Social Welfare (MoHSW) and ICF Macro. 2010. *Lesotho Demographic and Health Survey 2009.* Maseru: MoHSW.
Moultrie, T.A., S.S. Takudzwa, and I.M. Timæus. 2012. 'Birth Intervals, Postponement, and Fertility Decline in Africa', *Population Studies* 66(3): 241–58.
Mturi, A.J. 2003. 'Parents' Attitudes to Adolescent Sexual Behaviour in Lesotho', *African Journal of Reproductive Health* 7(2): 25–33.
Mturi, A.J., and W. Moerane. 2001. 'Premarital Childbearing among Adolescents in Lesotho', *Journal of Southern African Studies* 27(2): 259–75.
Nzioka, C. 2003. *A Baseline Study on the Magnitude of Abortion among Women of Childbearing Age in Lesotho.* Maseru: Ministry of Health and Social Welfare & World Health Organization.
Orderson, C. 2011. 'Annual Ruth First Memorial Lecture, 2010. University of the Witwatersrand: Voices from the Margin', *African Studies* 70(1): 156–65.
Radcliffe-Brown, A.R., and C.D. Forde 1950. *African Systems of Kinship and Marriage.* New York: Oxford University Press.
Romero-Daza, N., and D. Himmelgreen. 2004. 'The Sotho', in C.R. Ember (ed.), *Encyclopedia of Medical Anthropology*. New York: Springer, p. 957–64.
Rosenberg, S., R.F. Weisfelder and M. Frisbie-Fulton. 2004. *Historical Dictionary of Lesotho.* Lanham, MD: Scarecrow Press.
South Africa Demographic and Health Survey (SADHS). 1998. *Preliminary Report.* Pretoria: Department of Health, Medical Research Council, Demographic and Health Surveys Macro International Inc.
Sechefo, J.M. 1900. *Customs and Superstitions in Lesotho.* Rome: Anthropological Studies.
Shostak, M. 1982. *Nisa erzählt: Das Leben einer Nomadenfrau in Afrika.* Reinbek bei Hamburg: Rowohlt.
Silberschmidt, M. 2004. 'Masculinities, Sexuality and Socio-Economic Change in Rural and Urban East Africa', in S. Arnfred (ed.), *Re-thinking Sexualities in Africa.* Uppsala: Nordiska Afrikainstitutet, pp. 233–48.
Silberschmidt, M., and V. Rasch. 2001. 'Adolescent Girls, Illegal Abortions and "Sugar-Daddies" in Dar es Salaam: Vulnerable Victims and Active Social Agents', *Social Science and Medicine* 52(2001): 1815–26.

Singh, S., J.A. Durroch, L.S. Ashford and M. Vlassoff. 2009. *Adding it up: The Costs and Benefits of Investing in Family Planning and Maternal and Newborn Health*. New York: Guttmacher Institute and United Nations Population Fund.

Timaeus, I.M., and T.A. Moultrie. 2008. 'On Postponement and Birth Intervals', *Population and Development Review* 34(3): 483–510.

Tuoane, M., I. Diamond and N. Madise. 2003. 'Use of Family Planning in Lesotho: The Importance of Quality of Care and Access', *African Population Studies* 18(2): 105–32.

Tuoane, M., N.J. Madise, and I. Diamond. 2004. 'Provision of Family Planning Services in Lesotho', *International Family Planning Perspectives* 30(2): 77–86.

UNAIDS. 2013. *HIV and AIDS Estimates*. Geneva. Retrieved 1 February 2017 from http://www.unaids.org/en/regionscountries/countries/lesotho.

UNFPA. 2012. *Final Country Programme Document for Lesotho*. New York.

USAID 2006. *Adding Family Planning to PMTCT Sites Increases PMTCT Benefits*. Washington DC: USAID.

Van Balen, F., and M. C. Inhorn. 2002. 'Introduction. Interpreting Fertility: A View from the Social Sciences'. in M. Inhorn and F. van Balen (eds), *Infertility around the Globe: New Thinking on Childlessness, Gender, and Reproductive Technologies*. Berkeley: University of California Press, pp. 3–32.

Van Rijn, K. 2006. 'The Politics of Uncertainty: The AIDS Debate, Thabo Mbeki and the South African Government Response', *Social History of Medicine* 19(3): 521–38.

Warren, C., S. Phafoli, S. Majara and T. Tsukulu. 2008. 'Extending Prevention of Mother-to-Child Transmission through Postpartum Family Planning in Lesotho'. Maseru: Ministry of Health and Social Welfare & Population Council. Retrieved 27 February 2017 from http://citeseerx.ist.psu.edu/viewdoc/download?doi=10.1.1.518.4879&rep=rep1&type=pdf.

World Fertility Survey (WFS). 1977. *Lesotho Fertility Survey*. Princeton: Office of Population Research.

Chapter 9

'The Doctor's Way'

Traditional Contraception and Modernity in Cambodia

Eleanor Hukin

Introduction

Within the discipline of demography, the term 'traditional contraception' has come to have a specific meaning relating to nonsupply forms of birth control that rely on behaviour changes and can be practised without the need for supplies. The category encompasses withdrawal, lactational amenorrhoea, terminal and periodic abstinence (including fertility awareness-based methods).[1] At times, 'folk methods', such as the use of herbal medicines, charms and incantations to avoid pregnancy, are also grouped with 'traditional methods'. Placed in opposition to 'modern contraception', the term 'traditional contraception' becomes subsumed with other related words, such as 'outdated' and 'primitive' (Basu 2005). In thinking about how regional fertility transitions unfold, an intuitive expectation might be for a region to move from using no parity-specific fertility control to using traditional methods to limit childbearing and finally to a stage where modern methods are the prevailing means of managing births (Johnson-Hanks 2002). This pattern was observed in Europe, where the decline in marital fertility occurred through the uptake of traditional contraceptive methods and abortion (Watkins 1986); only later did modern methods become the dominant way to control family size. Evidence has shown that marital fertility declined, in Europe, first in groups of higher social status (from as early as the seventeenth century) before spreading to the wider population (Livi-Bacci 1986). Contemporary fertility transitions differ because of the widespread family planning programmes that provide and promote modern contraceptives. Nevertheless, there still remains an intuitive expectation for traditional methods to give way to modern methods. Bongaarts and Bruce (1995: 59), for example, based on data from non-European populations in the late 1980s, refer to 'the abandonment of traditional birth-spacing methods in more advanced countries' in discussing changes in the prevalence of unmet need that occur at various levels of socioeconomic development.

This chapter examines the use of traditional methods of contraception in Cambodia. In analysing patterns of contraceptive use and nonuse, it becomes clear that a significant proportion on women are rejecting modern methods and are instead relying on traditional contraceptive methods to regulate their childbearing. Given the expectations and observations found in the demographic literature, the pattern of traditional method use in Cambodia seems all the more counterintuitive. This chapter aims to outline and explain the pattern of traditional method use in Cambodia. It is only by examining the social context and meanings of contraception that the unexpected pattern can be made sense of and understood.

Research Design and Methods

The research design used a mixed methods approach. The quantitative and qualitative research methods were used chronologically. The first stage of the research involved quantitative analysis of secondary data from the Cambodian Demographic and Health Survey (CDHS) of 2005. I used the quantitative data to establish trends and patterns in contraceptive use, and analyse factors associated with those trends. This helped to set up the research problem by showing the patterns of contraceptive use in Cambodia, and revealed unexpected findings that then fed into new research questions, which were then explored through the qualitative aspect of the research. The second stage involved using qualitative methods: I conducted ethnographic fieldwork in Cambodia for a period of twenty-one months, including nine months of language learning. Whilst there are various possible strategies to combine quantitative and qualitative research in one study, I employed a sequential approach, with the second (qualitative) stage of the research elaborating on and expanding the findings of the first (quantitative) stage (Creswell 2002; Bryman 2008). What was learnt in the earlier stage was integrated into the second stage; this is one of the ways in which mixed methods studies have been used by social scientists (Axinn and Pearce 2006). This chapter on traditional method use forms part of a wider study that looked at women's and men's reproductive decision-making with a focus on their experiences of and meanings given to contraception, situating these understandings within the broader social context (Hukin 2014).

Quantitative Data

Secondary data analysis was conducted on data from the Cambodian Demographic and Health Survey (CDHS) of 2005. The Demographic and Health Surveys are large-scale, nationally representative household surveys that collect data on health, fertility and family planning, from reproductive-aged (15–49 years) women, with smaller samples of men. The CDHS programme has conducted over three hundred surveys in ninety countries since 1984 (ICF International 2014) and is a key demographic data source for low and middle-income countries. The CDHS was implemented or overseen by national ministries, UN bodies and USAID. Using SPSS software, I analysed descriptive statistics to examine trends in contraceptive use and binary logistic regression to analyse the factors affecting the likelihood of women using traditional as opposed to modern contraceptives. During analysis, sample weights were applied to the data to account for the oversampling of small areas and urban areas. The survey collected data from 16,823 women and 7,229 men (NIPH et al. 2006).

Qualitative Data

The qualitative data were collected during twenty-one months of ethnographic fieldwork from September 2008 to July 2010 in Siem Reap, northwest Cambodia. By this I mean long-term immersion in people's everyday lives, using a combination of methods (participant observation and interviews) and taking an iterative approach, continually reassessing my research strategy as new information challenged or supported tentative analyses and the appropriateness of my techniques. I spent nine months learning Khmer, Cambodia's national language, and the further twelve months focused on fieldwork. I employed one research assistant. The specific methods used were participant observation, informal interviews and recorded semistructured interviews with women and men, and healthcare providers. The data produced took the form of handwritten notebooks of fieldnotes and transcriptions of recorded interviews, which were later coded and analysed thematically. Interviews recorded in Khmer were simultaneously translated and transcribed into English. For the fieldwork, I chose two locations in Siem Reap province. I divided my time between a rural and an urban site, in and around Siem Reap town, and each week stayed three to four nights in each site.

A key advantage of an ethnographic approach is its openness to new information unknown at the outset of the study, making it ideal for crosscultural research such as this project where the worldview held by participants differs substantially from that of the researcher. An objective was to learn about contraceptive behaviour from the actors' viewpoints and to situate it within the context of everyday life. This entailed paying attention to a wide variety of matters that bear on the phenomena, in order to better understand meanings, actions, norms and attitudes (Becker 1996).

Participant observation is a method rarely used by demographic researchers (Randall and Koppenhaver 2004; Coast et al. 2007). This study provides an example of the value of this method for gaining a nuanced understanding contraceptive behaviour and, more generally, for explaining demographic phenomena observed at the population level that are only accessible through close attention to local contexts and lived experience. This study fits into a tradition of anthropological demography by bringing an ethnographic approach (in terms of epistemology and methods) in order to explain a typically demographic subject: contraceptive behaviour. Triangulating quantitative and qualitative findings, the results from the two types of data can both support and reinforce or contradict each other; in the case of this study, the qualitative findings both confirmed and offered an explanation for the pattern seen in the quantitative findings. In doing so, this study expands on the growing research that incorporates statistical analysis of large-scale surveys and qualitative microanalyses in order to enrich understanding of population questions (Obermeyer 2005).

Patterns of Traditional Method Use

Between 2000 and 2005, there was a substantial shift in the contraceptive method mix of Cambodia, with traditional contraceptive methods becoming increasingly popular. Figure 9.1 shows that only 5 per cent of married women were using a traditional method

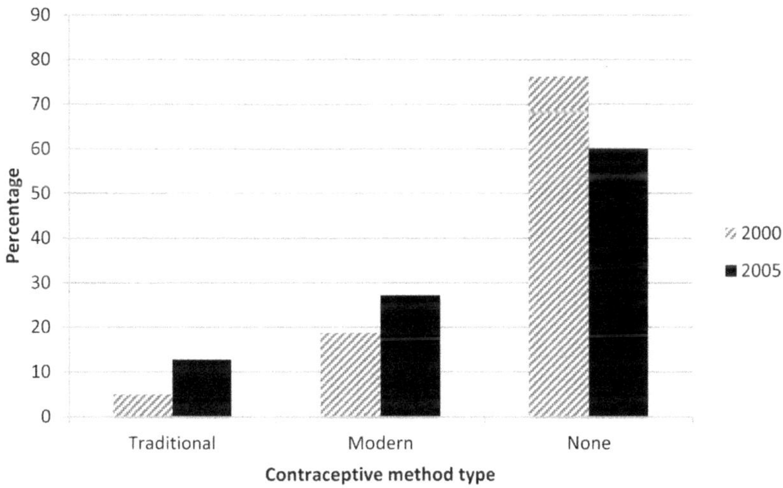

FIGURE 9.1 Contraceptive Method Type: Percentage of Married Women (Aged 15–49) in 2000 and 2005

Description: *n* 2000 = 9,071, *n* 2005 = 10,087
Source: NIPH et al. (2006)

in 2000, and by 2005 this had grown to 13 per cent. Since modern method use was also increasing during the same period, from 19 per cent to 27 per cent, it is difficult to see just how much traditional methods grew in comparison to modern methods.

To find out which method type increased the most, it is helpful to look at traditional method use amongst contraceptive users only (excluding nonusers), as shown in Figure 9.2. As a proportion of all the methods used, traditional methods increased from a fifth of users to nearly a third of all contraceptive users (21 per cent to 32.4 per cent). By 2005, a traditional method, withdrawal, had become the second most popular method, used by a fifth of all users. Whilst use of withdrawal and the daily pill increased in comparison to other methods, the proportions of contraceptive users relying on injectables or sterilization decreased over this period.

Demographic Variation in Method Type

The type of contraception used (traditional or modern) varies by demographic characteristics, with some groups having higher rates of traditional method use than others. Chi-squared tests confirmed that the associations seen between contraceptive type and various characteristics – age, education, residence and wealth – were statistically significant.[2]

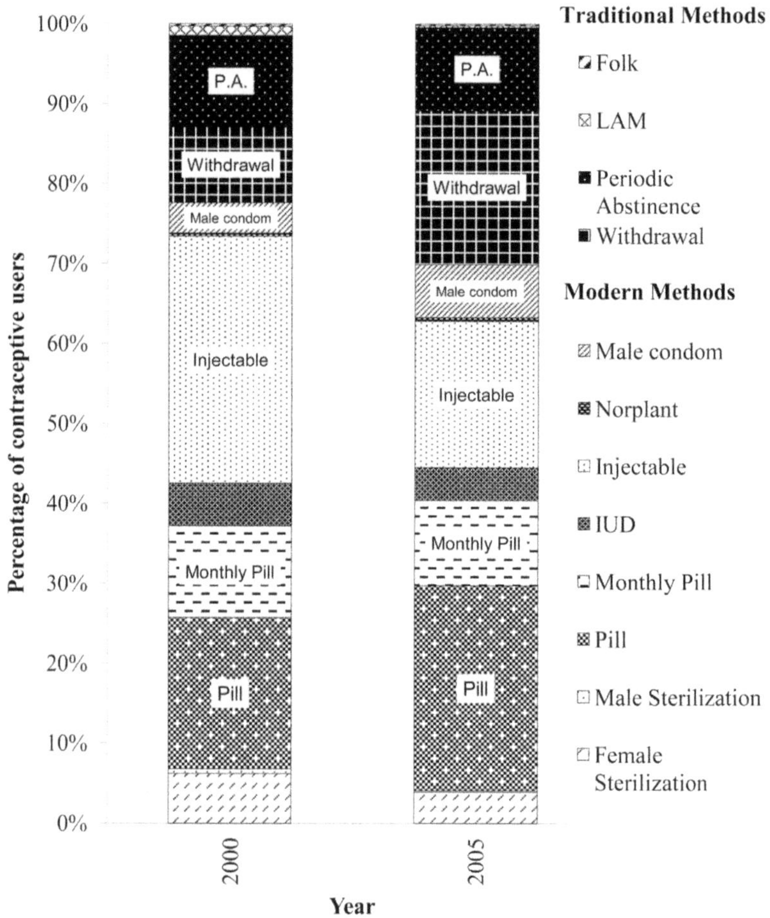

FIGURE 9.2 Contraceptive Method Mix: Percentage of Married Women (Aged 15–49) Using Each Contraceptive, amongst Contraceptive Users in 2000 and 2005

Description: n in 2000 = 2,159, 2005 = 4,033.
Source: NIPH et al. (2006)

Figure 9.3 shows that, as age increases, traditional method use increases until the 30–34 year age group (when it peaks and then gradually reduces, with a sharp drop for the eldest group). For education (measured as the highest level attended), the pattern is straightforward: each increase in education level sees an increase in traditional method use. For residence, use is higher for urbanites and by wealth level;[3] traditional method use increases fairly gradually with wealth, and then with a sharp increase between

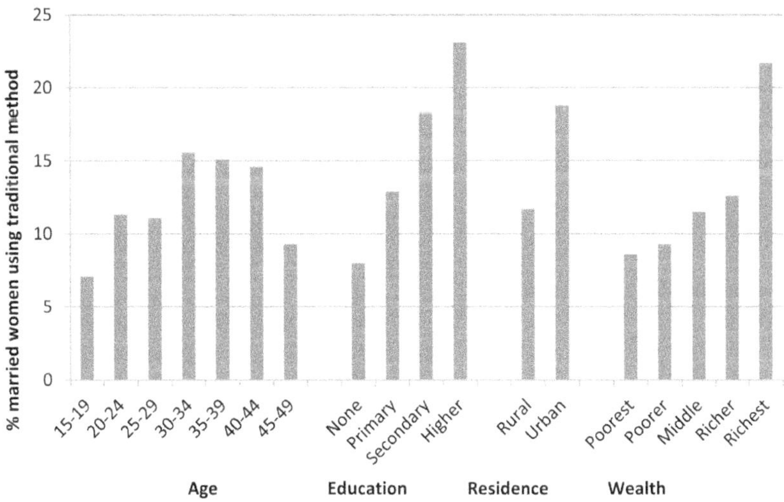

FIGURE 9.3 Traditional Contraceptive Use According to Age, Education, Residence and Wealth amongst Married Women (aged 15–49) in 2005

Source: NIPH et al. (2006)

the richer and richest wealth quintiles. In summary, women with higher levels of education, higher household wealth and living in urban areas use more traditional methods than their counterparts with less education and wealth, who live in rural areas.

Factors Increasing the Likelihood of Traditional Method Use

To explore further the factors associated with traditional method use, whilst controlling for confounding effects, binary logistic regression was used. This model tests the likelihood of using traditional contraceptive methods, amongst married women aged 15–49 years who use contraception (either traditional or modern). The response variable is whether women use traditional methods; modern contraceptive use is the reference category. Backwards elimination was used to specify the model. The variables entered into the base model were selected on the basis of theoretical interest in terms of the likelihood of affecting contraceptive use. Table 9.1 presents the result of the logistic regression. All variables remaining in the model were statistically significant.[4]

Due to the multicollinearity of wealth, residence and education, these three variables (or sets of dummy variables) had complex effects in this model. In order to make the results interpretable, interaction terms were included for 'wealth and education', 'wealth

TABLE 9.1 Logistic Regression of Factors Affecting Use of Traditional Contraception

Variables	Estimate	SE	Odds ratio
Age			
15–19	–0.24	0.27	0.79
20–29	–0.29***	0.09	0.75
30–44	0		1
45–49	0.54***	0.14	1.72
Number of living children			
None	0.81***	0.29	2.26
1–2 children	0		1
3–4 children	–0.14	0.09	0.87
5+ children	–0.34***	0.12	0.71
Religion			
Non-Buddhist	–0.80***	0.28	0.45
Buddhist	0		1
Medical care variables			
Permission	–0.38***	0.14	0.69
Distance	–0.20**	0.08	0.82
Health facility	–0.14*	0.07	0.87
Media influence			
Heard family planning message	0.20**	0.09	1.22
Wealth			
Richest	1.35***	0.52	3.87
Richer	1.23**	0.54	3.42
Middle	1.27**	0.55	3.55
Poorer	1.49**	0.58	4.42
Poorest	0		1
Education			
None	1.19**	0.54	3.27
Primary	1.19**	0.53	3.28
Secondary+	0		1
Wealth education interaction			
For richest			
None	–1.43**	0.60	0.24
Primary	–1.08**	0.54	0.34
Secondary +	0		
For richer			
None	–1.41**	0.60	0.24
Primary	–1.37**	0.56	0.25
Secondary +	0		
For middle			
None	–1.34**	0.61	0.26
Primary	–1.39**	0.57	0.25

Variables	Estimate	SE	Odds ratio
Secondary +	0		
For poorer			
None	–2.06***	0.64	0.13
Primary	–1.57***	0.60	0.21
Secondary +	0		
For poorest			
None	0		
Primary	0		
Secondary +	0		
Intercept	–1.76***	0.52	

Note: *p < .1; **p < .05; ***p < .01
Source: NIPH et al. 2006 (CDHS 2005)
Parameter estimates, standard errors and odds ratios from logistic regression models measuring effects of sociodemographic characteristics, medical care variables and exposure to family planning messages in the media on contraceptive use type, amongst currently married or in union women using contraception in 2005

TABLE 9.2 Odds Ratios for Wealth Differentials by Education

Groups	Odds ratios		
	For women with no education	For women with primary education	For women with secondary+ education
Richest	0.92	1.31	3.86
Richer	0.84	0.87	3.42
Middle	0.93	0.89	3.56
Poorer	0.57	0.92	4.44
Poorest	1	1	1

and residence' and 'education and residence'. Following this, residence was no longer found to be significant in the model, and so was removed. Other variables eliminated from the model after likelihood ratio tests included several other medical care variables. In order to interpret the effect of the interaction term for wealth and education, odds ratios were calculated separately (Tables 9.2 and 9.3).

This interpretation of results will focus on wealth and education as these are the most interesting findings. The effects of wealth on tradition method use are fairly complex, making it difficult to give a general statement. However, if the two extremes only are compared with each other (i.e. the richest and the poorest), it is possible to draw some more intuitive conclusions.

Table 9.2 presents the odds ratios[5] for the effect of wealth, at different education levels, on the likelihood of traditional method

TABLE 9.3 Odds Ratios for Education Differentials by Wealth

Groups	Odds ratios				
	For richest	For richer	For middle	For poorer	For poorest
None	0.78	0.80	0.86	0.42	3.29
Primary	1.12	0.84	0.82	0.68	3.29
Secondary +	1	1	1	1	1

use. For women with no education, the odds of the richest group are 0.92 times the odds of the poorest group. For women with primary education, the odds of the richest are 1.31 times the odds of the poorest. For women with secondary or higher education, the odds for the richest group are 3.86 times the odds of the poorest group. Overall, the difference between the richest and poorest is largest for women with secondary education. Also, the effect of increasing wealth changes direction (i.e. increases or decreases the risks), depending on the level of education: amongst the non-educated, being in the richest wealth group (rather than poorest) decreases the risks; amongst the primary educated, and even more so amongst the secondary educated, being in the richest wealth group increases the risks of traditional use compared to the poorest wealth group.

Table 9.3 presents the odds ratios for the effect of education, at different wealth levels, on the likelihood of traditional method use. In the richest group, having primary education increases the likelihood of traditional use (by 1.12 times) over having secondary or higher education, whereas having no education decreases that likelihood (by 0.78 times). In the richer, middle and poorer groups, having no education and having primary education both decrease the likelihood of traditional use in comparison to those with a secondary education. In the same comparison for the poorest group, having no or primary education increases the risks of traditional use by over three times (3.29).

In general, being more educated increases the likelihood of using traditional methods. However, this pattern varies by wealth quintile with two key exceptions: the pattern is inverted for the poorest group and, amongst the richest group, primary-educated women are more likely to use traditional methods than secondary-educated women. Within most wealth quintiles, there is very little difference between the effects of primary and the effects of no education, so the change appears to be taking place between primary and secondary schooling (the richest group differs here). In most cases, more education is having the effect of decreasing modern method use relative to traditional method use.

Residence is not significant after controlling for wealth and education (and interaction terms). On rerunning the model with the wealth variables removed, residence became significant. This suggests that residence acts as a substitute for wealth (as richer people tend to live in urban areas) and that it is wealth that is having the true effect on traditional method use. If we assume that rural women live further away from health facilities than urban women, this finding indicates that traditional method use is not something practised simply because these women live far from health facilities that supply modern methods. This interpretation is supported by the effect of the medical care variable 'distance being a problem': women who reported that in obtaining medical care for oneself, distance was a big problem; they had a decreased likelihood of using traditional methods relative to women who said distance was not a problem.

In summary, the effect of education was that being more educated, in general, increases the likelihood of using traditional methods. However, this pattern varies by wealth quintile with two key exceptions: the pattern is inverted for the poorest group and, amongst the richest group, those women having a primary education are more likely to use traditional methods than those with a secondary education. Within most wealth quintiles, there is very little difference between the effects of primary education and the effects of no education, so the change appears to be taking place between primary and secondary schooling (the richest group differs here). In most cases, more education is having the effect of decreasing modern method use relative to traditional method use.

Wealth has complex effects on the likelihood of traditional methods use, which vary by education level. The effect of increasing wealth changes direction (i.e. increases or decreases the risks) depending on the level of education: amongst the non-educated, being in the richest wealth group (rather than poorest) decreases the risks; however, amongst the primary educated, and even more so amongst the secondary educated, being in the richest wealth group compared to the poorest group increases the likelihood of using traditional methods.

Cambodia's fertility transition is well under way. The Total Fertility Rate (TFR) has fallen from an estimated 6.7 children per woman in the period 1962–70 to 3.4 in 2005 and to 3.0 in 2010 (Heuveline 1998; NIPH et al. 2006; NIS et al. 2011). Within society, certain groups have been the forerunners of this fertility decline (Heuveline

1998) and continue to have the lowest fertility rates. In 2005 urban women had a TFR of 2.8, whilst fertility in rural areas was 3.5 children per woman. Women with more education had lower fertility than those with less education: women with secondary or higher education had a TFR of 2.6, substantially lower than those with only primary (3.5) or no schooling (4.3). The greatest range in TFR is seen across wealth groups, where fertility ranges from 2.4 amongst the richest women to 4.9 amongst the poorest. This suggests that the greater preference for traditional methods amongst more educated wealthy women is not linked to an inability to achieve low fertility.

This analysis of CDHS data has revealed that, in general, wealthy, educated women have a greater preference for traditional methods than poorer, less educated women. Given the demographic literature referred to in the introduction, this pattern of contraceptive use seems counterintuitive. The following section of this chapter moves on to an analysis of qualitative data collected during fieldwork and provides an explanation for this unexpected result.

Explaining the Pattern of Traditional Method Use

Many participants in this research expressed a dislike or dissatisfaction with modern contraceptive methods based on their experience or fear of side-effects to their health (Hukin 2012). Amongst these women, traditional methods were often seen as providing a solution to the problem of avoiding pregnancy without jeopardizing one's health. Although women of all social backgrounds placed great importance on being healthy, their orientations towards how to be healthy differed, to some extent according to their socioeconomic group. Their actions differed according to their level of trust in biomedicine and belief in the indigenous health cosmology, but also their trust in the type of biomedicine they could access. Amongst upper-class women I found a lack of trust in the Cambodian health system; although they had a strong faith in biomedicine's efficacy, they were not confident that they could access the best of it easily. When affluent people in Siem Reap become seriously ill, they travel abroad to seek treatment in Vietnam, Thailand or Singapore. They regard the health system in Cambodia, both public and private, as inferior. They also do not necessarily have blind faith in biomedicine, using it selectively and often combining this type of health-seeking behaviour with religious acts as a way to cure illness or maintain health.

Many daily rituals are oriented to preserving health and happiness in one's family – from the daily lighting of incense, sacrificing offerings and praying to much larger calendar and lifecycle rituals. People of all socioeconomic levels often take action on the advice of fortune tellers and *kru*, 'religious teachers or gurus'. Wealthy urbanites are likely to first seek treatment for illness from a pharmacy or clinic, but, in light of the perceived health risks of modern methods, many prefer to control their fertility with a nonsupply contraceptive method. Using a traditional method enables women to manage their childbearing at the same time as avoiding the perceived risks of modern contraceptives. The following sections examine different methods of traditional contraception in turn before discussing abortion and the use of multiple strategies to control childbearing.

Periodic Abstinence as 'the Doctor's Way'

The only fertility awareness method that I came across in my field sites was the calendar (or rhythm) method. The method requires that a woman monitor her menstrual cycle and calculate the days she is fertile. Then she must either abstain from sexual intercourse or use another method during the fertile days.[6] Far from being classified as a 'traditional method' as demographers would, it was often referred as *kbouern pairt*, 'the doctor's way'[7]. People who used this method had learnt it from healthcare providers, usually a midwife. It was seen as a method suitable for educated women (*neak jeh dung* – 'knowledgeable people'). There was a general consensus among the people I spoke to (including the general population and family planning providers such as midwives and pharmacists) that this was a method only for 'knowledgeable people'. Some even said that it was only for those who had studied medicine. It was not seen as an option for illiterate (or rural) women, who were said to be more well-matched with a method like the IUD or injection, which required little monitoring of time or one's body and only infrequent action:

> Counting days [periodic abstinence]? I think . . . [we] don't have that [in this village]. Some they read according to the book and do in line with that, but us here, not many of us read like those who read books. They read the method, how to do it in the book, when is the time . . . this month . . . this day . . . that day . . . yes they have [that method]. The people who have ever studied to be a *pairt* (medic/doctor), they know, but the normal people; who is going to know about that? They mostly protect by pill or injection.
> (Female, 44 years, 3 children, rural site)

> Well to say how it is, some poor people are not very clever. [Research assistant interrupts: 'Some poor families are illiterate.'] They don't know how to count days. They don't understand the way to do it, not clearly. So that's why they like to use the scientific methods like the IUD or injection: done in one time. It is easier than natural methods, avoiding from mistakes as well. They might try to use a natural method but then have a mistake and get pregnant, so after that they change to use something like IUD or injection.
> (Female, 42 years, 3 children, urban site)

The calendar method was seen as being more challenging than other methods, but suitable for women whose daily lives already involved an awareness of the clock and the calendar, such as teachers or civil servants. Women in my rural field site, mostly farmers or shopkeepers, whose lives did not revolve around the clock and the calendar, perceived the method as something that would not fit with them. Some pointed out that women who used 'the doctor's way' were women who were familiar with the Gregorian/international calendar, which is used in Cambodia for civil purposes. The other calendar system used in Cambodia is the Khmer lunisolar calendar, on which religious events are based. Many rural women only follow the lunisolar calendar, which is important for observing the weekly *tngai sel* 'holy day' and larger religious festivals. In my rural site, women often kept track of the month by looking at the waxing and waning of the moon, not necessarily using a written calendar. Some explained their use of the Khmer calendar and unfamiliarity with the 'foreign calendar' as being part of the reason why they could not use the day counting method.

There is also an issue of men's cooperation affecting the possibility of using the calendar method or withdrawal. Fertility awareness-based methods require the women's partner to cooperate by agreeing to abstain or use another method during the fertile period (WHO and CPP 2007: 239). Alternatively, it requires sexual autonomy on the part of the woman to be able to control when she has sex (Johnson-Hanks 2002). Some thought this type of cooperation varied between socioeconomic groups, while others emphasized that this was down to the individual couple's relationship:

> Poor people they don't know how to use the natural methods so that's why they go to do the injection. The people who are at the countryside, they are uneducated so they don't know how to use the natural methods, particularly because of the man's feeling. But

> the people who live in the city (*'neak psar* – market people') if they decide to 'release' they will release [i.e. they are able to control ejaculation]. But in the countryside they cannot control their minds at the end of sexual intercourse or they are drunk. And some men, they are really eager to have sex every day (*l'mowp*) [so cannot abstain]. Yes some people they like to sleep with their wife a lot . . . But us people who live in the city, normal people [rich people] they have their wife earn a living, not have lots of children. They are educated so they can control their mind and they have to do the job as well.
> (Female, 51 years, 6 children, urban site)

> We use natural methods for couples who understand each other. But for people who live at countryside they drink beer or they cannot control their minds. According to our mind – if we don't understand each other so we cannot do this method too. I don't mean rich people only [can do it] but the most important thing is it's up to the family. Some they don't understand, even rich or poor, they think about their feeling only so we can say it depends on the people.
> (Female, 38 years, 2 children, urban site)

As well as being considered to be a method suitable only for certain types of couples (who communicate and cooperate with each other), the calendar method fits with dominant Khmer ideals of femininity: of being self-disciplined and in control. Disciplined, in this sense, means being in control of one's bodily disposition, movement, speech and emotions, and in Khmer literature is associated with Khmer ideals of virtuous women (Ledgerwood 1990). This is something articulated in schools and in advice from parents and elders about how girls should behave, and in the didactic codes for women, the *Chbap Srei* (Rules for Women), for example, not laughing loudly, being messy or uncontrolled in one's movements. In the same way the norm is for women to be responsible for household budgeting, and for controlling the number and timing of births. The decision on having children may be made jointly, but then it is very much seen to be the woman's job to ensure that things go to plan. In the interviews, women who had had unplanned pregnancies and abortions often spoke of being 'blamed' and 'scolded' by their husband. Men likewise frequently commented that it was up to their wife to organise contraception:

> According to my observation, it is only the woman who finds out about the method to protect from having a child. Men, they don't care about it. If their wife is ignorant about contraception, in the family they might have a lot of children. The man won't trouble himself with that. If us women didn't go out and find some method

> for ourselves to improve the standing of living of our families and waited for the men to do it . . . not likely. [They] don't bother themselves with that.
> (Female, 38 years, 2 children, urban site)

> No, you don't use withdrawal all the time, you use day counting too. Most important is to ask the wife, if she says we can [have sex] then we can. Important is: it's 'on' the wife [it is her responsibility]. The husband is not important, he doesn't know, because sometimes he gets drunk . . . Importantly, it is up to the wife.
> (Male, 24 years, 1 child, urban)

Because the calendar method is associated with biomedicine in a positive way (modern and scientific, but without side-effects) and is associated with education (being only for 'knowledgeable people'), it has come to be seen as something modern. In this way it correlates with identity ideals aspired to by wealthy, educated, urban women. It was in no way thought of as a 'traditional method' of contraception, but rather something for urban, well-informed, modern, educated women. As a method that conforms to these gendered norms and duties, and distinguishes the educated from the uneducated, not to mention having the advantage of maintaining one's health (and beauty), the calendar method has become increasingly popular for elites. This is confirmed by both the CDHS findings above and my qualitative findings. The push factors away from using modern methods and the pull factors towards non-invasive (or 'non-supply') methods both contribute to the pattern observed in survey data, and therefore explain why the odds of using traditional methods (over modern methods) are greater for wealthy, educated women than poor, uneducated women.

Withdrawal as 'Our Own Way'

Unlike periodic abstinence, withdrawal was not associated with being scientific and educated, and I did not come across any health workers who advised people how to use it, as was the case for the calendar method.[8] However, like periodic abstinence, it did share the association of being a healthy way to delay or prevent births. I met women of all wealth levels who used or had used this method, but it was seen by some as being a method for the less educated, particularly if used as the only method:

> [People who use withdrawal] don't have knowledge, they are not *neak jeh dung* knowledgeable people, they just know 'no water no baby'.
> (Female, twenties, NGO health education worker)

Unsurprisingly, given the nature of this method, it was often emphasized that this method required the husband to commit to it, thus it was said to be either entirely the husband's decision to do this or, more often, that the husband and wife had agreed together to use this birth control strategy. I do not want to give the impression that Cambodian men are all extremely well behaved and obedient towards their wives' choices regarding traditional method use, but rather that this is one of the limiting factors on the use of such methods: in order for the couple to practise withdrawal or abstinence, the husband has to cooperate. If the husband refuses to use this method, or gets drunk and cannot control himself, or is unwilling to be abstinent during his wife's fertile period, then traditional methods will not be used. This quote is from a woman asked about any obstacles that put her off modern contraceptives, such as expense or having to travel to obtain them:

> No I don't think about that. But the important thing is my health. I don't think about it being expensive or making a journey . . . But they say if you use it, it doesn't affect your health, they spread out the information. But really/actually, in our couple we can discuss and use this method [withdrawal], so we use it. But if we didn't have this method, we would use another one, IUD or . . . But our family can talk together. If they don't agree, you must do something yourself like IUD or the pill. It's not important about the price, or anything, just health.
> (Female, 36 years, 2 children, urban site)

When interviewees were questioned about which methods of contraception they had heard of, people tended not to spontaneously include withdrawal as a contraceptive method, only including it in the category of contraception (*gar bunyea gomnert*, 'birth delayer') when prompted. It was often referred to as 'our own way' or 'my husband has his own way', thus separating it from other methods of contraception. Colloquially, it is referred to as *jat tuk graw beang*, 'pour the water outside the pot', and usually causes some amusement when discussed, probably because it is directly related to the act of sex and, unlike condoms, has not been widely discussed and advertised in the media and public life. The separation of withdrawal (as 'our own way') from other methods of contraception and the fact that it is still rather taboo in conversation (evidenced by the embarrassed laughter) raise the possibility that this method is underreported in survey responses. This was found to be the case in Sri Lanka, where modern methods were open for discussion, but traditional methods were not, leading to an underestimation of contraceptive prevalence (Gajanayake and Caldwell 1990).

Abstinence

In Cambodia, abstinence is a behavioural choice that occurs within specific social contexts and times that call for a person to *dtorm* or 'abstain' from certain behaviours for religious or cultural reasons. Buddhist monks and nuns abstain from sex continually, as do some Buddhist lay people and some *kru khmer* (traditional healers) on *tngai sel* (holy days). These lay men and women tend to be elders, beyond reproductive age for women, who have taken the ten precepts of Buddhism. In this context, the prohibition on sex is one of a number of religious proscriptions that entail a more ascetic, abstemious life. Such self-denial and restraint is a part of religious discipline, so whilst permanent or 'terminal' abstinence is seen as the norm for the elderly, it makes sense that periodic abstinence (the calendar method) is seen as acceptable for younger (i.e. reproductive-aged) people. Furthermore, abstinence is also expected before marriage. For married couples of reproductive age, the traditional context for abstinence is during the postpartum period and during menstruation.

Postpartum abstinence continues to be observed by both urban and rural women in my field sites. The length of time varies considerably according to how disciplined women, or their husbands, can be and their strength of commitment to the beliefs justifying the traditionally longer postpartum abstinence (i.e. much longer than the recommendations they reported from healthcare providers of 1.5–4 months). Some women reported waiting a few weeks and others a year – the average was said to be three to six months. The justification was to protect health at a time when women are said to be *sorsay kjay*.[9]

Of major importance in this recuperation period, widely recognized as a dangerous time, is the need to protect against *dtoah* (relapse). The category of *dtoah* captures a range of postpartum health problems and is said to potentially cause death. Abstaining from sex is one of several activities elders advise should be avoided in order to prevent *dtoah* – others include heavy lifting, excessive physical work, cold showers and eating certain foods. Having sex too soon after birth is said to cause a particular type of *dtoah*, *dtoah kbal domnaik* (head of the bed relapse).[10]

A common theme in women's discussions of postpartum abstinence was the difficulty in managing husbands who did not want to abstain for as long. Abstinence was perceived as being good for the woman, but of no benefit for the man. Others acknowledged that women too sometimes could not wait as long as was advised by elders. The traditional lengthy postpartum abstinence period, grounded in traditional Khmer medical reasoning (of the dangers of *dtoah* for *sorsay kjay* women), remains, but has now been modified and amalgamated with biomedical advice to abstain, initially to recover from birth and then to spread out childbearing. Some interviewees, particularly rural women, justified the postpartum abstinence in traditional Khmer medical theory, whilst others, often urban, discussed it within the frame of 'doctor's advice'. It was common for both rural and urban women to know that doctors recommend not having children spaced too closely together because of the harmful effects on the mother's health.

In addition to the postpartum sex taboo, sex during menstruation is also proscribed. Women said this could cause health problems such as damage the womb, transmitting germs and worsening their complexion. This fits with of other examples of blood being considered polluting that I came across during fieldwork.[11]

The traditional contexts within which terminal abstinence and periodic abstinence occur range from religious proscription, amongst clergy and lay people, to maintaining health following birth and during menstruation. None of the reasons for abstaining in these contexts is primarily or explicitly connected to avoiding pregnancy. However, they do show that the idea of abstaining from sex is a long-accepted behavioural choice in Cambodia in certain contexts. Therefore, it should be no surprise that when a couple wants to postpone or limit childbearing, periodic abstinence is seen by many as an acceptable and legitimate way to do so.

Other Traditional Methods

As a proximate determinant of fertility, breastfeeding affects fertility. In Cambodia, as elsewhere (Randall 1996), it is not practised consciously as a way to control fertility. Whilst breastfeeding was widespread amongst research participants, no one discussed breastfeeding as a way to intentionally avoid pregnancy. However, women were aware that the absence of menstruation postpartum meant that they were unlikely to become pregnant. Folk methods of contraception were rarely mentioned by informants, but included pressing the lower abdomen in an attempt to remove fluid after intercourse and *coitus intercrura*. The latter method has been found to be more commonly used than is reported in surveys, often because it is not asked about (Caldwell et al. 1987). These two methods were reported to me from a woman who had had side-effects from several modern methods and now used these methods and withdrawal. Several people also reported that drinking large quantities of traditional medicine (*tnam Khmer*) was a way to avoid pregnancy. The traditional medicine drunk during the postpartum period to restore the *sorsay* (*tnam sorsay*) was said to delay pregnancy. The traditional medicine used as an abortifacient (discussed below) was said to lead to permanent sterility in some women if consumed in sufficient quantities. Both were said to work by drying out and withering the uterus (*svet sbown*), and neither was said to be reliable.

Abortion and Multiple Strategies of Birth Avoidance

Strategies for avoiding pregnancy were at times complex, multiple and dynamic, changing throughout women's life courses as priorities and situations shifted. Several interviewees reported using multiple methods simultaneously, usually to make pregnancy prevention more reliable. In discussions of traditional methods and their effectiveness, some reported the possibility of resorting to abortion if they did become pregnant. Women paid close attention to their menstrual cycle, knowing when to expect their period and using this as confirmation they were not pregnant. Rural women (mostly) knew when to expect their period based on the stage of the moon, for example, three days after the full moon, and urban women more often kept track of the date on a calendar. Some interviewees described how they would buy a pregnancy test if their period was overdue and if this were positive, they would 'swallow a tablet', meaning use medical abortion pharmaceuticals.

Medical abortion drugs (mifepristone and misoprostol) are readily available in Siem Reap and can be bought over the counter at several pharmacies for around $10 (but sometimes more) for a single procedure. Women usually buy the drug in a pharmacy, not knowing even the name of it, simply telling the seller in the pharmacy that they are pregnant and want to abort, or that they 'want to bring back their period'. Recourse to these drugs was not confined only to users of modern contraception. Many of the women who talked about this strategy were users of withdrawal or day counting for fear, or experience, of side-effects and health risks from modern methods. Although aware that medical abortion itself also carries side-effects and health risks, the difference is, they explained, that using the abortion pill is a one-off event, whereas a modern method (mainly referring to the pill or injection) requires regularly consuming chemicals over a long period of time. It was this repeated, continuing long-term use of invasive methods that concerned people. Factored into the risk of abortion was the possibility that it would never be needed and their method would protect them from pregnancy.

In Cambodia, as in other Buddhist countries such as Thailand, abortion is seen as a sin and for this reason some interviewees stated they would not consider it for themselves. However, many people agreed that there were circumstances, particularly if a family had many children and were living in poverty, when this would be to some extent justified. Abortion was simultaneously said to be *tomadar* [normal] and *baap* [a sin], and when asked about perceptions, the common first response was that it was 'not good' because it was 'bad for the woman's health' and, second (sometimes only on probing), respondents said that it was a sin according to Khmer religion and went against Khmer tradition.

The uncertainties related to health risks and side-effects associated with modern contraceptive methods mean that many women are put off using them altogether, whilst others use them but feel worried about the consequences. Few really want to be using invasive (supply) methods, but for some women, the need to avoid pregnancy (and the greater reliability of modern methods) means they are willing to accept the perceived health risks. Part of this relates to socioeconomic status. Of the women I spoke to, wealthier and more educated women were more likely to know that they had the option of a (relatively) safe abortion, either a medical or surgical abortion, if they accidentally became pregnant through the failure of their contraceptive method. They knew where and how to obtain one and, importantly, they knew they could afford it. I would speculate that this knowledge of having a fallback of a safe option is another contributing factor as to why traditional method use is higher for more educated and wealthier women. They know they are using a 'less effective method', but they know that if need be, they have the option of an affordable safe abortion. In contrast, poorer women were much less confident in their ability to access a safe abortion if they need one. And I would speculate that this often pushes the poorer women to seek more effective methods than traditional contraception. Having decided they do not want another child at that time, they are less willing to risk the possibility of an abortion, knowing that a biomedical, safe abortion is out of their reach. One of the interviewees reinforced what I had been thinking about this link between wealth, traditional methods and abortion when I asked about why rich people might prefer traditional methods:

> Well I would say, the rich people have money, if anything happens they can have an abortion. The rich people they can get rid of it, easy. But when you don't have money, you have to use contraception. (Female, 28 years, 1 child, urban site)

Traditional methods of abortion continue to be performed in Cambodia by *chmop* (traditional birth attendants), although not all *chmop* know how or are willing to do it. The procedure involves a type of deep massage of the pregnant woman's lower abdomen followed by drinking Khmer medicine, which is said to 'heat' her and 'melt' the foetus, making the woman abort. The medicine is drunk for three days, by which time the abortion should mainly be over, then the woman is advised to look after herself in the same way as a postpartum woman. Only in the rural field site was this practised, and some women stated they had found it to be a reliable way to manage their childbearing, having had several such abortions over their lives. Other women told of dreadful experiences, where life-saving biomedical interventions were needed. Still, several informants felt they trusted this 'natural' 'Khmer' method of abortion over biomedical options, aware that biomedical options were not completely safe (particularly those accessible to them, given their lack of knowledge and finances).

As well as these types of abortion, women may seek help from a *pairt*. The term *pairt* refers to someone with biomedical training and tends to be used for medical personnel of all levels, including doctors, nurses and midwives, and even clinic receptionists. Women are unlikely to know what level of *pairt* they are dealing with and whether abortion is legal or illegal. Cambodia has some of the most liberal abortion laws in Asia (Potdar et al. 2008). Abortion is legal in the first twelve weeks of pregnancy upon the request of the women, and with restrictions at later stages (RACHA 1997). However, few people I spoke to knew this, with many thinking it was illegal. This is likely to drive people to unnecessarily seek unsafe abortions rather than going to legitimate providers of safe abortions.

Contraceptive use involves a dynamic decision-making process. Different contraceptive methods were not only seen as 'suiting' some women and not others, but it was also acknowledged that over the course of a particular woman's life, different contraceptives would become more or less appropriate. The pros and cons of each method need to be repeatedly weighed up depending on the circumstances. The effectiveness and reliability of modern methods was valued when pregnancy would be socially or economically more costly, as this quote from a young woman illustrates:

> With a natural one [i.e. a 'traditional' contraceptive method] sometimes we have a mistake, then it's very difficult. But if you are young, so you can use that. For example, you have just only one child, then you have a mistake and have two children. It's not too bad. But if you are old, you don't want any more.
> (Female, 25 years, no children, urban site)

The issue of effectiveness was also discussed by participants as being dependent not only on the method but also on the user. And this was another factor contributing to whether a particular method 'suited' a woman. Some women commented that the pill was no more effective than day counting, since it was easy to forget to take it; likewise, even obtaining a repeat injection could also be forgotten or mistimed. This highlights that the effectiveness and reliability of different contraceptives is open to interpretation.

Discussion

Through quantitative analysis of CDHS data, an initially surprising finding was revealed: wealthy, educated women had a greater preference for traditional methods than poorer, less educated women. Using qualitative, ethnographic findings, the chapter has provided an explanation for this unexpected result. It became clear that the relationship between socioeconomic status and notions of health was important for understanding the pattern. Whilst Khmer women of every social class placed importance on being healthy, how they acted to maintain or gain good health and avoid ill-health depended on both their conceptualization of a healthy female body and also their capacity, financial and otherwise, to achieve good health. Differing paradigms of health exist simultaneously in Cambodia and the ideas that cluster around these conceptual frameworks support different contraceptive regimes, i.e. a preference for traditional, modern or no contraceptive methods. These different frameworks revolve around attitudes to, and trust in, biomedicine in general and the Cambodian health system in particular. But they are also grounded in people's pragmatic realities – what they know, what they can do and what they can afford.

The ethnographic findings showed that the use of traditional methods varies by social class, in part because such methods were perceived as not appropriate for everyone. One way in which people chose to avoid the side-effects and health worries of modern methods was to use a behavioural method, either day counting or withdrawal. Interestingly, day counting was thought of as 'the doctor's way' and therefore as modern and scientific. This meant it was considered suitable for educated women, who tended to be wealthier. It was presumed that the method could only be used by people familiar with the Gregorian ('foreign') calendar, so rural, illiterate or poor women were seen as (and saw themselves as) unsuitable candidates for this method. The type of relationship a couple had and the willingness of men to cooperate in 'natural methods' were said by some to also relate to social class.

A body of literature, largely produced by anthropological demographers, has drawn attention to a few seemingly counterintuitive cases of traditional method preference in unexpected sectors of society, namely elite, educated, urban women. Johnson-Hanks has pointed out that 'women's contraceptive practice often achieves social goals beyond averting pregnancy' (2002: 231). In Cameroon, periodic abstinence was used by over half of contraceptive users and by practising it, users were asserting a modern, educated and disciplined self. The method conformed to identity ideals aspired to within the local gendered system of honour (Johnson-Hanks 2002). Also taking an anthropological demographic approach, Bledsoe has argued that in West Africa, contraception has been with the aim of having as many children as possible rather than of limiting the number of children (Bledsoe et al. 1998; Bledsoe 2002). Women used contraceptives to rest their bodies and space births in order for subsequent pregnancies to be successful and remain healthy. Bledsoe describes how this relates to a local concept of aging quite different from a Western linear model of passing time; instead, aging is viewed as contingent upon the events and difficulties, including obstetric episodes, endured.

Basu (2005) offers an explanation for the similar pattern of traditional method use found in India, arguing that 'traditional contraceptives' are better described as 'ultramodern contraceptives', whereby 'modern' (highly educated, urban) women are using traditional methods and 'traditional' women are using modern methods.

She shows how two paradigms of modernity operate simultaneously in India, and both support different contraceptive regimes. Amongst higher socioeconomic groups, a 'back-to-nature' approach to a healthy body incorporating elements of the Ayurvedic medical system is seen as both nationalistic and modern. Within this framework, noninvasive traditional methods are viewed as desirable. This theory has been re-examined by Husain et al. (2012), who find traditional method use amongst Indian elites associated with son preference. Once the desired number of sons has been attained, users change from traditional methods to more effective modern methods (Husain et al. 2012).

My research complements and adds to this body of literature. In Cambodia, women who are wealthier and more educated are more likely to use traditional contraception than those who are less wealthy and less educated. What demographers call 'traditional contraception' is actually thought of as being the most modern and is used by the most 'modern' (i.e. educated, wealthy) women in Cambodia. This counterintuitive pattern can only be made sense of when viewed within the specific cultural system of meaning. In explaining the pattern of contraceptive use in Cambodia through relating it to the broader social processes in which it is embedded, the study also shows the value of anthropological ways of thinking about and researching demographic problems.

Meeting the Unmet Need for Modern Contraception

Traditional methods tend to be viewed negatively in the arena of family planning. A key report by UNFPA and the Guttmacher Institute (Singh et al. 2009), which provides global estimates of the global of unmet need for contraception,[12] focused on the unmet need for *modern* contraceptives rather than the standard definition of the unmet need for *contraception* (either traditional or modern). It placed users of traditional methods into the group of women with unmet needs. This estimate has since been used to advocate increased spending on family planning at the recent London Family Planning Summit, a key advocacy event the global family planning movement, and in academic literature on the subject (Cottingham et al. 2012: 173; Shiffman and Quissell 2012: 181). Whilst the authors of the original report (Singh et al. 2009) are careful to use the term 'unmet need for modern contraception', subsequent writers who cite their estimate instead give the figure as the number of women with an 'unmet need for family planning' (Cottingham et al. 2012: 173; Shiffman and Quissell 2012: 181). But should meeting this unmet need for *modern* methods be a priority if women are satisfied with traditional methods?

Much of the focus on promoting modern over 'traditional' methods is based on the assumption that modern methods are more effective at preventing pregnancy. This is questionable when we compare rates of unintended pregnancies published by the World Health Organization (WHO). The WHO's family planning handbook (WHO and CPP 2007) gives contraceptive effectiveness measures that place fertility awareness methods above some modern methods, such as female condoms and diaphragms, and traditional methods are far more effective than using no method at all. Furthermore, it is debatable whether effectiveness at preventing pregnancy should be the single factor with which to judge contraceptive methods (Johnson-Hanks 2002). Women and men have competing demands and desires, from work to relationships to personal wellbeing. They are likely to judge their contraceptive use in terms of how effectively it allows them to achieve all of these aims, rather than only in terms of biomedical effectiveness. In Cambodia, as elsewhere, some women decide modern methods are not the most effective at meeting their needs and instead choose to use day counting or withdrawal. Instead of the international community and providers focusing on uptake of modern methods, perhaps policy-makers and programmers should ensure they provide services and education to support both traditional and modern methods, given that in numerous contexts outlined here, some women at least are satisfied with traditional methods.

An implication of the findings of this chapter regards the diffusion of family planning attitudes and behaviours. Demographic debates have established the importance of the diffusion of innovative behaviours within cultural groups in accounting for regional patterns of fertility transitions (Coale and Watkins 1986; Cleland and Wilson 1987). That a sizeable proportion of Cambodia's elites are currently choosing to use traditional methods where modern methods are accessible to them raises the possibility that such behaviour may diffuse and be taken up more widely amongst the rest of the country's population. This provides further support for the suggestion that policy-makers and family planning providers should ensure that couples interested in such methods are able to use them as effectively and reliably as possible, and that they receive family planning counselling in these methods as well as modern methods.

Conclusion

What benefit can an anthropological analysis bring to the study of demographic phenomena? Perhaps the most important contribution is the ability to capture an emic perspective; that is, the viewpoint of those whose behaviour is the subject of the study. This can bring fresh insight and allow a refocusing of concepts and categories taken for granted but not universally held. From a strictly demographic viewpoint, it seems problematic and puzzling that wealthier, more educated women should be choosing traditional methods over modern methods. Yet anthropological analysis, incorporating far more wide-ranging issues than is typical of demographic analyses, has revealed that women's active choice to use these methods was far from illogical. Furthermore, it showed that the term 'traditional' method contrasts with the meanings attached to these methods in the Cambodian context.

'Traditional' is a value-laden concept, signifying characteristics that do not fit with the meanings ascribed to such methods in Cambodia. Use of the term by demographers is a misrepresentation that contributes to an inaccurate understanding. Furthermore, it potentially has real-life effects as generations of family planning providers, government planners and international donors understand the term 'traditional' and, taking on board the signified meanings, view such methods as inappropriate, ineffective, of the past and to be discouraged. This is problematic if women who are satisfied with their 'traditional method' are pushed to switch to a modern method and the concomitant risk of unwanted side-effects. The term 'behavioural methods' is a more fitting replacement for 'traditional methods'; it distinguishes the same methods (withdrawal, rhythm and lactational amenorrhea) from modern methods, without the inaccurate preconceived ideas that are attached to the term 'traditional'. These findings from Cambodia, together with others from Cameroon (Johnson Hanks 2002), Italy (Gribaldo et al. 2009) and India (Basu 2005), suggest that it is time for demographers to update their terminology.

Eleanor Hukin is a demographer and anthropologist with expertise in reproductive and maternal health in LMICs. She gained her Ph.D. in Demography from the London School of Economics conducting ethnographic research into the unmet need for contraception and currently works as a Technical Advisor at Options Consultancy Services.

Notes

1. Fertility awareness-based methods (such as calendar and symptom-based methods) rely on detecting a woman's fertile period and abstaining or using another method during that time.
2. Folk method cases have been combined with traditional method cases as the frequencies for folk were so low (only eight cases).
3. This wealth index is an indicator of the socioeconomic status of the respondent's households. It is not based on consumption or income, but is a composite indicator based on information collected on the dwelling and household characteristics, consumer goods and assets (NIPH et al. 2006: 22).
4. For the medical care variables, women were asked whether various issues were a problem or not – for example: 'When you are sick and want to get medical advice or treatment, is each of the following a big problem or not? Getting permission to go to a health facility.' For the media influence variable, women were asked if they had heard a family planning message in the media in past twelve months.
5. An odds ratio of less than one indicates the effect of the dummy variable makes traditional method use less likely, in comparison to the reference category. Similarly, odds rations of more than one make traditional method use more likely.
6. The term 'periodic abstinence' refers to situations where sexual intercourse is purposely abstained from for a limited period of time. It usually describes periods of abstinence within a sexually active relationship. This may be practised as a way to avoid becoming pregnant or for reasons unrelated to avoiding pregnancy, for example postpartum abstinence that is concurrent with breastfeeding. In this section I discuss periodic abstinence used for pregnancy prevention. In the section below entitled 'Abstinence', I discuss periodic abstinence (during the postpartum period and menses) when the reasons stated for abstaining are not primarily related to pregnancy prevention.
7. *Kboern* means a body of theories or principles.
8. It is possible that they did advise some people on use of withdrawal, but were not admitting it to me, perhaps thinking this would seem unmodern or incorrect.
9. *Sorsay* is a collective term for all vessels and fibres in the body, including nerves, veins and tendons. *Sorsay kjay* means 'unripe *sorsay*' and refers to the weakened state of a woman's body after birth; all postpartum women are described as being *sorsay kjay*. During birth, a woman's *sorsay* are strained and exerted, from pushing and using up all her strength and energy; this is said to result in a cold state. Traditionally during this period, a woman lies on a raised bed over burning embers of charcoal (*ang plerng*, 'fire roasting'), the purpose being to return her

body to a balanced state of hot/cold equilibrium and to help her breast-milk to flow.

10. This was said to potentially lead to convulsions and death. One *chmop* (traditional birth attendant) described the symptoms as locked jaw, stiffness, trembling, pale face, dry and peeling skin and weight loss. Sometimes the symptoms do not show immediately, but months or years later.
11. For example, the ceremony practised by some families in my rural field site seven days after a child is born. The ceremony was primarily seen by members of the community as a way to apologize to the *chmop* (traditional birth attendant). The couple offers the ceremony in her honour as a way to pay back the debt they owe her, as during the birth she was in a low position of service to the birthing mother and became polluted with the mother's blood.
12. Unmet need for contraception is a key international indicator for family planning and reproductive health. It refers to women who state that they do not wish to become pregnant again or for at least two years, and who are not using contraception.

References

Axinn, W., and L. Pearce. 2006. *Mixed Method Data Collection Strategies*. New York: Cambridge University Press.

Basu, A.M. 2005. 'Ultramodern Contraception', *Asian Population Studies* 1(3): 303–23.

Becker, H. 1996. 'The Epistemology of Qualitative Research', in R. Jessor, A. Colby and R. A. Shweder (eds), *Ethnography and Human Development: Context and Meaning in Social Inquiry*. Chicago: University of Chicago Press, pp. 53–71.

Bledsoe, C. 2002. *Contingent Lives: Fertility, Time and Aging in West Africa*. Chicago: Chicago University Press.

Bledsoe, C., F. Banja and A. Hill. 1998. 'Reproductive Mishaps and Western Contraception: An African Challenge to Fertility Theory', *Population and Development Review* 24(1): 15–57.

Bongaarts, J., and J. Bruce. 1995. 'The Causes of Unmet Need for Contraception and the Social Content of Services', *Studies in Family Planning* 26(2): 57–75.

Bryman, A. 2008. *Social Research Methods*. New York: Oxford University Press.

Caldwell, J., K., Gaminiratne, P. Caldwell, S. Silva, B. Caldwell, N. Weeraratne and P. Silva. 1987. 'The Role of Traditional Fertility Regulation in Sri Lanka', *Studies in Family Planning* 18(1): 1–21.

Cleland, J., and C. Wilson. 1987. 'Demand Theories of the Fertility Transition: An Iconoclastic View', *Population Studies* 41(1): 5–30.

Coale, A., and S.C. Watkins (eds). 1986. *The Decline of Fertility in Europe: The Revised Proceedings of a Conference on the Princeton European Fertility Project*. Princeton: Princeton University Press.
Coast, E., K. Hampshire and S. Randall. 2007. 'Disciplining Anthropological Demography', *Demographic Research* 16(16): 493–518.
Cottingham, J., A. Germain and P. Hunt, 2012. 'Use of Human Rights to Meet the Unmet Need for Family Planning' *The Lancet* 380(9837): 172–80.
Creswell, J.W. 2002. *Research Design: Qualitative, Quantitative, and Mixed Method Approaches*. London: Sage.
Gajanayake, I., and J. Caldwell. 1990. 'Fertility and its Control: The Puzzle of Sri Lanka', *International Family Planning Perspectives* 16(3): 97–111.
Gribaldo, A., M. Judd and D. Kertzer. 2009. 'An Imperfect Contraceptive Society: Fertility and Contraception in Italy', *Population and Development Review* 35(3): 551–84.
Heuveline, P.H. 1998. '"Between One and Three Million": Towards the Demographic Reconstruction of a Decade of Cambodian History (1970–79)', *Population Studies* 52(1): 49–65.
Hukin, E.F. 2012. 'Contraception in Cambodia: Explaining Unmet Need', Ph.D. dissertation. London: London School of Economics and Political Science.
Husain, Z., S. Ghosh and M. Dutta. 2012. '"Ultramodern Contraception" Re-examined: Cultural Dissent, or Son Preference?' *Asian Population Association Conference*, Bangkok, 26–29 August 2012, Bangkok: Asian Population Association.
Hukin, E.F. 2014. 'Cambodia's Fertility Transition: The Dynamics of Contemporary Childbearing', *Population and Development Review* 40(4): 605–28.
ICF International. 2014. 'The DHS Program Demographic and Health Surveys', *The DHS Program*. Retrieved 1 February 2017 from http://www.dhsprogram.com.
Johnson-Hanks, J. 2002. 'On the Modernity of Traditional Contraception: Time and the Social Context of Fertility', *Population and Development Review* 28(2): 229–49.
Ledgerwood, J. 1990. 'Changing Khmer Conceptions of Gender: Women, Stories, and the Social Order', Ph.D. dissertation. New York: Cornell University.
Livi-Bacci, M. 1986. 'Social-Group Forerunners of Fertility Control in Europe', in A.J. Coale and S.C. Watkins (eds), *The Decline of Fertility in Europe*. Princeton: Princeton University Press, pp. 182–200.
NIPH (National Institute of Public Health), NIS (National Institute of Statistics) and ORC Macro. 2006. *Cambodia Demographic and Health Survey 2005*. Phnom Penh and Calverton.
NIS (National Institute of Statistics), Directorate General for Health and ICF Macro 2011. *Cambodia Demographic and Health Survey*. Phnom Penh and Calverton.

Obermeyer, C.M. 2005. 'Reframing Research on Sexual Behaviour and HIV', *Studies in Family Planning* 36(1): 1–12.

Potdar, R., T. Fetters and L. Phirun. 2008. 'Initial Loss of Productive Days and Income Among Women Seeking Induced Abortion in Cambodia', *Journal of Midwifery and Women's Health* 53(2): 123–29.

RACHA (Reproductive and Child Health Alliance). 1997. *Cambodian Abortion Law* (unpublished translation). Phnom Penh: Author.

Randall, S. 1996. 'Whose Reality? Local Perceptions of Fertility versus Demographic Analysis', *Population Studies* 50(2): 221–34.

Randall, S., and T. Koppenhaver. 2004. 'Qualitative Data in Demography: The Sound of Silence and Other Problems', *Demographic Research* 11(3): 57–94.

Shiffman, J., and K. Quissell. 2012. 'Family Planning: A Political Issue', *The Lancet* 380(9837): 181–85.

Singh, S., J.E. Darroch, L.S. Ashford and M. Vlassoff. 2009. *Adding it up: The Costs and Benefits of Investing in Family Planning and Maternal and Newborn Health*. New York: Guttmacher Institute and UNFPA.

Watkins, S.C. 1986. 'Conclusion', in A.J. Coale and S.C. Watkins (eds), *The Decline of Fertility in Europe*. Princeton: Princeton University Press.

WHO and CPP (Center for Communication Programs at Johns Hopkins Bloomberg School of Public Health). 2007. *Family Planning: A Global Handbook for Providers*. Baltimore and Geneva: CPP and WHO.

Chapter 10

Demographers on Culture

Fertility, Nuptiality, Family Structures

Yves Charbit and Véronique Petit

The theme of culture, as a fundamental *métier* of anthropology, implicitly underpins discussion of the many specific instances of conjuncture and difference addressed in this book. As demographers sensitive to the anthropological dimension of demographic behaviour, however, we would like to reflect more explicitly on this theme, as it is often treated as a kind of black box – best left unopened – in demographic research. In reviewing a number of aspects of fertility, nuptiality and family, we shall consider how the supposedly mysterious contents of the box can be dealt with readily, to the advantage both of demography and of anthropology. As part of this, it is very important to note that some crucial clarifications only become possible once demographic measurement is brought to bear on cultural practices. Fertility, nuptiality and family structure are, after all, subfields of research in which demographers have some expertise – and not only because these issues lend themselves to measurement.

A good starting point is Marshall Sahlins' introduction to *Culture in Practice*, in which he refuses to regard 'polygynous households' as an abstraction. Quoting White, who in 1949 classified polygyny as a 'cultural trait', he observes that it might equally be considered as a 'social form'. Sahlins immediately follows this statement with the observation that the distinction between culture and society is unacceptable, and this leads him to propose 'a comprehensive sense of culture': 'the culture concept encompasses any and all forms of human practice, including social relationships thereof, everything constituted and organized symbolically' (2005: 16).

A standard is thus set. Demographers working in the field of population and development are on notice that they cannot content themselves with 'pure' measurement. Not contextualizing polygamy is tantamount to not explaining anything since, as we shall see, polygyny (and fertility levels consequent on this marriage form) does not occur independently of other marriage options, and is not constant across the life course. To measure polygyny in the abstract is merely to play with an imaginary statistical dynamics. In contrast, anthropology, as is widely recognized, often provides its most perceptive insights when it comes to major events of the lifecycle. This was shown clearly by David G. Mandelbaum's pioneering *Human Fertility in India: Social Components and Policy Perspectives* (1974). The complementarity of anthropology and demography is also obvious in other early works of, say, Edward Evans-Pritchard (1994), Claude Meillassoux (1970, 1977) or Pierre Clastres (1972). The significance of demographic behaviour in developing countries has, from this solid starting point, become a major matter of concern for anthropology, as is evident in the important volume *Anthropological Demography: Toward a New Synthesis* (Kertzer and Fricke 1997). Yet that volume mainly gathered contributions by anthropologists, only a few demographers daring to go beyond the narrow limits of their discipline.

In research completed in Sub-Saharan Africa, the Caribbean and Southeast Asia, we have aimed at narrowing the gap between demography and anthropology. As demographers concerned with the epistemological issue of causality at the individual level, we support Sahlins' view that the problem of cultural determinism must be addressed; that is, the relationship between individual action and cultural order cannot remain a black box (Sahlins 2005). Since demographers rely massively on individual quantitative data, they immediately bump into a crucial problem when working on 'culture' as a causal determinant of men's and women's individual behaviour: how to connect the micro- and macro-levels? The double nature of culture, as defined by Sahlins, impacts on both levels: demographic behaviour is at once enacted in the actions and projects of particular human beings, which take the wider form of a structure or system of collective comprehension. At the micro-level, demographers usually regard culture as identified by one or more of the many characteristics of the individuals they survey, and rely on a few quantitative indicators, usually spoken language, religion or ethnic belonging, which they aggregate. At the macro-level, demographers commonly use culture, taken as category, as a residual factor – or, worse, as a magic wand – and it is here that culture becomes a black box where the hidden truth lies (Kertzer and Fricke 1997: 18).

Far too many demographers are not able to look seriously at culture as a macro-level phenomenon, except by making brief ritual reference to the alternative between traditional and modern. At best, they may add inverted commas to both adjectives, but this is just paying preventive lip service to foreseeable objections fired at them by sociologists and anthropologists. In Hammel's and Friou's words, 'in the Notestein tradition, one might only have to achieve "modernisation"' (whatever that is), and let social actors mysteriously adapt, without our understanding just what they are adapting too' (1997: 192, note 3). Earlier, Hammel had severe but well-deserved words for the use of culture in demographic works: 'culture in demography seems mired in structural functional concepts that are about 40 years old, hardening rapidly and showing every sign of fossilization' (1990: 456; see also Levine and Scrimshaw 1983: 667). Although more than three decades have elapsed since Hammel's remarks, major demographic survey programmes in the world today remain reliant on fossilized notions of culture, as we shall note below.

We would suggest that demographic methodologies are nevertheless irreplaceable as a means of demonstrating how and why adaptation and change are occurring, but that this requires careful integration of anthropological and demographic concepts and methods. The following sections draw examples from our work in the Caribbean and in Sub-Saharan Africa, leading to discussion of some epistemological conditions for a better treatment of culture.

The Demography of Cultural Practices

Has demography really nothing to say about culture? Its contribution cannot be dismissed when it comes to one of its strengths, which is to provide solid quantitative data – granting, of course, the need to keep a critical eye on potential biases in the indicators used. Hammel and Howell credited demography as 'cutting across and unifying the sub-disciplines of anthropology as few other topics do' (1987: 141). Assessing the validity of this sweeping generalization would take us too far, but a few points should be stressed here.

The first concerns certain structural patterns, especially family typologies. The family in both developing and industrialized countries has often been assumed to tend inevitably towards the Western nuclear model (e.g. Goode 1963), though it has in fact taken a great variety of forms. For instance, in Western countries, with the rise of individualism and the evolution of women's status, divorce has led to the phenomenon of family reconstructions. In parallel, personal choices and social constraints made or endured by women have led them to have children outside of marriage, further weakening it as an institution. Meanwhile, in West Africa and many other parts of the world, the extended family remains widespread and solidly entrenched – despite the pressure exerted by Western television series that display *ad nauseam* families in which women and men are assumed to act on an equal basis, forming a nuclear couple with a couple of kids in the midst of cosy middle-class comfort. These are images duly received by African viewers glued to their TV sets. Yet a convergence of cultural factors in Africa continues to favour fertility higher than in the West, with households encompassing several reproductive units. These factors include: the weight of elders' authority; the inferior status of women; the powerful economic rationality of labour-intensive agriculture systems dependent on the free manpower of children and women; the economic solidarity of villages in taking on agricultural work (the practice of 'helping hands'); and strategies of alliance and social prestige gained through marriages.

Quantifying the frequency of these different forms of family structure and, above all, their evolution over several decades can be achieved only with the help of censuses and household surveys. Contrary to all expectations, this has enabled demographers to demonstrate that the size of households in Africa has increased *more* in urban areas than in rural areas. This result runs counter to the accepted view that modernization is associated, if not explained, by urbanization, hence the fertility of urban women is expected to be lower than that of rural women. It is further carelessly asserted that urban households in consequence are smaller. There lies a crucial confusion here between the family, as a biological unit, and the household, as an economic unit. The size of the former is determined by mortality (notably at young ages), marriage (age at marriage being a major determinant) and fertility (e.g. whether or not the couple uses contraception). However, when we turn to the family as an economic unit, an altogether different logic is at play and another crucial factor comes to the fore – geographical mobility or, more particularly, rural exodus. The larger size of urban households arises from the doubling-up of two subpopulations: an influx of adults in search of urban jobs together with an increase in children fostered by heads of households (the so-called practice of *confiage*). Because the economy and memberships of urban households remain part of wider kin structures linking villages and towns, it is often more realistic to see members as belonging to at least two residential units, sometimes separated by great distances (cf. Davis 2004: 302). In sociological terms, family networks continuously link families in places of origin with their extensions in urban areas.

The second point also concerns the way in which demographers are able to tackle cultural issues with a strong social dimension and, more particularly, how measurement provides specific comparisons necessary to assess anthropological observation. Here, the standard example is that of polygamy. As Walters describes in her chapter in this volume on East Africa, throughout the period of colonization, the evangelization of 'African tribes' condemned polygamy and promoted monogamy and fidelity. Religious teaching focused on the promiscuity and immorality of polygamous couples, with the stigmatization of venereal diseases in central Africa, and increased sterility associated with it, adding powerful arguments. However, with the distribution of antibiotics and the retreat of syphilis and gonorrhoea, the risk of declining fertility and of a shortage of labour associated with plural sexual relationships and pathological sterility gave way to a diametrically opposed argument: polygamy *increases* fertility. What can demography contribute when confronted with such an imbrication of cultural, social and economic arguments – especially in the charged moral context in which in which Western agencies aimed at controlling an African sexuality assumed to be natural and unrestrained?

Demographers first quantified the relative frequency of monogamous and polygamous households. Ironically, this provided grist to the mill of social scientists working in the West, since the sexual promiscuity supposed to be an African characteristic could be observed just as well in countries where polygamy did not exist. Further, by measuring the gap between the average ages of men and women, they gave an undeniable foundation to the thesis that polygamy should be analysed as a means of control exercised by older men over their juniors; by monopolizing available women (which men's wealth, in effect, allowed them to buy), they simultaneously captured the two priceless economic resources of female labour and, above all, potential offspring.

But, more subtly, demographers also made it possible to clarify the debate on the comparative fertility of monogamous and polygamous women. Initially, in a simplistic discourse that once again mixed economic with cultural factors, the expected fertility of women in polygamous unions was supposed to be higher than that of monogamous women, given the incentive that the more children a woman could have, the greater her share in the rights and goods these children produced – not to mention the prestige linked to the capacity to give birth to many children. These motivations reiterated the central value of fertility in Africa. However, there is a problem with this classic anthropological argument: how do we know whether each of the births counted is genuinely attributable to polygamy?[1] Polygamy and monogamy are not fixed attributes; they evolve over time. For instance, women categorized as participating in a monogamous union find themselves mechanically attributed the status of 'first wife' when the husband takes a second, the family then becoming polygamous. To measure the comparative fertility of monogamy and polygamy, we need to attribute each birth to the marital status in which a woman found herself at a given moment. To achieve this, a detailed typology is necessary that not only distinguishes between 'always monogamous' and 'polygamous' women, but also *amongst* polygamous women, i.e. separating those who were first wives and those entering the household directly as second or later co-wives. 'First wives' therefore constitute an intermediate category between the two others since they usually will have had part of their offspring in a monogamous situation. It is in this way possible to measure without bias the fertility of polygamy and monogamy or, put differently, to control for the impact of vital conjunctures leading to polygamy.

Better still, this analysis makes it possible to control for another confounding factor, the risk of divorce linked to the central cultural and social value of fertility, which places great pressures on women. A wife must attempt to give birth to her first child relatively soon after marriage since, culturally and economically, that is what her husband, their parents and the whole society expect of her. Survey questionnaires enable us to track the timing of births in a marriage, for example, by giving information on the date of the first birth and that of the marriage. Where the difference between the two dates exceeds five years, a wife is commonly suspected of not being able to conceive a child. She then runs the risk of being joined by a co-wife and finding herself in a polygamous situation. However, combining data on potential sterility with the three-part typology of marital fertility mentioned above opens up a further and different perspective: the dynamics of unions cannot be summed up only by a polygamy/monogamy alternative, as there is a third possibility, that of divorce or repudiation for suspected sterility.[2]

Regarding all of these points, it is clear that demography can concur readily with anthropology's holistic vision by providing critical measures that require a sharpened differentiation of local practices of family and household formation, types of marriage and the reproductive patterns characteristic of each. We have conceptualized this and other problems of linking behaviour to longitudinal analysis in the framework of comprehensive demography. Individuals have a wide range of responses, both demographic (marriage rate, birth rate, migration) and non-demographic (pluri-activity, village strategies of inter-ethnic negotiations) to counter the problems incurred, for example those due to poverty.

Towards Parity between Demographic and Anthropological Approaches

The two research themes of the extended family and polygamy show the specific contribution demography is able to make when it brings well-defined measurement and strictly quantitative data to bear in sociological debates. Unfortunately, demographers too often content themselves with hooking their carriage to the end of the train, without then taking the trouble to walk up the corridor to find out what sort of locomotive is pulling it. The real test for interdisciplinary research is for demography and anthropology to play equal parts. A good example is provided by instances in which data and analysis are organized along the very lines of anthropological arguments.

In the Caribbean, a folk saying states 'looking for bread finding meat'.[3] It is generally argued that in these societies, where machismo is of great cultural importance and where women are caught in a system of unstable mating patterns, and poor women seek to 'give a child' to the current partner, hoping that he will thence be anchored to the household and contribute to its expenses. Predictably, men tend to disappear when a pregnancy occurs. Turning to demographic evidence, it is helpful to compare women involved in two broad categories of relationship: so-called unstable or 'visiting' unions; and married or common law wives who are involved in much more stable partnerships and who are generally economically better off. The usual expectation in the literature, following on the folk saying, is that women with visiting partners will have higher fertility than stable unions. The quantitative evidence, however, runs counter to this expectation (see also Pauli, this volume), even as there is popular acceptance that extramarital pregnancy is a regular consequence of powerful gender differences, such as machismo, as cultural values. Indeed, there can be little doubt that such expectations of higher fertility exist locally, as women in new partnerships are likely to behave in conformity to unequal gender relations. However, even if such premises are correct, the conclusion is wrong, since what ultimately matters for a pregnancy to occur is sexual exposure. And while sexual exposure is frequent in a stable couple, it is often far less so for a single woman, especially if she is poor, overworked, older or less sexually appealing. Such women are likely to experience long periods of sexual solitude and hence lower fertility. In the Caribbean, time spent out of any sort of union amounts to more than 20 per cent of their reproductive lifespan, a result observed in all the available representative sample surveys (Charbit 1987). Likewise, the vulnerability of young women recounted in several earlier chapters is consistent with this pattern: strategies for women in unstable relationships reflect themes of financial insecurity, gender inequality and spousal entrapment, which in turn constrain reproduction not only as women adjust their contraceptive use to suit the needs of a given relationship, but consciously practise sexual abstinence and postponement (Kroeker and Hukin), consider abortion (van der Sijpt) or suffer infertility due to health problems (Bochow).

The current and much-needed emphasis on interdisciplinarity here bears fruit both for demographers and for anthropologists. For the former, in contrast to a tendency to focus more or less exclusively on national demographic trends in marriage age or the spread of contraception, we see that beneath such patterns, there exist major differentials in the fertility of subpopulations as different groups define themselves by contrasting patterns of nuptiality. This is, of course, a longstanding observation of historical demographers (e.g. Hajnal 1982), where findings on European fertility differentials between class groups again may conflict with popular stereotypes. The importance of different patterns of nuptiality for understanding fertility outcomes, and of clarifying the role of evolving class and other power relations as they shape experience over time are themes that unite the African, and Central and Southeast Asian case studies presented here with this history.

On the anthropological side, purely biological components of demography, such as monitoring time out of wedlock, caution against hazardous conclusions drawn from locally popular cultural constructs. In the Caribbean case, matrifocal households, as defined by anthropological research (sometimes also called 'grand-mother families', e.g. of two generations of women, both single, with young children), are supposed to be very frequent. Yet survey data for Guadeloupe, Martinique, Jamaica, the Dominican Republic, Haïti, Trinidad and Tobago, and Guyana, and published census data for Cuba and Puerto Rico, as well as isolated surveys in Barbados, Jamaica, Martinique and Providencia, have revealed a stunning but consistent proportion of two-thirds of nuclear households and less than 5 per cent of matrifocal families. As noted by some anthropologists, it is likely that ethnographic work suffered from selection bias. Further, mothers having had children from one, two or even three or more men, thus following a pattern of what we called *pluripaternité* (multiple sequential fatherhood), are by no means in the majority. In Guadeloupe and Martinique, for instance, surveys revealed that 69 per cent of children were born from a woman's relations with a single father. Data of this kind – which might or might not show the same pattern –would provide an important basis for assessing the nuptiality and fertility patterns described in the several contemporary African societies described in the preceding chapters.

In sum, the minimum and yet irreplaceable contribution of demographers is to adequately measure in a given society the sociocultural models identified by anthropologists, especially when addressing issues of fertility, nuptiality and family structure. Underlying this contribution is the capacity of demographic measurement to blend cross-sectional and cohort analysis, thus combining what anthropologists and linguists sometimes refer to as synchronic and diachronic perspectives. On the one hand, contextualized measurement enables demographic changes, usually observed in a short or medium-term timespan, to be understood with respect to often less labile, long-term cultural patterns. On the other hand, demographic cohort or longitudinal analysis enables the experience of a sequence of generations to be compared, something that the data presented by Pauli and others in this volume show is crucial to understanding how fertility trends are evolving differentially in the several subpopulations of women and their families.

Unfortunately, a word of caution must be introduced here, particularly in the context of prevailing demographic survey programmes in the developing world. In sharp contrast to efforts made in some World Fertility Surveys of the 1970s, attempts at contextualization have been drastically impoverished in succeeding rounds of the current mainstay of developing world survey research, the Demographic and Health Surveys (DHS). Top priority is now given to measuring levels and trends of fertility with particular reference to the prevalence of modern methods of contraception. Hammel's and Friou's remark, cited earlier, that demographers tend automatically to ascribe any adaptation to modern interventions – without inquiring into how or why such changes are occurring – thus remains a telling criticism. In consequence, the contribution that mainstream survey demography may make to sociology – and even more to the anthropology of cultural variation in fertility, nuptiality and family systems – has hopelessly shrunk. This is amply demonstrated by the several chapters in this volume that refer to DHS data (Pauli, Bochow, Kroeker, Hukin, and Randall, Mondain and Diagne): DHS fertility measures can provide them with only a kind of ballpark figure, a national-level, cross-sectional measure of total fertility per woman that takes no account of constraints on reproduction arising from the family and marital systems described above, and particularly of how these constraints vary over time. In consequence, in these chapters DHS data are revealed giving a misleading picture of the processes and significance of reproductive change. DHS data can thus become an obstacle, rather than an aid, to understanding. As a number of critical studies (Szreter et al. 2004) have shown, anthropological demographers can do better than to follow demographers' habit of relying on loose definitions of cultural or economic categories, whilst comfortably crouched behind their datasets.

Conclusion

Mainstream demographic analyses of fertility, nuptiality and migration in developing countries suffer from epistemological weaknesses, and awareness is clearly necessary to better define field research and analyse data. By way of conclusion, four general points can be made.

First, explaining individual behaviour entails questioning oneself as to its rationality, not in terms presupposed by the researcher and his or her culture, but that makes sense for the actors. Let's start from the elementary idea that culture governs our perception of reality and moulds the responses of actors to the contextual changes with which they are confronted. In order to explain behaviour, and not simply describe it as most demography tends to do, we have proposed a research strategy with the goal of building a comprehensive demography. An inspiration here is Max Weber, whose work leads to a radically different approach to that of Durkheim (Petit 2013). Durkheim, through his systematic attempt to objectify behaviour (including demographic behaviour), has had a huge and profound influence on demographic research since its nineteenth-century formation. Comprehensive demography offers a new agenda for research on population and development, with major implications for fieldwork. It allows exploring behaviour, and the value systems and beliefs underlying it, not only on the level of individuals but also on meso- and macro-levels. This is demonstrated in our work on fertility, nuptiality, migration and reproductive health issues in different contexts: Senegal, Mauritius, Mali, Burundi, Vietnam, Guinea-Conakry and Djibouti (Petit 2016).

Second, as demographers are incorrigibly empiricist, they try obsessively to document how and why changes take shape in the ethos of individuals and groups. In a paper published in 1992, Karen Mason criticized demographers' so-called cultural theories, pointing out 'invalid equations' commonly made between cultural processes, ideational processes and fertility decisions. Ideational changes, for instance, the desire to have lower fertility, can occur without any cultural change and may have little to do with couples knowing possible methods to have fewer children. Of course, at some point in time, both ideational changes and techniques are likely to be integrated into popular culture. As Hammel (1990: 467) put it, culture may be understood as 'a transitory and negotiated set of understandings . . . a constantly modified and elaborated system of moral symbols'. A key problem for the researcher is to place conjuncture and difference in an *adequate* temporal scale that shows how the many merely ideational adjustments in the way in which life course events are seen can be disentangled from more fundamental cultural change.

Most of the difficulties can be overcome by adopting a typology of responses to changes (Charbit and Petit 2011). This enables several levels of analysis regarding the compromises formulated by the actors when confronted with potential or open conflicts between their cultural values and contextual changes, whether economic, social or political. Population programmes provide a classic example of contextual change. Some programmes (e.g. in

Mexico and India) have attempted to impose male sterilization campaigns. With respect to fantasies linked to virility, one possible compromise for the husband who has been vasectomized is to justify his acceptance of sterilization by economic arguments: 'we'll no longer be overburdened by children'. But insofar as female sterilization would have led to exactly the same result, the response is clearly a rationalization. When comparing the proportions of men and women sterilized, this becomes a real question, the issue being to know why the sterilization of women is better accepted than that of men. Here, analysis of gender-based differences would be particularly illuminating.

Third, the implicit assumption that individual characteristics of surveyed individuals are 'explanatory factors' must be seriously reconsidered. Religion, for example, is defined for survey purposes as an individual characteristic and is largely reified. As Walters' historical reconstruction (Chapter 2, this volume) shows, in Africa individuals change religions or put into effect a syncretism of the value systems to which they have been subjected, opening up avenues both of continuity and change in their marriage, reproductive and other arrangements. Religion is thus not an attribute indicative of a given disposition, but a multifaceted vehicle for individual and group agency. Likewise, changes of ethnic affiliation and the construction of other new identities may occur under the pressure of changing relations of domination, as in the Tajik examples discussed in Roche and Hohmann's chapter; as they show, families and their members may simply ignore attributed ethnic affiliations, forming other principal subpopulation units suited to their reproduction and nuptiality preferences (see also Brown 2015). Or take the 'status of women'. This is usually defined on the basis of their level of education, profession and area of residence, but these are *neither necessary nor sufficient conditions* for their status to be higher or lower, because the status of women as revealed by the ethnography of sexuality, nuptiality and family dynamics is ignored, while it is probably at least as decisive (Johnson-Hanks 2015; van der Sijpt, this volume). This approach to defining status, which equates it only with a few standardized sociodemographic and economic characteristics, ignores all other levels of analysis. This, in turn, limits the way in which demographers are able to explore gender relations, usually confining it to comparing women's opinions and behaviour (for instance, on the use of reproductive health services) with their partner's, using data drawn from male and female samples. Again, a lack of contextualization results in a poor contribution to the analysis of gender relations. An important methodological implication follows: a woman's status simply cannot be assessed through data collected using only a demographic questionnaire of individuals (cf. Kreager and Schröder-Butterfill 2014). Such a limited approach is in any case unnecessary, as Randall and her colleagues (this volume) show – thus contributing helpfully to a wider body of research on fertility and on family planning in Senegal (Charbit et al. 1994; Petit and des Robert 2004), Mauritius (Hillcoat-Nalletamby 2002) and Guinea (Petit 2016), which demonstrates how these issues can be approached on the basis of contextualized assumptions in which fertility decisions made by women are bound up in potential gender conflicts and family dynamics that reflect the conjuncture of broader community, regional and national contexts.

Fourth, published analyses of individual behaviour presuppose in most cases a *homo economicus*-type rationality that is very rarely discussed at the epistemological level in the works of demographers, even as other rationalities – social, cultural or political – are not taken into account. Consistent with the utilitarian philosophy underlying this assumed pure economic rationality of the actors, population policies rest on the implicit hypothesis that populations and social groups willingly agree to them, while in reality, power relations govern the scope of people's choices and possible decisions. In this book a diversity of historical power structures is noted that continues to shape the contemporary scene: apartheid (Pauli), *homo sovieticus* (Roche and Hohmann), Catholicism (Walters) and the economic and institutional legacies of British colonialism (Bochow and Kroeker). This very effectively dissolves the convenient ahistorical premise that individual and group action is conditioned only by purely economic and contraceptive utility. The complex issue of historical legacies, which cannot be dealt with adequately within the scope of this chapter, takes us back to the origins of demography and to population doctrines. In the sixteenth and seventeenth centuries, long before the rise of economics, a founding conceptualization of population as one of the bases of a prince's power was laid down by political and moral philosophers (Charbit 2010). The subsequent development of population policies rests upon an implicit hypothesis that has evolved as central to the Western logic of the social contract since the eighteenth century, namely, that what is good for the nation is also good for the individual. The specific demographic argument, constantly hammered in the promotion of population programmes, is that the adoption of modern contraception by the bulk of the people is the key to increasing GDP per head. However, another logic has been proven far more relevant: that in the developing world, people may not at all see clearly why they should erode their main reliable economic asset, the family labour force, just to comply with a government policy of low fertility. Lower fertility must make sense in relation to such assets, and it may even be that the words 'national economic growth' mean little or nothing on their own. Latent or overt conflicts like this are likely to shape, and to explain, the failure of family planning projects.

Put in a nutshell, given the 'epistemological crisis of demography' (Fricke 1997: 248), anthropological demography opens up new and promising avenues for research. The uniqueness of the methodological contribution of demography to population and development issues – and to anthropological research on them – should not be underestimated. However, the emergence of anthropological demography has enabled a fruitful interdisciplinary dialogue between anthropologists and demographers on the four epistemological issues we have noted, and this is especially important in view of the fact that, until recently, the two camps scored high on the scale of misunderstandings and quarrels.

Yves Charbit, Professor Emeritus of Demography at Paris Descartes University, created and headed the *Centre Population et Développement* (CEPED). He has published twenty-two books and sixty-two peer-reviewed articles on international migrations, family, nuptiality, reproductive health, theories and doctrines of population.

Véronique Petit is Professor of Demography at Paris Descartes University and a member of CEPED. She is a specialist on population and development, notably in Sub-Saharan Africa. In *Counting Populations. Understanding Societies* (Springer, 2013), she advocates a comprehensive approach to demography in light of anthropological demography.

Notes

1. Erica van der Sijpt's chapter, based on her Cameroonian ethnography, provides excellent examples of just how tenuous attribution of paternity can be and how factors determining marital status change across the life course.

2. Although childlessness may be due to no more than a curable temporary infertility, women usually do not benefit from such a benevolent attitude.
3. A detailed and extensively referenced version of the following discussion is provided by Charbit and Petit (2011).

References

Brown, M.J. 2015. 'Collective Identities, Shifting Population Membership, and Niche Construction Theory: Implications from Taiwanese and Chinese Empirical Evidence', in P. Kreager, B. Winney, S. Ulijaszek and C. Capelli (eds), *Population in the Human Sciences: Concepts, Models, Evidence.* Oxford: Oxford University Press, pp. 331–60.

Charbit, Y. 1987. *Famille et nuptialité dans la Caraïbe.* Paris: PUF.

———. 2010. *The Classical Foundations of Population Thought, from Plato to Quesnay,* Milton: Springer.

Charbit, Y., B. Mane and S. Niaye. 1994. 'Equipements communautaires, santé et planification familiale en milieu rural', in Y. Charbit and S. Niaye (eds), *La population du Sénégal.* Paris : DPS/CERPAA, pp. 295–317.

Charbit, Y., and V. Petit. 2011. 'Toward a Comprehensive Demography: Rethinking the Research Agenda on Change and Response', *Population and Development Review* 37(2): 219–39.

Clastres, P. 2006 [1972]. *Chronique des Indiens Guayaki.* Paris: Plon.

Davis, P.J. 2004. 'Re-contextualizing the Female-Headed Household: Culture and Agency in Uganda', in S. Szreter, H. Sholkamy and A. Dharmalingam (eds), *Categories and Contexts: Anthropological and Historical Studies in Critical Demography.* Oxford: Oxford University Press, pp. 295–321.

Evans-Pritchard E.E. 1994 [1968]. *Les Nuer: description des modes de vie et des institutions politiques d'un people nilote.* Paris: Tel-Gallimard.

Fricke, T. 1997, 'Culture Theory and Demographic Process: Toward a Thicker Demography', in D.I. Kertzer and T. Fricke (eds), *Anthropological Demography: Toward a New Synthesis.* Chicago: University of Chicago Press, pp. 248–278.

Goode, W.J. 1963. *World Revolution and Family Patterns.* New York and London: Free-Press of Glencoe, Collier-Macmillan.

Hajnal, J. 1982. 'Two Kinds of Pre-industrial Household Formation System', *Population and Development Review* 8(3): 449–94.

Hammel, E.A. 1990. 'A Theory of Culture for Demography', *Population and Development Review* 16(2): 455–85.

Hammel, E.A., and N. Howell. 1987. 'Research in Population and Culture: An Evolutionary Framework', *Current Anthropology* 27(2): 141–60.

Hammel, E. A. and D. S. Friou. 1997. 'Anthropology and Demography: Marriage, Liaison, or Encounter?', in D.I. Kertzer and T. Fricke (eds), *Anthropological Demography: Toward a New Synthesis.* Chicago: University of Chicago Press, pp. 175–200.

Hillcoat-Nalletamby, S. 2002. *La contraception à l'Ile Maurice: politique nationale, pratiques individuelles.* Paris: L'Harmattan.
Johnson-Hanks, J. 2015. 'Populations are Composed One Event at a Time', in P. Kreager, B. Winney, S. Ulijaszek and C. Capelli (eds), *Population in the Human Sciences: Concepts, Models, Evidence.* Oxford: Oxford University Press, pp. 238–56.
Kertzer, D.I., and T. Fricke. 1997. 'Toward an Anthropological Demography', in D.I. Kertzer and T. Fricke (eds) *Anthropological Demography: Toward a New Synthesis.* Chicago: University of Chicago Press, pp. 1–35.
Kreager, P., and E. Schröder-Butterfill. 2014. 'Cultural Variations in Daughter Preference in Rural Indonesia', in T. Devasahayam (ed.), *Gender and Ageing: Southeast Asian Perspectives.* Singapore: Institute of Southeast Asian Studies, pp. 150–73.
levine, R.A., and S.C.M. Scrimshaw. 1983. 'Effects of Culture on Fertility: Anthropological Contributions', in R.A. Bulatao and R. Lee (eds), *Determinants of Fertility in Developing Countries,* vol. II, New York, Academic Press, pp. 666–95.
Mandelbaum, D.G. 1974. *Human Fertility in India: Social Components and Policy Perspectives.* Berkeley: University of California Press.
Mason, K.O. 1992. 'Culture and the Fertility Transition: Thoughts on Theories of Fertility Decline', *Genus* 48(3–4): 1–13.
Meillassoux, C. 1970. *Anthropologie économique des Gouro en Côte d'Ivoire.* Paris: Édition Mouton, Ecole Pratique des Hautes Etudes.
———. 1977, *Terrains et théories,* Paris: Éditions anthropos.
Petit, V. 2013. *Counting Populations, Understanding Societies.* Dordrecht: Springer.
———. 2017 (forthcoming). *The Theory of Change and Response. From Fieldwork to Theory.* Dordrecht: Springer.
Petit, V., and M.-L. des Robert. 2004. *Entre résistance et changement la planification familiale en milieu rural sénégalais.* Paris: L'Harmattan.
Sahlins, M. 1985. *Islands of History.* Chicago: University of Chicago Press.
———. 2005. *Culture in Practice.* New York: Zone Books.
Szreter, S., H. Sholkamy and A. Dharmalingam (eds), *Categories and Contexts: Anthropological and Historical Studies in Critical Demography.* Oxford: Oxford University Press.

Chapter 11

Vital Conjunctures Revisited

Jennifer A. Johnson-Hanks

Viewed from enough distance, fertility decline is remarkable in its uniformity. Over a period of only a couple of hundred years, and largely in conjunction with economic development, urbanization, political transformation and cultural change, fertility has declined in most parts of the world from something like 5–7 children per woman down to something more like 1–3 children per woman. Along with the concomitant declines in mortality, fertility decline has had dramatic consequences for women, who might today spend 5 per cent of their adult lives pregnant or breastfeeding, in contrast to the 50 per cent common in many places a century ago. Everywhere, it seems, fertility decline is accompanied by social changes that make family a less central institution, but state, school and corporation more central ones. Everywhere, it seems, fertility decline is associated with a rise in individualism and a rejection of tradition.

However, when viewed a little more closely, fertility decline loses this apparent uniformity. On shorter timelines and smaller scales, it is fertility decline's *heterogeneity* that becomes remarkable. The poorest countries all have high fertility and the richest ones all have low fertility, but for *most* countries – all those in between the extremes of income – the predictive power of income on fertility is very low. In Asia, countries with the highest labour force participation for women have the lowest fertility, while in Europe, the reverse is true. In Western Europe, fertility decline has been associated with increases in age at first birth, whereas in Eastern Europe, age at first birth has remained flat or even fallen as fertility declined. Democratization is not a good predictor of fertility decline, nor is militarization or gender equity in education. Whether we look across times and places, or across different 'communication communities' (Szreter 1996) within a specific time and place, we find that what we call fertility decline is not a single social process at all, but merely an amalgam of different processes that all result in lower age-specific fertility rates for at least some subgroups over at least some ages. We find communication communities with very low fertility in nearly all high-fertility countries and vice versa; we find pockets where abortion is commonly practised within countries where it is rare; we find subpopulations with high rates of late, nonmarital childbearing within countries where early, marital childbearing is the norm. In short, we find structured, important exceptions to almost any large-scale generalization we observe.

This mismatch across different scales makes fertility decline a particularly interesting topic for interdisciplinary research. Juxtaposing the similarities across cases at the large scale against the heterogeneity at smaller scales sharpens our understanding of both. Add to this contrast the fact that fertility is essential for population replacement and almost everywhere given considerable cultural elaboration, and the importance of the interdisciplinary study of fertility declines becomes clear. Fertility defies the distinctions of biology and culture, individual and communal, agency and structure. While 'who bears children when' is the object of intense political debate and even direct manipulation, the analysis of reproduction cannot be only political. While childbearing is richly embedded in symbolic systems, its analysis cannot only be semiotic. While numbers of births over time have significant consequences for population size and structure, its analysis cannot be only formally demographic. But how can we work across these different scales and perspectives? In particular, how can we reintroduce variation, difference and context into the study of fertility decline? That is the challenge that is taken up in this timely and important volume.

Kreager and his collaborators begin this project with two contemporary approaches to cultural demography. The first is compositional demography, which focuses on differences in fertility, migration and mortality that 'reflect the varying composition, structure and social position of subpopulations, which open up differing access to social, economic and political hierarchies, and the differing advantages and disadvantages that go with them' (Kreager, this volume, page 2 of draft). Compositional demography has a deep historical foundation, as Kreager (2008) has so elegantly shown. Its contemporary form has been developed most richly in Britain, by scholars including Kreager himself (2011), Elizabeth Schröder-Butterfill (2015) and Simon Szreter (for example, Szreter and Garrett 2000). This work builds on the nuanced study of population change that emerged out of the Cambridge Group for the History of Population starting in the 1960s. Its deeper roots go back to the Manchester School, from Gluckman forwards, and its rich attention to case studies and structured social difference. Compositional demography makes the radical – and radically right – assertion that we cannot understand population variation or change apart from the social worlds in which it occurs. A 10 per cent decline in fertility at the national level is not at all the same thing if it occurs uniformly or through a 50 per cent decline in fertility in 20 per cent of the population. The populations we observe are composed out of distinctly different subpopulations: composition matters enormously.

The second approach to cultural demography on which the authors draw is my own model of vital conjunctures, in which a duration of uncertainty in a life or lives arises when multiple potential futures are in play, and therefore when multiple aspects of social experience that might otherwise intersect only minimally become mutually relevant in a visible way. An unintended pregnancy, a surprising job offer or even an impending college graduation can open up a duration of uncertainty and possibility that conjoins otherwise unrelated aspects of life (see Johnson-Hanks 2002, 2006). The framework of vital conjunctures builds on the work of social theorist Pierre Bourdieu, who uses the term 'conjunctures' to refer to the specific kinds of contexts in which social reproduction and social change can both occur.[1] In cultural demography, a focus on vital conjunctures pushes us to think about the consequences of context and time for demographic outcomes. For decades, demographers (especially in the United States) have sought to parcel out the associations between demographic outcomes and a laundry list of individual characteristics: race, income, religion, religiosity, education, employment status, share of household labour, risk aversion, depressive symptoms and so on. As Abbott (1988) has argued, this habit of mind treats the social world as an endless series of regression equations. But social life is not organized that way, and the association between any characteristic and any outcome is at best indirect. Vital events occur in specific conjunctures; individual characteristics might influence which woman finds herself in which conjuncture, or how she reacts to it when she is there, but the characteristics do not cause the outcomes and they cannot account for them.

The chapters offered here by Kreager and his collaborators contain a great deal of rich material and creative thinking, and they push us to think about vital conjunctures in new ways. In particular, how are conjunctures connected to composition? To what degree does our answer to that question depend on scale or scope? Problems of scale and scope become particularly important as the kinds of lived uncertainty that make up vital conjunctures expand, becoming endemic as a normalized 'state of exception',[2] as has happened over the last decades in so much of the world. As long as uncertainty and alternate possible futures are experienced only at the level of a small number of interrelated people, we can continue to imagine conjunctures without a coherent model of composition. But as conjunctures expand, compositional demography becomes an essential framework for understanding difference and change.

I approach these questions in three steps. First, I describe the concept of vital conjunctures. Second, I discuss what happens when conjunctures expand, either in scale or in time, as we are observing in much of the contemporary world. In this section, I suggest how these kinds of expansions point to the connection between conjunctures and composition, and to the ways in which compositional demography can improve on my own conjunctural approach. Finally, I consider how these two frameworks in unison can contribute to research on difference and diversity in population studies, and to studies of fertility more broadly.

Vital Conjunctures

Much of the time, people go through their daily lives with a sense of the future and a feeling of trajectory. Young people are in school in order to get degrees and jobs; young adults are working to save money for a car or a house or a wedding. We often have the feeling that we know 'where we are going' and what the future will be like. This feeling is often completely illusory, but it is nonetheless useful in organizing daily life and helping people make sense of their place in the world. As Randall, Mondain and Diagne suggest in their chapter in this volume, many of the most important domains in our lives are rich in uncertainty and ambivalence. Yet, we usually live with the illusion of clarity.

But sometimes this illusory clarity breaks down. Something happens that calls this clear road into question, and the future becomes visibly uncertain. At that point, the trajectory ahead becomes murky, with multiple paths appearing possible. Each path may suggest a radically different – even incommensurable – future. In the duration when these multiple potential futures are open, multiple domains of life that in the ordinary times would continue along partially independent of each other all become mutually intertwined. The duration during which multiple potential futures are in play is the vital conjuncture. For example, a young woman nears the end of her schooling and is applying for jobs in a variety of cities. The young man she has been dating isn't sure if he wants to move. Will he follow her and maybe even marry her? Or maybe it is time to break up? Where will she live? What job will she have? All at once, all these questions are on the table. Her choice of work becomes entwined with her choice of partner; her potential futures multiply and, for some time, her present is dominated by these multiple futures.

Alternatively, a young woman unexpectedly finds herself pregnant. Or she fails her exams and her parents refuse to pay the tuition for her to repeat the grade. Or she is offered an unexpected scholarship to a prestigious but faraway school. Each of these might open up a vital conjuncture, and the conjuncture would stay open until she regains that sense – illusory or not – of knowing the trajectory of the future. In all cases, a vital conjuncture is the zone of possibility that emerges around specific periods of potential transformation in a life or lives. It is a temporary configuration of possible change, a duration of uncertainty and potential. Vital conjunctures are particularly critical durations where more than usual is in play, and the futures at stake are significant.

In 2002 and 2005, I thought about the structure of conjunctures mostly through their horizons – that is, the social aspirations and values through which the individual actors construe them. This idea is echoed in a creative way in Walters' chapter in this volume, which develops the compelling framework of 'moral demography'. And, indeed, the horizons of the conjuncture are certainly important for how it is navigated – they provide the meaning and motivation. But the chapters here show that there are two other important kinds of structure that I did not focus on then, but that are at least as important.

The first of these concerns the tools, or resources, or means at hand that are available for use in responding to the conjuncture.

Hukin makes this point amply clear in her chapter on 'traditional' contraception in Cambodia, where the class stratification of access to abortion in turn structures the use of contraception. Similarly, in southern Cameroon, where abortion is illegal, safe abortions are available – but at a high cost and only if you come with references. Doctors who perform them after hours will only do so for someone they are confident will not report them. Who you are, what you have and who you know can dramatically recast your range of possible futures and therefore the structure of the conjuncture.

The second important form of structure that I previously ignored is the distribution of conjunctures themselves. Who finds themselves in what kind of conjuncture? Again, as with the resources at hand for their resolution, this is not at all equal. There is considerable variation in terms of who finds themselves confronting what kinds of structured zones of uncertainty. We see this elegantly expressed in Bochow's discussion in this volume of class, ethnicity and reproduction in Botswana. While elites and nonelites continue to share a cultural imaginary of successful womanhood, and continue to view infertility or subfecundity in similar ways, they face very different probabilities of experiencing the conjuncture of infertility in the first place.

Thus, the first way that these chapters offer a connection between vital conjunctures and compositional demography is through structures and resources. In several of the chapters, we can see clearly that in addition to the horizons of future possibility that their participants imagine, and to which they orient their action, vital conjunctures also have a great deal of old-fashioned 'morphology', as Halbwachs (1938) uses the term: they are structured by social institutions and resources, which are differentially available to different subpopulations. We thus need compositional demography to make sense of conjunctural action.

There is a second connection between conjunctures and composition, too, through scale and time. In my earlier formulation, vital conjunctures are outside of normal time – they are 'unsettled times' in Ann Swidler's (1986) language. Normal or 'settled' time entails the expectation that there is a trajectory through which the present leads into the future in some reasonably orderly way, so that the temporary break of a vital conjuncture stands in contrast to a background of relative certainty. But that is not always the case. In some contexts, uncertainty becomes so pervasive that the suspension of taken-for-granted futures that defines a vital conjuncture becomes, instead, the normal condition. It is to this possibility that we now turn.

The Expansion of Conjunctures

In this section, I discuss what happens when vital conjunctures expand in terms of time and scale. The cases I have considered tend to be both individual – in the sense that they happen to one person or a small number of people – and temporary, in the sense that these durations in which multiple futures are in play are relatively short. They have discernible ends, after which 'normal life' resumes. But, of course, conjunctures can dilate over both these dimensions. They can scale up, so that the household or neighbourhood or community or country is in a conjuncture. Conjunctures can also extend in terms of time, so that the suspension of the readily imagined future becomes not a state of exception, but the normal background against which fleeting sensations of certainty may be measured.

The first kind of expansion – in scale – requires in a first instance relatively little revision of the basic idea of a conjuncture. As long as the group of people over whom the conjuncture is distributed shares some sense of the future and in some real sense participates together in a frame of construal, and therefore the imagining of horizons, an expansion in scale changes little conceptually. Conjunctures are at any scale social phenomena, and their basic dynamics can still hold at a larger social scale.

At the same time, there are two important differences between individual vital conjunctures and conjunctures at larger social scales. The first concerns the role of intention and intentional action. With an individual vital conjuncture, it is easy to imagine the resolution of the conjuncture as coming as a result of a choice or decision of the individual at the centre of the conjuncture. At an aggregate scale, however, it is rarely the case that the resolution of the conjuncture comes about as a clear effect of the intentional action of a specific person or persons.[3] More common are unintended consequences, cascading effects and unexpected but collective resolutions. William Sewell on the French Revolution; Marshall Sahlins on the apotheosis of Captain Cook; Pierre Bourdieu on the process of marriage among the Kabyle and in Béarn in southwest France: in all of these cases, conjunctures are resolved partially outside of the intentional projects of the actors participating in them.

This may indeed be a compelling reason for us to think more, not less, about larger-scale conjunctures. Sometimes at the individual level, we can read intention and strategy where it is not really there or, at least, not there in the way we assume. Similarly, we can attribute to intention what came about by chance or structural forces. Focusing on larger scales makes these analytic errors harder. The push towards structure and morphology is also reflected in the second important difference between small-scale and large-scale conjunctures. At the smallest scales, all the effects of composition are invisible, because composition influences not what happened within the conjuncture, but rather who is in which conjunctures when – a set of processes that are outside of the core analytic framework suggested for individuals' vital conjunctures. When conjunctures expand in terms of scale, their distribution across social groups becomes a critical question. Thus, fundamental issues of population composition necessarily enter into the analytic frame.

Therefore, as conjunctures expand in terms of scale, the core idea remains the same, but the analysis becomes necessarily richer, more structural and in closer dialogue with compositional factors. This is seen clearly in the several chapters in this volume in which political economy, culture and social change rub together in a variety of productive ways. However, further issues arise when we think about conjunctures expanding in the temporal dimension. A number of authors have described contemporary life in Africa as marked by a sense that everything is temporary and provisional; the dissolution of long-term stability and of coherent long-term trajectories is experienced as a real possibility, even an apparent likelihood. An example, remarked by Cooper and Pratten (2014), is the delay of 'full adulthood': the ongoing curating of multiple possible futures shifts as the accumulation of 'wealth in people' that classically defined African social aspirations is replaced by individuals' own 'wealth in prospects'. In this volume, the reproductive control exercised by Basotho female household heads (described in Kroeker's chapter), the proliferation of subgroup statuses that shape Gbigbil pregnancy outcomes (see van der Sijpt's chapter) and the way in which Tswana couples use their position in professional strata to disguise AIDS-related infertility (see Bochow's chapter) are all cases in point. In each, choices made in individual vital conjunctures may decide an immediate reproductive issue, but without resolving a more widespread institutional uncertainty. More specifically, while the desire for stable marriages remains in all of these societies, in reality such choices no longer effect a reliable trajectory to successful adult status and sustained childbearing. The authors find no sign of a change in this situation anytime soon.

In short, under conditions of longstanding uncertainty, conjunctures no longer punctuate 'settled' normal time. When conjunctures expand in terms of time, the state of exception itself becomes normal, producing potentially different modes of short-term action, without entirely reinstating previously normative life trajectories or giving rise to clear new ones. This state has been described as one of suspended action, of interstitial pause, of persistent temporariness (see Dalsgard et al. 2014). The concept of vital conjuncture will therefore require further consideration before we can determine how, or even whether, it applies usefully to all provisional states. On the one hand, a vital conjuncture is defined in part by its end – by the fact that, at some point, multiple alternative futures are resolved in favour of one imagined trajectory. On the other hand, where people are in a state of continuing suspended action, normative models of a future trajectory may appear permanently withdrawn. Without a potential conclusion, the fact that multiple domains of ordinary life are brought into mutual relevance becomes immaterial. Without a potential conclusion, the fact that imagined futures orient action may become irrelevant.

Thus, whereas the framework of vital conjunctures can easily accommodate conjunctures that expand in terms of scale, it may be less well suited to account for periods of uncertainty that seem to expand indefinitely in terms of time. Yet periods of suspension have their limits. It may take decades before the significance of suspended action becomes clear. People may nonetheless go on viewing their vital conjunctures as events that should, as much as possible, be used to re-establish normative trajectories. The chapter on Tajik fertility by Roche and Hohmann provides a useful instance of this, especially as the former Soviet sphere is one in which 'states of exception' and 'suspended action' have been found applicable, and the processes involved are clearly long term in nature. Over an extended period, from the 1920s until independence, the Soviet state carried out a series of radical interventions in what is now Tajikistan, especially from 1947, when local populations experienced complete upheaval: forced relocation, elimination of elites and property, artificial ethnic reclassification, attempts to break down family solidarity by the imposition of work brigade structures and so forth. By the 1970s, however, local populations had regrouped, using the brigade structure as a framework within which traditional family and, more particularly, sibling-based fertility variation was reasserted. As Roche and Hohmann describe, despite even further upheaval during the civil war in the 1990s, this reassertion of normative vital trajectories articulated in a new subpopulation base continues to be sustained today. Yet this could hardly have been foreseen during the upheaval, when the suspension of family norms was being enforced, and the subpopulation units and their recruitment were still in the process of forming.

However, compositional demography only partly resolves the problem of theorizing 'states of exception' in which reproduction is subject to generalized uncertainty. As the Tajik example suggests, some social phenomena are visible only in retrospect. And it is difficult to anticipate the suspension of reproductive norms. The case of strongly gendered subpopulations, described here for a Senegalese context by Randall and her colleagues, while stable in the short term, could well become subject to the uncertainties described in the other African chapters. At present, men and women share in the local Islamic prescription of patriarchy and high fertility, while women privately practise contraception. Men for the present can publicly profess local Islamic norms, while carefully turning a blind eye to what their wives are doing. Is such an arrangement sustainable? Whatever the answer, the course of fertility and the vital conjunctures in which it is arbitrated cannot be followed without tracking how subpopulations with different solutions to this situation emerge within the two gendered groups. Conjunctures and composition thus jointly suggest a framework for thinking about heterogeneity in fertility and beyond.

Conjunctures and Composition

Compositional demography draws attention to the fact that 'population' is never pre-given, but is always the product of acts of classification, inclusion/exclusion and partial alignments between groups. That is, population is always a political product, even where it is not explicitly a political project. While deployed today in novel ways, compositional demography is not a new idea. As Kreager (2015: 30–31) explains, from Aristotle to Rousseau, population was understood as 'composed of shifting factional sub-populations' or open and shifting networks: 'The population of a state, in short, was defined by sets of memberships, their important structural features being human relationships, not quantum or trends – populations built . . . via networks that form and sustain ties that make for effective action.' By focusing attention on the social and political processes through which populations are constituted, compositional demography offers a way of connecting theories of action to aggregate rates. In this way, compositional demography offers a compelling resolution to one of the most central conundrums in social theory, at least since Quetelet (1869): why and how do individual actors, who experience their actions as personal and freely chosen, nonetheless reproduce population rates with such striking regularity?

Compositional demography, as expressed through the chapters in this collection, resolves Quetelet's conundrum by reframing it. The conundrum is ill-formed, they suggest, because it skips from individual to high-level aggregate without attending to the intermediate structure. Patrick Heady's chapter, for example, demonstrates that low fertility in Europe cannot be understood in a framework that includes only individual-level and national- level variables. There is an intermediate, community level, that of 'social pressure and social support', which 'means that the system as a whole has certain properties that may not be deducible from the attitudes of the individuals within it' (page 25 of draft). Thus, the conundrum is not about how individual actors reproduce population rates, but rather how communities – perhaps Szreter's term 'communication communities' is apposite here – coordinate and orient action, making certain choices easy and others hard, and certain demographic outcomes more probable and others less so. Over the last century, many demographers have sought to model population dynamics without understanding social dynamics; compositional demography insists that this has been a fool's errand.

Compositional demography offers compelling tools for thinking about the social structures, factional alignments, networks and communities through which people are connected and how their forms of action are oriented. However, a comprehensive understanding of the intersection of population and culture still requires a theory of demographically relevant action. That is the contribution of a conjunctural approach. In this volume, Walters proposes a framework of 'moral demography', which 'operates in the space between the individual and the social, at the interface where populations are made by a series of micro-events arising from individual-level decisions themselves shaped by and shaping the macro-hegemonic context' (page 3 of draft). In other words, she suggests that we treat conjunctural action as the mechanism through which compositional change occurs and conversely treat population composition as a – or even *the* – key force structuring the conjunctures in which action occurs. This, I think, is exactly the right approach, and the nuance and innovation of Walters' chapter gives me great optimism that the approach will be fruitful.

If populations are structures of interrelated subgroups, then the processes of subgroup recruitment and loss are at the heart of population dynamics. Differential fertility and mortality rates may matter (see Hout et al. 2001), but are not the dominant processes. Instead, subgroups emerge and grow out of individual events in which people are selected into and out of categories, classes and groups. These acts of selection may take a variety of forms, from self-selection by voluntary affiliation to structural selection as membership in one (or more) class or category. Understanding the processes of recruitment and loss that have given rise to recognized subpopulation categories and classes provides the contexts in which events of selection may occur. These acts of selection may occur in visible, dramatic ways (like religious conversion or migration), but may also be small and quotidian (like whether you stay after class to chat with your classmates). In any case, subpopulations are social constructs, not only in the abstract sense that they are discursive objects, but also in the concrete sense that they are constructed through sequential events of social selection. The units and boundaries emerge, change and disappear as an aggregate consequence of small-scale events: population composition depends on conjunctural action.

But conjunctures also depend on composition in at least two ways. First, conjunctures are not evenly distributed across social space. Who faces an unintended pregnancy, an unexpected promotion that entails a long-distance move or a spiritual experience that makes conversion to a different religion feel intuitive? The prevalence of these kinds of vital conjunctures – circumstances in which major acts of selection become feasible – varies considerably across different subgroups in a population. Faculty members pretty commonly face conjunctures like job offers in faraway places, parental health crises and divorces; they only very rarely face vital conjunctures around unwanted pregnancies or narcotics arrests. People who regularly attend evangelical churches face different opportunities for selection into and out of population subcategories than do people who regularly attend neuroscience conferences or who regularly attend blues bars.

Population composition also matters for conjunctures because it shapes how people respond to the conjunctures in which they find themselves. Again, this happens in two ways. Our communication communities provide us with the schemas for action and horizons of possibility through which we navigate conjunctures, at the same time as our group memberships shape the resources – material and otherwise – to which we have access. Confronted with a similar conjuncture, people who regularly attend evangelical churches are likely to react differently than people who regularly attend neuroscience conferences or who regularly attend blues bars. Compositional factors matter for both the distribution of conjunctures and the responses within them. As Walters notes, the events shape the contexts, which shape the events.[4]

Conclusion

I began these reflections with the fact that fertility patterns at the largest scales appear simple and coherent, but that the harder we look at them, the less clear they appear. But as we think about composition and conjuncture, a new kind of clarity starts to emerge. While fertility is not well predicted by economic or political variables at the national level, there is a great deal of meso-level structure in fertility heterogeneity. Social groups are structured in myriad little ways that coordinate individual-level fertility outcomes. Within specific subpopulations, people are likely to find themselves in similar kinds of conjunctures and to resolve them in similar ways, whether directly related to fertility or not. Finding housing in the same housing market; managing work–family tradeoffs within the same workplaces; confronting expectations from the same opinion leaders; seeking contraception from the same doctors: within communities, people's actions are aligned as they find themselves struggling against the same challenges, using shared systems of meaning and value to give sense to those struggles. A great strength of this volume is how abundantly the chapters show the concrete ways in which context and social networks matter for fertility. They demonstrate that the fact that context matters is not reason to give up on comparative understanding; we can understand fertility *through* variation and context, not in spite of it.

As Susan Watkins (1991) has shown, from the middle of the nineteenth century to the middle of the twentieth, European fertility not only fell, but also became far less variable within countries. As the mechanisms through which communication communities were sustained changed – from local gossip networks to national media – the synchronizing effects of social communication on fertility came to apply over larger areas. Today, national boundaries still matter, but smaller-scale variation is coming to matter in a different and more potent way. In the United States, neighbourhoods are becoming more homogeneous by income and political affiliation. At the same time, technology enables people to hear only the news they want and only the views with which they already agree. Following a composition and conjuncture framework, we would predict that fertility practices would also start to diverge. And anecdotally, that is precisely what is happening. Over the next decade, we will be able to see more clearly whether this anecdotal pattern emerges as a demographically perceptible one. In this book, Kreager and his colleagues offer us a compelling approach to fertility heterogeneity; the contexts in which it will be useful are legion.

Jennifer Johnson-Hanks is Professor of Demography and Sociology at the University of California, Berkeley. Her work focuses on the relationship between demographic rates and cultural practices, particularly as regards childbearing in Sub-Saharan Africa. She is author of *Uncertain Honor* (2006) and coauthor of *Understanding Family Change and Variation* (2011).

Notes

1. For example: 'Practices can be accounted for only by relating the objective structure defining the social conditions of the production of the habitus which engendered them to the conditions in which this habitus is operating, that is, to the conjuncture which, short of a radical transformation, represents a particular state of this structure' (Bourdieu 1977: 78).
2. The phrase 'State of exception' was coined by the political philosopher Carl Schmitt and is developed by Giorgio Agamben (2005). It is one of a range of terms used by scholars of contemporary Africa, the former Soviet sphere and post-9/11 America to talk about what happens to social life and individual life projects in times of extended and comprehensive uncertainty.
3. One set of cases in which individual intentional action can lead to the resolution of a larger-scale conjuncture is that of 'stand-offs', as so elegantly analysed by Robin Wagner-Pacifici (2000).
4. Of course, some variant of this basic idea is shared across nearly all major theories of social action (for example, Bourdieu 1977; Giddens 1979).

References

Abbott, Andrew. 1988. 'Transcending General Linear Reality', *Sociological Theory* 6(2): 169–86.

Agamben, G. 2005. *States of Exception*. Chicago: University of Chicago Press.

Bourdieu, P. 1977. *Outline of a Theory of Practice.* Cambridge: Cambridge University Press.

Cooper, E., and D. Pratten (eds). 2014. *Ethnographies of Uncertainty in Africa.* London: Palgrave Macmillan.

Dalsgard, A.L., M.D. Fredricksen et al. (eds). 2014. *Ethnographies of Youth and Temporality: Time Objectified.* Philadelphia: Temple University Press.

Giddens, A. 1979. *Central Problems in Social Theory: Action, Structure, and Contradiction in Social Analysis.* Berkeley: University of California Press.

Halbwachs, M. 1938. *Morphologie sociale.* Paris: Librairie Armand Colin.

Hout, M., A. Greeley and M.J. Wilde. 2001. 'The Demographic Imperative in Religious Change in the United States', *American Journal of Sociology* 107(2): 468–500.

Johnson-Hanks, J. 2002. 'On the Limits of the Life Cycle in Ethnography: Toward a Theory of Vital Conjunctures', *American Anthropologist* 104(3): 865–80.

———. 2006. *Uncertain Honor: Modern Motherhood in an African Crisis.* Chicago: University of Chicago Press.

Kreager, P. 2008. 'Aristotle and Open Population Thinking', *Population and Development Review* 34(4): 599–629.

———. 2011. 'The Challenge of Compositional Demography', *Asian Population Studies* 7(2): 85–88.

———. 2015. 'Population theory – A Long View'. *Population Studies* 69(Suppl. 1): 29–37.

Quetelet, A. 1869. *Physique Sociale, Ou Essai sur le développent des facultés de l'homme.* Gilly: Academie Royale de Belgique.

Schröder-Butterfill, E. 2015. 'Networks, Strata and Ageing: Towards a Compositional Demography of Vulnerability', in P. Kreager, B. Winney, S. Ulijaszek and C. Capelli (eds), *Population in the Human Sciences: Concepts, Models, Evidence.* Oxford: Oxford University Press, pp. 257–91.

Swidler, A. 1986. 'Culture in Action: Symbols and Strategies', *American Sociological Review* 51: 273–86.

Szreter, S. 1996. *Fertility, Class and Gender in Britain, 1860–1940.* New York: Cambridge University Press.

Szreter, S., and E. Garrett. 2000. 'Reproduction, Compositional Demography, and Economic Growth: Family Planning in England Long before the Fertility Decline', *Population and Development Review* 26(1): 45–80.

Wagner-Pacifici, R. 2000. *Theorizing the Standoff: Contingency in Action.* Cambridge: Cambridge University Press.

Watkins, S.C. 1991. *Provinces into Nations: The Demographic Integration of Western Europe, 1870–1960.* Princeton: Princeton University Press.

Index

www.ingramcontent.com/pod-product-compliance
Ingram Content Group UK Ltd.
Pitfield, Milton Keynes, MK11 3LW, UK
UKHW021009120926
8556IPUK00029B/369

9 781785 336041